The 361 Classical Acupuncture Points

Names, Functions, Descriptions and Locations

Other Related Titles from World Scientific

Acupuncture Understood: Rediscovering Traditional Five Element Healthcare
by Stuart Lightbody
ISBN: 978-981-4583-77-0
ISBN: 978-981-4583-78-7 (pbk)

Acupuncture: Theories and Evidence
edited by Hong Hai
ISBN: 978-981-4452-01-4

Evidence-Based Acupuncture
edited by Tang-Yi Liu and Ping-Chung Leung
ISBN: 978-981-4324-17-5

'May the spirit of the Dao spread far and wide...'

Published by

World Scientific Publishing Co. Pte. Ltd.
5 Toh Tuck Link, Singapore 596224
USA office: 27 Warren Street, Suite 401-402, Hackensack, NJ 07601
UK office: 57 Shelton Street, Covent Garden, London WC2H 9HE

Library of Congress Cataloging-in-Publication Data
Names: Lightbody, Stuart, author.
Title: The 361 classical acupuncture points : names, functions, descriptions and locations / Stuart Lightbody.
Other titles: Three hundred sixty one classical acupuncture points
Description: Hackensack, NJ : World Scientific, [2020] | Includes bibliographical references and index.
Identifiers: LCCN 2019036813 | ISBN 9789811201257 (hardcover)
Subjects: MESH: Acupuncture Points
Classification: LCC RM184.5 | NLM WB 369.5.M5 | DDC 615.8/92--dc23
LC record available at https://lccn.loc.gov/2019036813

British Library Cataloguing-in-Publication Data
A catalogue record for this book is available from the British Library.

ISBN 978-981-120-125-7

For any available supplementary material, please visit
https://www.worldscientific.com/worldscibooks/10.1142/11307#t=suppl

Typeset by Stallion Press
Email: enquiries@stallionpress.com

Printed in Singapore

The 361 Classical Acupuncture Points

Names, Functions, Descriptions and Locations

Stuart Lightbody

World Scientific

NEW JERSEY • LONDON • SINGAPORE • BEIJING • SHANGHAI • HONG KONG • TAIPEI • CHENNAI • TOKYO

Disclaimer

It is the responsibility of the practitioner, relying on experience and knowledge of the patient, to make diagnoses and to formulate the best treatment for each individual patient and to take all appropriate safety precautions. To the fullest extent of the law, neither the publisher nor the author assumes any liabilities for any injury and/or damage.

About the Author

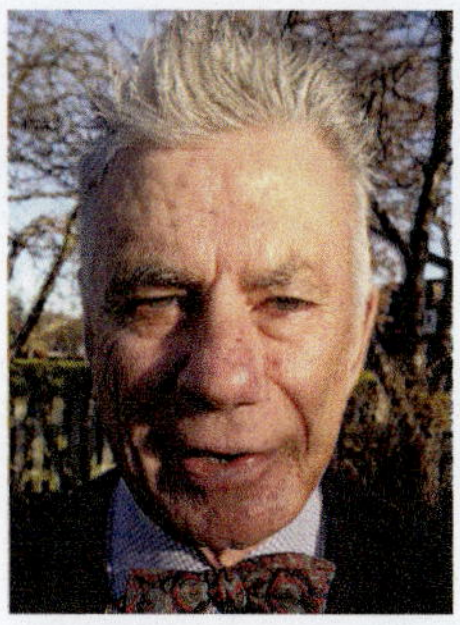

Stuart Lightbody holds a Licentiate, Bachelor and Masters qualification in Classical Acupuncture and is a member of The British Acupuncture Council (Overseas) and has been in practice since 1979. He was a member of the teaching faculty at the College of Traditional Acupuncture from 1982 to 1992.

He has written extensively on Preventive Medicine and Acupuncture for the *Daily Express* and is the author of "Acupuncture Understood: Rediscovering Traditional Five Element Healthcare" (World Scientific).

He is the Acupuncture contributor to Men's Health Matters (Vermilion/ Ebury Press), the Hamlyn Encyclopaedia of Complementary Health and The Hamlyn Encyclopaedia of Child Health (Reed International Books Limited).

Contents

Foreword

For a student of Acupuncture, the mid 70's were a time of discovery, wonderment and exhilaration as a whole new perspective on life and the inner workings of the human being was placed before us. The syllabus at the College I attended was a work in progress, and although improvements were continually being made it was still somewhat haphazard in its *modus operandi* and would bear little resemblance to the well regulated colleges we have today. However a strong sense of purpose prevailed and, with it, a sincere desire to bring into the public domain this wonderful system of medicine.

The course included influences from past teachers such as Soulie de Morant, Jacques Lavier, Felix Mann, Roger de la Fuÿe (de la Filye), and Wu wei-ping and bringing it all alive were the lectures by Professor JR Worsley whose emphasis on the importance of the Spirit of the Points and the need to understand and treat the patient at the deepest level shone through.

It was during these times that a seed was planted in my mind for this book and, although it has taken several decades for it to come to fruition, its purpose still remains the same: to provide a valuable contribution to the Acupuncture world, especially its students and practitioners, as they strive in their noble endeavour to serve the needs of their patients. It is to them that this book is dedicated.

In it I have tried to crystallise the wisdom and knowledge from the past and, together with my own experiences, to provide insight into the meaning of the Points, their position on the body and their effects upon the body, mind and particularly the spirit of the patient.

Because of the condensed nature of the text and therefore its limitations, space has been allocated within each Point section so that the student/practitioner may record their own insights, understandings, observations and reflections with regard to their effects. The information in it should only be used in accordance with pulse findings and other traditional methods of diagnosing the root cause of the patient's energetic imbalance. It is not intended as a symptomatic substitute for the holistic approach. A sincere respect, appreciation and understanding of these Points seems to me essential in bringing about that unique connection between the heart of the practitioner and their patient. Guo Yu(Kuo Yiu), a physician from the Han dynasty, puts this understanding well when he states that "the word medicine embodies the idea of attention .... a kind of spirit connects the physician's heart with their hand and this is something I know but cannot explain".

The dedicated Acupuncture practitioner who has the privilege to access these inner treasures should not take that good fortune lightly. Just one Point can change a person's life for the better — it happened to me in 1975 and I am still very thankful for that.

Stuart Lightbody

Acknowledgements

Sincere thanks and acknowledgements go to those teachers at what was then the College of Chinese Acupuncture (UK) and to its founder Professor J R Worsley. Those teachers included David Arditti, Meriel Darby, Angela and John Hicks, Julia Measures, Peter Mole, Allegra Wint, Judy Becker Worsley, and Ron Wray.

Thanks also go to Richard Bertschinger, Pam Bone, Peter Eckman, Alan Hext, Linda Howden, Claude Larre, Bill Mueller, Stephen Paul, Elizabeth Rochat de la Vallée, Beryl Williams and to those Acupuncture luminaries from antiquity whose wisdom and knowledge in the form of their texts, odes, commentaries and treatises continue to inspire and educate us today.

A special debt of gratitude, however, goes to Dr Leanne Langlois whom I was extremely fortunate to meet whilst part-way through gathering information on each of the 361 Points. It is because of the specialist knowledge gained from her Doctorate qualification in Physiology, her years as an acupuncture practitioner and Point location teacher, together with her formidable attention to detail, that the pictorial accuracy and verbal descriptions of the Point locations are of such a high standard. This, combined with the excellent graphics produced by Dave Pugh, has helped create a wonderful resource for both student and practitioner irrespective of the tradition studied.

Finally, as with my first book "Acupuncture Understood", sincere thanks and gratitude go to my wife Ruth who has been there as a profound source of inspiration, guidance and support throughout the years of its compilation.

Heart

- **Emperor of the Kingdom — Supreme Controller**
- **Sovereign of all the Organs**
- **The Heart Governs the Blood and houses our higher consciousness, the Shen**

Heart

HT 1 — Utmost Source (Extreme Source, Utmost Spring, Supreme Spring)
Entry Point. First Aid for heart failure or fainting (massage or needle).

This point can enhance a person's clarity of consciousness and reconnect them with their true self, the Shen, the perpetuator of good in a person. Consider in cases of long-term emotional stress or sadness (sadness or over-excitement takes its toll on the Heart). Utmost Source can often have an immediate effect, enabling a patient to regain their mental and emotional equilibrium. We need to guard our 'still place' within so our Spirit remains intact. Propriety, the Heart's virtue, upholds our inner 'mandate of Heaven'. For numbness or extreme tenderness on the tip of the tongue, speech troubles, hysteria, over-impulsiveness or lack of vision.

HT 2 — Blue Green Spirit (Green Spirit)

Consider for the spiritual revival of the Supreme Controller. Can be used to revitalise the Mind and the (Ling) Spirit. Usually forbidden to needle, and thus is an under-used point. Consider using moxa. It can help expand and relax the chest. It can also be effective for frontal or generalised headaches. Blue Green is nature's intense, vibrant hue.

⊥	Δ		Location
5	5	Just posterior to the lower border of the pectoralis major muscle where the arm attaches to the torso	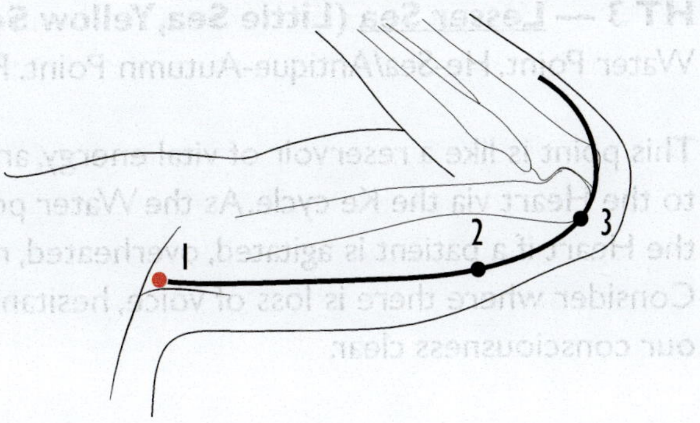
X	5	Do not use during pregnancy **3 cun** proximal to flexure of elbow In groove formed by medial border of the biceps brachii muscle and humerus	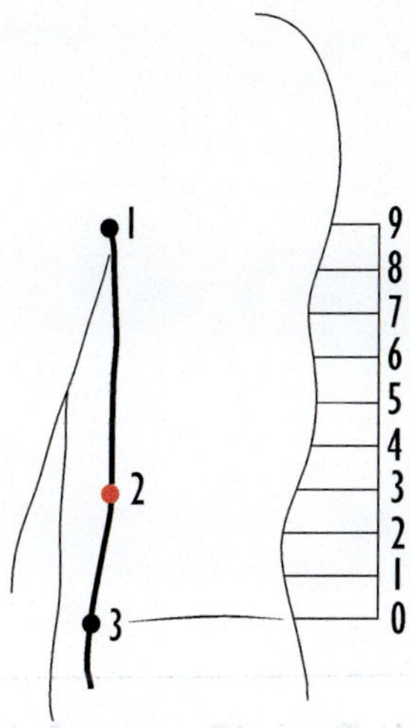

Heart

HT 3 — <u>Lesser Sea</u> (Little Sea, Yellow Sea, Lesser Yin Sea)
Water Point. He-Sea/Antique-Autumn Point. First Aid: Exhaustion.

This point is like a reservoir of vital energy, and is commonly used to transfer Qi from the Kidneys to the Heart via the Ke cycle. As the Water point, it controls Fire and helps to soothe and calm the Heart if a patient is agitated, overheated, restless, having difficulty sleeping or is exhausted. Consider where there is loss of voice, hesitant speech or forgetfulness. This point helps in keeping our consciousness clear.

HT 4 — <u>Spirit Path</u> (Route of the Spirit, Spirit Way)
Metal Point. Jing-River/Antique-Late Summer Point.

The Spirit in this context refers to the Ling Spirit: hidden, serene, mysterious, receptive (as in Ht 2). The Metal should be the temperature of the Earth. If it is too cold it may result in physical rigidity, arthritis of the elbow or wrist, or an inability to bend the hands and wrists. If it is too hot it may manifest as cardiac pain or palpitations. Consider using this point if the Spirit is weakened or broken, or when a patient is sad or miserable. For loss of inner direction and purpose in life. Reconnects us with the Father and lends structure. Useful with Ht 7, to help encourage the patient back on their harmonious path or "Way of the Dao".

⊥	Δ		**Location**
3-5	3-7	Halfway between the lateral edge of the tendon of the biceps brachii muscle and the medial epicondyle of the humerus	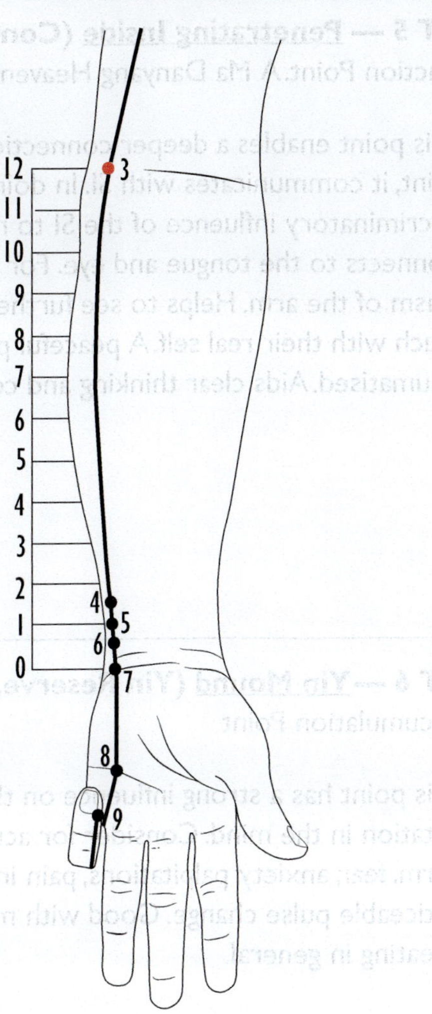
3	3-5	Between the tendons of Flexor Carpi Ulnaris and Flexor Digitorum Superficialis **1.5 cun** proximal to Ht 7 On ulnar artery	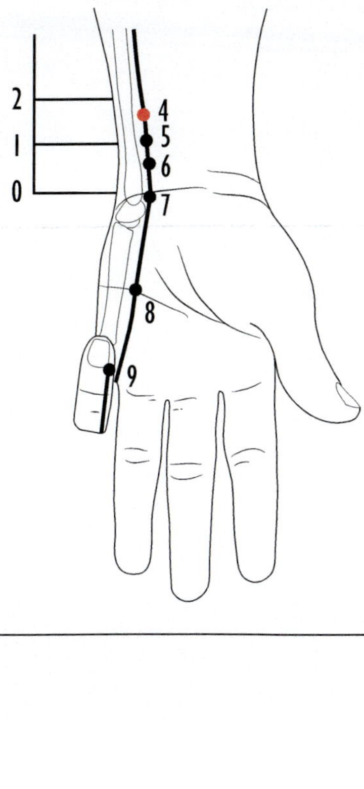

Heart

HT 5 — Penetrating Inside (Communication with the Interior)
Junction Point. A Ma Danyang Heavenly Star Point. 'Audacity point'.

This point enables a deeper connection to be made with the patient. Being the junction point, it communicates with SI. In doing so, it harmonises these two Officials and brings in the discriminatory influence of the SI to maintain the Heart's virtue and thus the 'Mandate of Heaven'. Connects to the tongue and eye. For stuttering and speech disorders, palpitations, neuralgia or spasm of the arm. Helps to see further beyond the mask — enables the patient to be more in touch with their real self. A peaceful point that gives strength and stability to a person shocked or traumatised. Aids clear thinking and communication. Helps maintain emotional harmony.

HT 6 — Yin Mound (Yin Reserve, Stone Palace, Yin Cleft)
Accumulation Point

This point has a strong influence on the mental state of a person because of its ability to calm agitation in the mind. Consider for acute conditions affecting the Heart such as hysteria, shock, alarm, fear, anxiety, palpitations, pain in the chest, sudden dumbness or insomnia. Can produce a noticeable pulse change. Good with moxa. Helpful for night sweats (together with Kid 7) and for sweating in general.

⊥	Δ		Location
3	3-5	Between tendons of Flexor Carpi Ulnaris and Flexor Digitorum Superficialis **1 cun** proximal to Ht 7 in the same channel as Ht 4	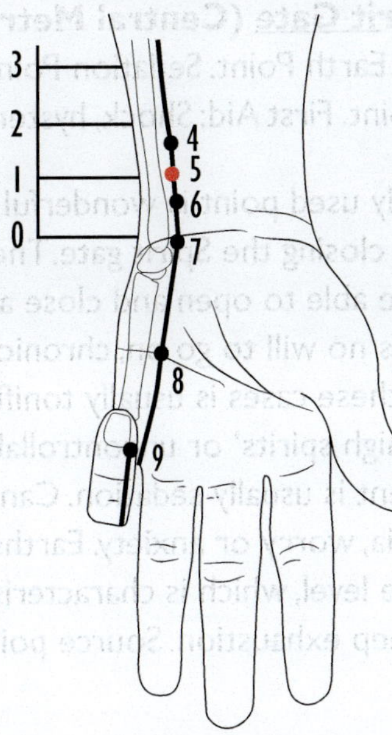
3	3-7	Between tendons of Flexor Carpi Ulnaris and Flexor Digitorum Superficialis **0.5 cun** proximal to Ht 7 in the same channel as Ht 4	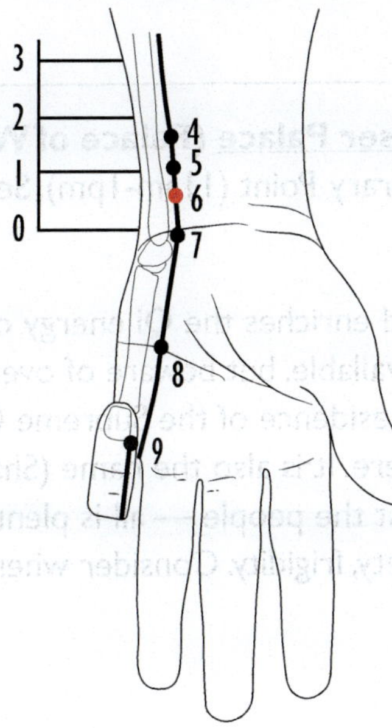

Heart

HT 7 — Spirit Gate (Central Metropolis)
Source Point. Earth Point. Sedation Point. Shu-Stream/Antique-Summer Point. 'Courage Point', Shokanten Point. First Aid: Shock, hysteria, electric shock, heart failure, extreme anxiety.

This frequently used point is wonderful for calming and steadying the Spirit of the Heart. It helps in opening or closing the Spirit gate. The Shen should be able to flow unhindered, therefore this gate should be able to open and close appropriately for its function to be fulfilled. Consider where there is no will to go on, chronic sadness or lack of spirit, indicating the gate may be closed; treatment in these cases is usually tonification. The patient may be experiencing hallucinations, 'exceedingly high spirits' or uncontrollable talkativeness, indications that the gate may be stuck open; treatment is usually sedation. Can be effective for palpitations, arrhythmia, effects of a broken heart, insomnia, worry or anxiety. Earths and strengthens the Heart when it is jittery. Consider for shock at some level, which is characterised by uncontrollably bursting into tears, desperation, panic, hysteria or deep exhaustion. Source points affect the Yuan Qi and thus the patient's constitutional wellbeing.

HT 8 — Lesser Palace (Palace of Weariness, Lesser Treasury, Little Storehouse)
Fire Point. Horary Point (11am-1pm). Seasonal Horary Point — Summer. Ying-Spring/Antique-Spring Point.

Revitalises and enriches the Qi energy of the Heart. Helps in getting the maximum benefit from what Fire is available, but beware of overheating. Lesser Palace can also mean the House of the Emperor or Residence of the Supreme Controller (Fire is its home) — everything is good, pure, and healthy here. It is also the name (Shao Fu) of the Chinese Official who stores and distributes goods amongst the people — all is plentiful here. Helpful for fear, fear of meeting people, agitation, heartfelt anxiety, frigidity. Consider where there are vivid dreams involving fire or heat.

HT 9 — Little Rushing In (Lesser Surge, Lesser Rushing)
Wood Point. Tonification Point. Exit Point. Jing-Well/Antique-Winter Point

This point can regulate the amount of Qi flowing into the Heart. If deficient: there may be a white vaginal discharge, expressionless voice, low energy levels or difficulties with speech. If in excess: there may be hypertension, palpitations, an unsteady pulse, red vaginal discharge, fearful dreams, or dreams associated with fire or smoke. This point brings the 'Hun' to the Shen, and aids in maintaining and sharpening penetrative thought. Brings a surge of energy to the meridian.

⊥	△		Location
3	5-7	On proximal radial corner of pisiform bone	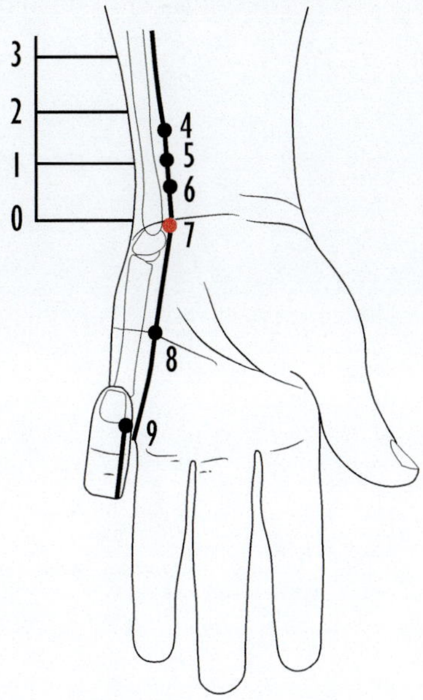
2-3	3-5	Between 4th and 5th metacarpal bones In depression proximal to the head of the 5th metacarpal Point usually lies just proximal to the distal palmar crease (do not use crease as definite marker — bones are more important)	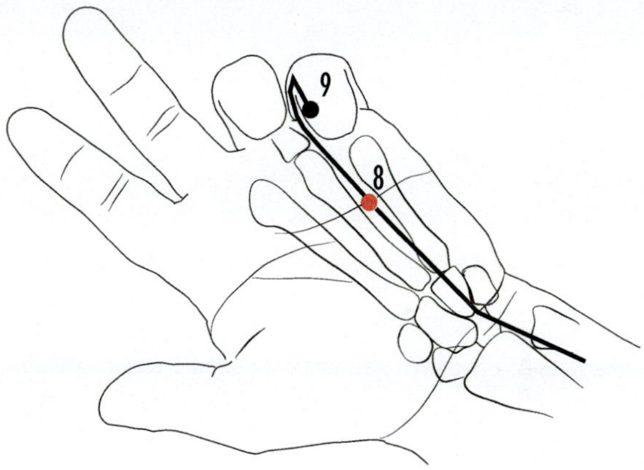
1	3-5	Radial nail point of 5th digit	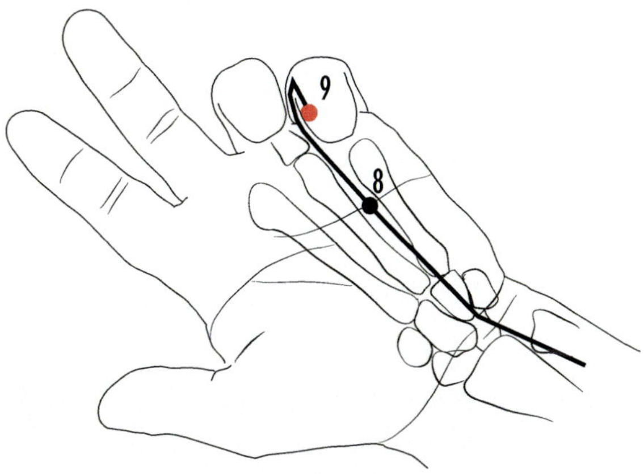

Small Intestine

- **Separator of the Pure from the Impure — Secretary to the Emperor**
- **Responsible for making things thrive —Transformer of matter**

Small Intestine

SI 1 — <u>Lesser Marsh</u> (Little Marsh)
Entry Point. Metal Point. Jing-Well/Antique-Winter Point.

As a distal point, it can be used for symptoms such as asthma, bronchitis, torticollis or tinnitus (the SI connects to the neck and ear). Helps clear mental fog and gives clarity to the mind. As the Metal and Entry Point, it brings quality to SI and enables discernment of what is appropriate and correct. Consider for a SI CF who is severely depressed, suicidal, insecure, immature, or overly sarcastic. For periodic breast swelling or mastitis. Promotes lactation. A marsh in this context is valued as an area of fertility and nourishment (e.g. for those living in rice-producing communities).

SI 2 — <u>Forward Valley</u> (Front Valley)
Water Point. Ying-Spring/Antique-Spring Point.

This point cleanses, bathes and moistens the Small Intestine. It can help to balance secretions in the Kingdom. Transformation and separation are made difficult without fluidity (e.g. sifting of thoughts or separation of nutrients from our food). A deficiency of Water can manifest as a redness of the skin, or as dry, red or inflamed eyes. An imbalance in secretions can also cause disturbances in the ear such as tinnitus. Consider for an inability to lift the arms or grasp objects, and for inflammation of the finger joints.

SI 3 — <u>Back Ravine</u> (Back Stream)
Wood Point. Tonification Point. Shu-Stream/Antique-Summer Point. 'Vitality Point'.
Opening Point of Du Mai. Coupled Point of Yang Qiao Mai (Heel Vessel).

Consider this point if Wood's influence is lacking within the Small Intestine. This may manifest as emotional instability, night sweats, hearing problems, or slow recovery after shock or surgery. When used with Bl 62 it affects the Du Mai and thus the spine, the lower back and kidneys, and helps invigorate the mental faculties. Consider for stiff neck, or pain in the fingers or joints. Has the Small Intestine stopped giving birth to new ideas, or starting new tasks? The patient could be stuck, unable to mature or sort themselves out. This Official acts like a 'secretary' — a discriminating influence for the Emperor. This point relieves muddle and mental 'stagnation' as it aids in the separation of the pure from the impure — thus supporting the processes of decision-making and sorting things out. It can also help in illuminating an appropriate way forward in a person's life.

⊥	△		Location
I	3-5	Ulnar nail point of 5th digit	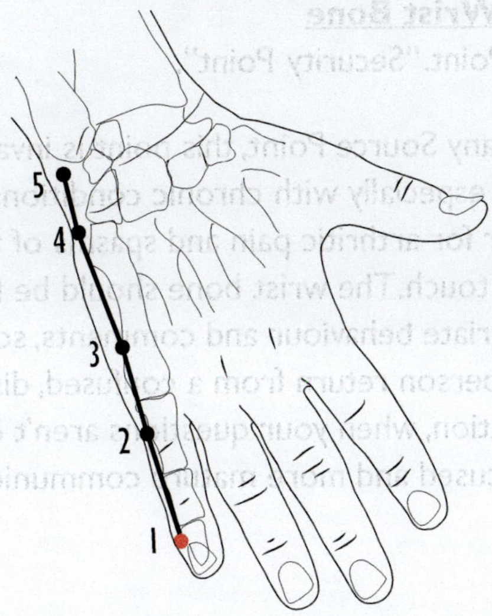
I	3-7	Distal to flare of base of proximal phalanx of 5th digit At end of metacarpo-phalangeal crease (form a loose fist to see) Traditionally located at the change of skin colour	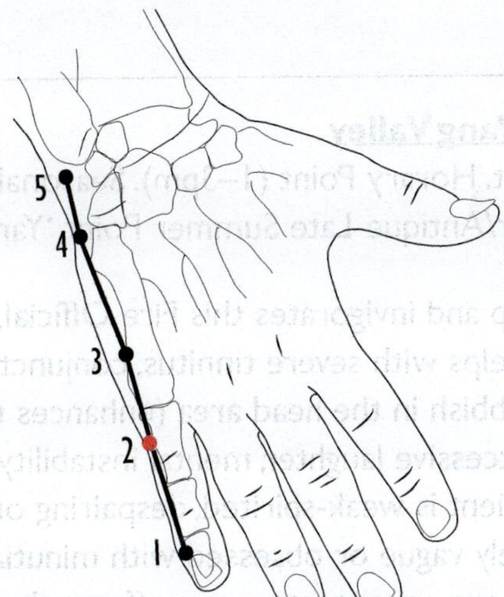
3	3-7	Proximal to metacarpo-phalangeal joint of 5th digit At the flare of the head of the 5th metacarpal bone At ulnar end of distal palmar crease Traditionally located at the change of skin colour	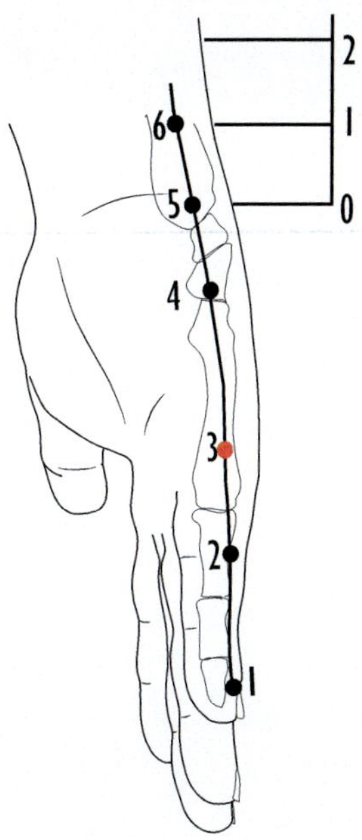

Small Intestine

SI 4 — <u>Wrist Bone</u>
Source Point. "Security Point".

As with any Source Point, this point is invaluable when you are wary of over-stimulating or over-sedating, especially with chronic conditions. This is because of their in-built self-regulating quality. Consider for arthritic pain and spasms of the fingers or wrists, or where there is dullness of sense of touch. The wrist bone should be flexible so we can reach out and touch. Consider for inappropriate behaviour and comments, sometimes of a sexual nature (lack of discrimination). Helps a person return from a confused, disjointed, muddled place, particularly noticeable during conversation, when your questions aren't clearly answered or the subject is suddenly changed, to a clean, focused and more mature communication with other people.

SI 5 — <u>Yang Valley</u>
Fire Point. Horary Point (1–3pm). Seasonal Horary Point — Summer.
Jing-River/Antique-Late Summer Point. 'Yang vitality point'.

Shakes up and invigorates this Fire Official, thus bringing out its inherent potential: aids mental clarity. Helps with severe tinnitus, conjunctivitis or skin eruptions, particularly on the face, as it clears rubbish in the head area (enhances the separation of pure from impure). Consider for high fevers, excessive laughter, mental instability (mind out of control) or excessive talking or, conversely, if the patient is weak-spirited, despairing or unable to cope. For SI-type people who are either excessively vague or obsessed with minutiae. Helps clarify what is correct in relationships so they can be more consistent — not off one day and back on the next. Can be effective for arthritis in the wrists and fingers.

⊥	△		Location
3	3-7	Between 5th metacarpal bone and Hamate bone (can't normally feel) Superior to abductor digiti minimi when the fingers are abducted Traditionally located at the change of skin colour	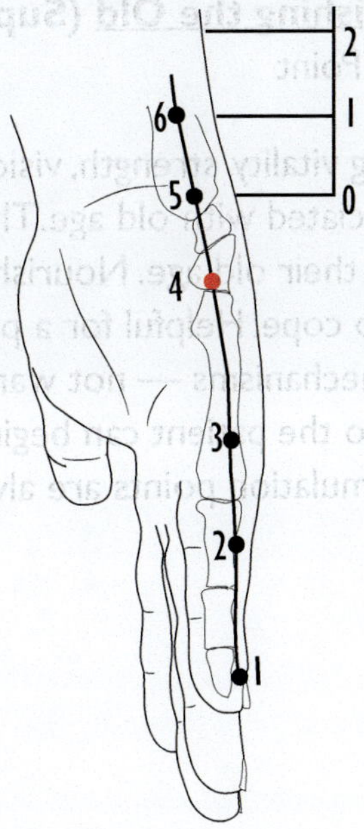
2	3-7	Medial aspect of wrist flexure Between triquetral bone and Styloid process of Ulna	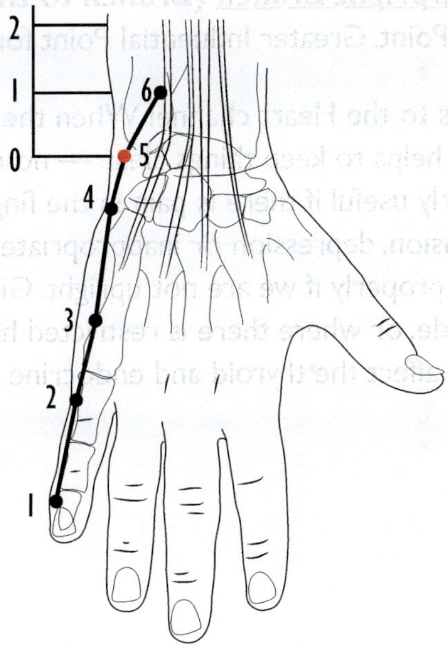

Small Intestine

SI 6 — <u>Nourishing the Old</u> (Supporting the Old)
Accumulation Point

For diminishing vitality, strength, vision and hearing, bloodshot eyes, stiff or painful joints — all problems associated with old age. The Chinese name for this point, 'Yang Lao', means to care for our parents in their old age. Nourishes Body, Mind and Spirit. Helps keep cynicism at bay. Gives the strength to cope. Helpful for a problem that a patient has been trying to cope with for years. Poor coping mechanisms — not wanting to cope. Consider following with the Wood point (SI 3 Back Ravine) so the patient can begin to move on in their life. For confusion, muddle or a lack of maturity. Accumulation points are always beneficial for chronic conditions.

SI 7 — <u>Upright Branch</u> (Branch to the Upright)
Junction Point. Greater Influential Point for the head and neck. 'Equilibrium point'.

Connects to the Heart channel. When the Heart is upright and correct it has virtue. The Small Intestine helps to keep things clear — no confusion. For an inability to grasp or hold an object. Particularly useful if there is pain in the fingers, forearm or elbow. Consider for psychopathic apprehension, depression or inappropriate conduct, especially of a sexual nature. We cannot separate properly if we are not upright. Gives support and balance when a person is leaning over to one side, or where there is restricted head rotation, or a patient is 'in their head' (i.e. confused). Is said to affect the thyroid and endocrine systems.

⊥	Δ		Location
3	3-5	Posterior-medial surface of forearm Between tendon of Extensor Carpi Ulnaris and the groove on the Medial surface of head of ulna Between the head of ulna and styloid process Point lies between upper border of tendon of Extensor Carpi Ulnaris and the groove in the Ulna Approx **1 cun** proximal to SI 5 but anatomy takes precedence	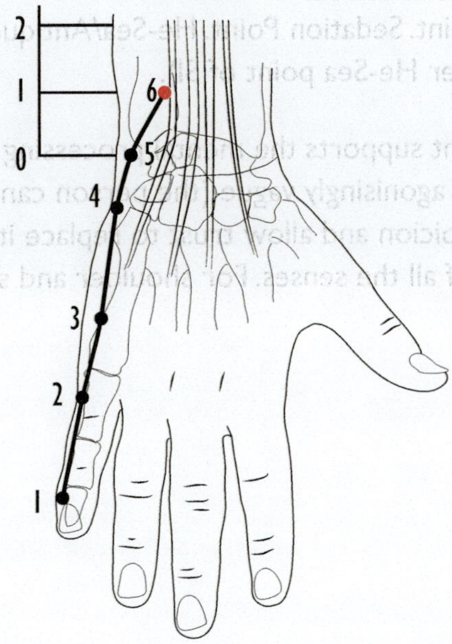
3	3-7	Forbidden from 6th month of pregnancy Posterior surface of forearm **5 cun** proximal to SI 5 Between medial border ulna bone and lateral border of Extensor Carpi Ulnaris muscle	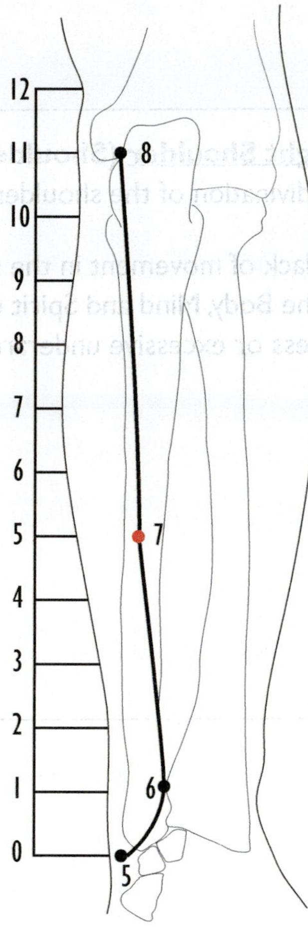

SI 8 — <u>Small Sea</u>
Earth Point. Sedation Point. He-Sea/Antique-Autumn Point. Has a connection with St 39 (which is the Lower He-Sea point of SI).

This point supports the mental processing of the Small Intestine which can become obsessed with detail or agonisingly vague (the person can't discriminate). Earth brings stability to Fire and helps to ease suspicion and allow trust to replace it. Consider when the whole body/psyche/soul is dulled; dulling of all the senses. For shoulder and scapula pain. Has a local effect on the elbow.

SI 9 — <u>Upright Shoulder</u> (Shoulder Virtue, Shoulder Divination)
'Enquiring by divination of the shoulder' (i.e. palpation)

Consider for lack of movement in the shoulder, or numbness there due to the effects of Wind. Helps to rid the Body, Mind and Spirit of impurities. For all shoulder problems. Beneficial for tinnitus, deafness or excessive underarm perspiration.

⊥	△		Location
2	3-5	Halfway between the Olecranon process of the ulna and the medial epicondyle of the humerus. In the humero-ulnar joint.	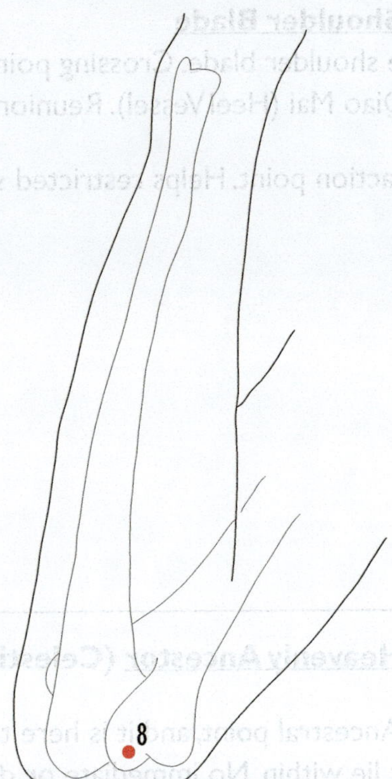
5-7	X	Posterior torso, posterior aspect of shoulder Inferior to shoulder joint Just inferior to the posterior border of the deltoid muscle Approx **1 cun** directly superior to the meeting point of the upper arm and the torso	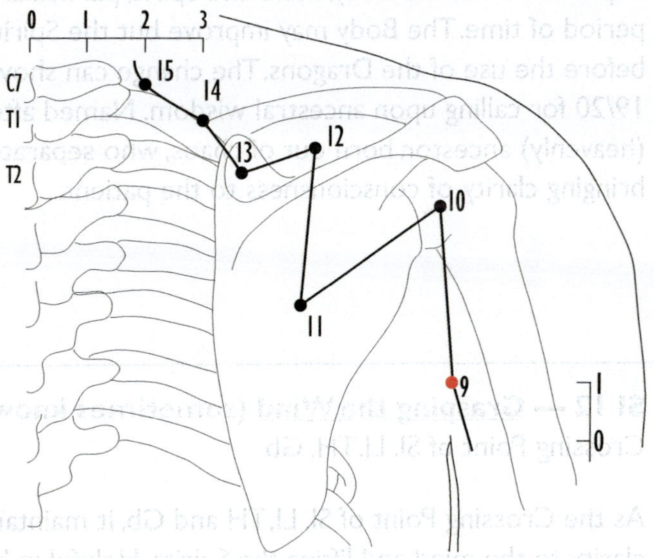

Small Intestine

SI 10 — <u>Shoulder Blade</u>
AEP of the shoulder blade. Crossing point of SI, Yang Wei Mai (Linking Vessel) and Yang Qiao Mai (Heel Vessel). Reunion Point of LI, TH, Gb.

Cleansing action point. Helps restricted shoulder movement. Consider for frozen shoulder.

SI 11 — <u>Heavenly Ancestor</u> (Celestial Ancestor, Celestial Gathering)

This is an Ancestral point, and it is here that we can call upon the help and guidance of the wise elders that lie within. No immediate or dramatic change, but slow, steady, positive change. Strongest spiritual point on the SI meridian; we are going to the Spirit of the Small Intestine here. Eliminates impurities from the Body, Mind and Spirit, particularly if the patient has been on drugs for a long period of time. The Body may improve but the Spirit remains in a quagmire — consider this point before the use of the Dragons. The change can show in the clarity of the pulses. Similar to Du 19/20 for calling upon ancestral wisdom. Named after a star, but is also said to refer to a mythical (heavenly) ancestor, born out of chaos, who separated the heavens from the earth, thus analogically bringing clarity of consciousness to the patient.

SI 12 — <u>Grasping the Wind</u> (sometimes known as 'Clutching at Straws')
Crossing Point of SI, LI, TH, Gb

As the Crossing Point of SI, LI, TH and Gb, it maintains the purity of Body Mind and Spirit, bringing clarity to the mind and lifting the Spirits. Helpful in bringing about cohesion when a person feels scattered, confused or disorganised. Consider for frozen shoulder. Moxa can be very effective here for deficient or cold conditions. Can help if there is an inability to lift the arms.

<table>
<tr><th>⊥</th><th>△</th><th></th><th>Location</th></tr>
<tr><td>5-7</td><td>3-7</td><td>Forbidden from 6th month of pregnancy
Posterior torso, posterior aspect of shoulder
Superior to the posterior axillary crease
In a depression that is just inferior to the neck of the Acromion of the scapular spine
Approx 1 cun medial to TH 14</td><td>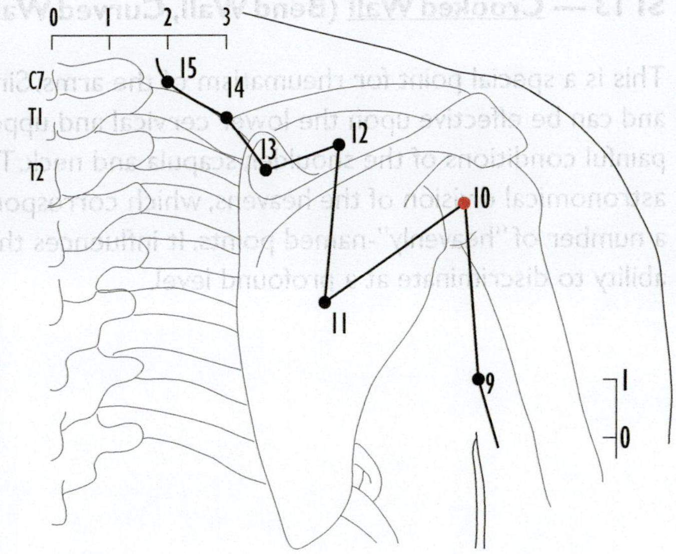
</td></tr>
<tr><td>5</td><td>5-7</td><td>On the scapula bone
At the centre of the infraspinous fossa of the scapula</td><td>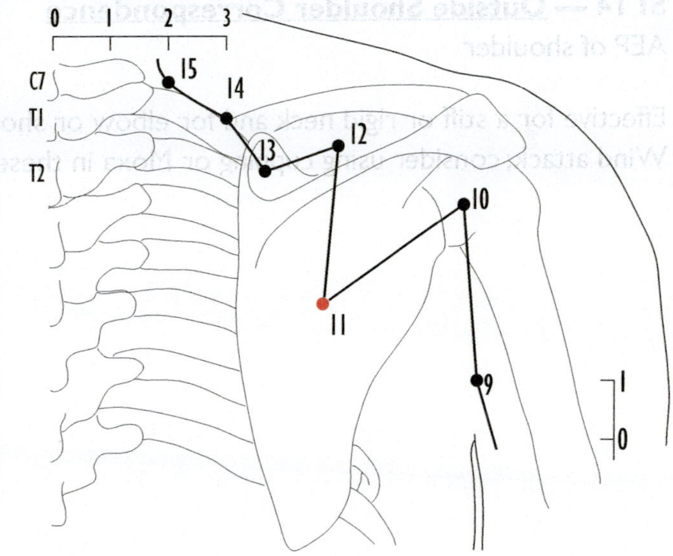
</td></tr>
<tr><td>5</td><td>7</td><td>Superior to scapula spine
At the centre of the supraspinous fossa of the scapula
Directly superior to SI 11
In a depression formed when arm is raised</td><td>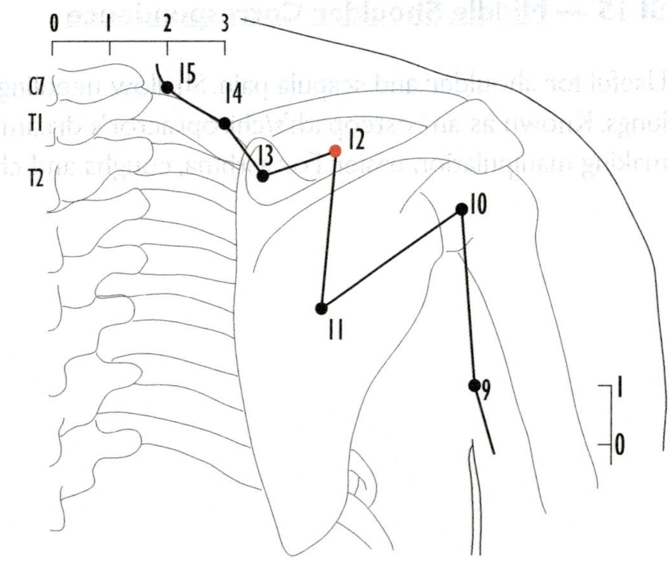
</td></tr>
</table>

Small Intestine

SI 13 — <u>Crooked Wall</u> (Bend Wall, Curved Wall)

This is a special point for rheumatism of the arms. Similar to the cleansing action of SI 9 and SI 10, and can be effective upon the lower cervical and upper thoracic vertebrae. Use for chronic or painful conditions of the shoulder, scapula and neck. Thought to be the name of an ancient Chinese astronomical division of the heavens, which corresponds to this area of the body where there are a number of "heavenly"-named points. It influences the deeper part of the human being and the ability to discriminate at a profound level.

SI 14 — <u>Outside Shoulder Correspondence</u>
AEP of shoulder

Effective for a stiff or rigid neck and for elbow or shoulder problems. Can be useful for chills and Wind attack; consider using cupping or Moxa in these instances.

SI 15 — <u>Middle Shoulder Correspondence</u>

Useful for shoulder and scapula pain. Shallow needling is required, as the point lies close to the lungs. Known as an "osteopath's/chiropractor's dream" — makes muscles pliable and drains toxins, making manipulation easier. For asthma, coughs and chills. Consider Moxa and cupping here.

⊥	△		Location
5	3-7	Posterior torso Medial end of the supraspinous fossa of the scapula Approx midway between SI 10 and the spinous process of the 2nd thoracic vertebra	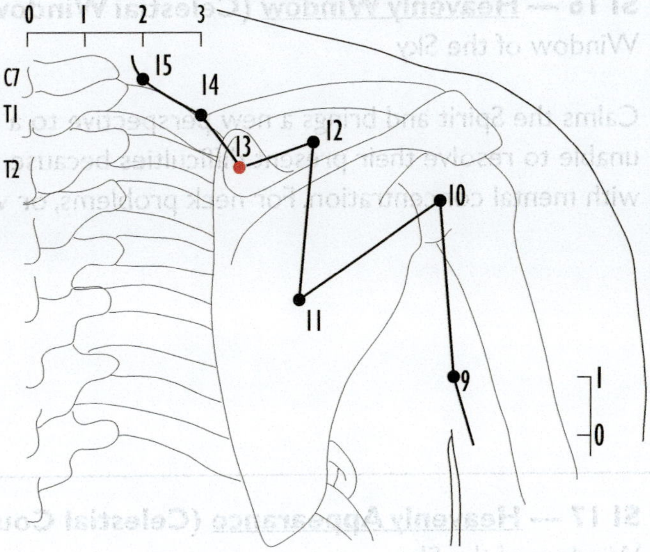
6	3-10	Level with Intervertebral space between T1 and T2 vertebrae **3 cun** lateral to the posterior median line Level with Du 13 (which is between T1 and T2)	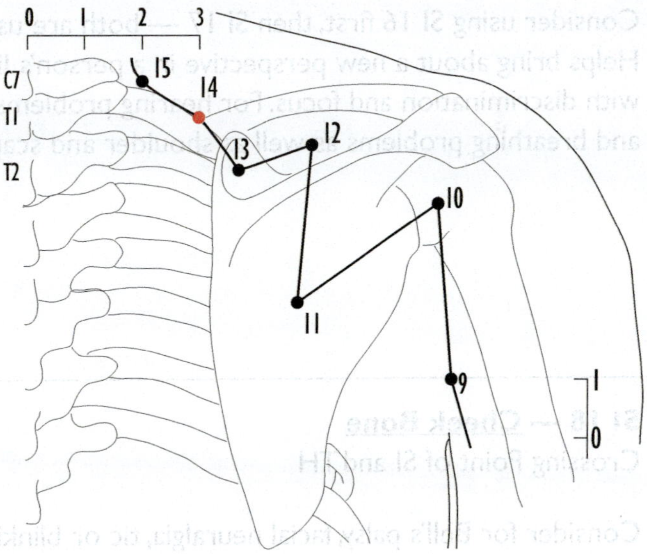
3-6	5-10	Level with Intervertebral space between C7 and T1 vertebrae **2 cun l**ateral to the posterior median line Level with Du 14 (which is between C7 and T1)	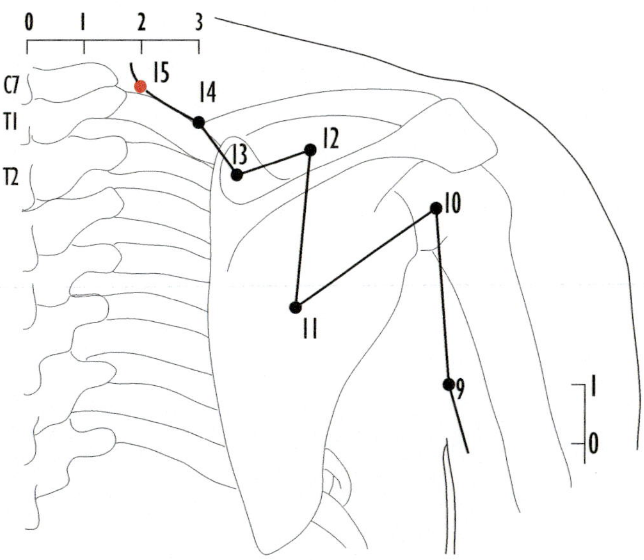

Small Intestine

SI 16 — <u>Heavenly Window</u> (Celestial Window)
Window of the Sky

Calms the Spirit and brings a new perspective to a person who has lost hope and vision, or who is unable to resolve their present difficulties because they cannot separate pure from impure. Helps with mental concentration. For neck problems, or where there is sluggishness or lethargy present.

SI 17 — <u>Heavenly Appearance</u> (Celestial Countenance)
Window of the Sky

Consider using SI 16 first, then SI 17 — both are used to treat the Spirit. For mental imprisonment. Helps bring about a new perspective in a person's life. Enhances clarity of consciousness. Helps with discrimination and focus. For hearing problems such as tinnitus or deafness. Also for asthma and breathing problems as well as shoulder and scapula pain.

SI 18 — <u>Cheek Bone</u>
Crossing Point of SI and TH

Consider for Bell's palsy, facial neuralgia, tic or blinking eye. Also for tooth and jaw problems.

⊥	Δ		Location
3	3	Lateral surface of neck Posterior border of sternocleidomastoid muscle On a contour with the laryngeal prominence, St 9 and LI 18	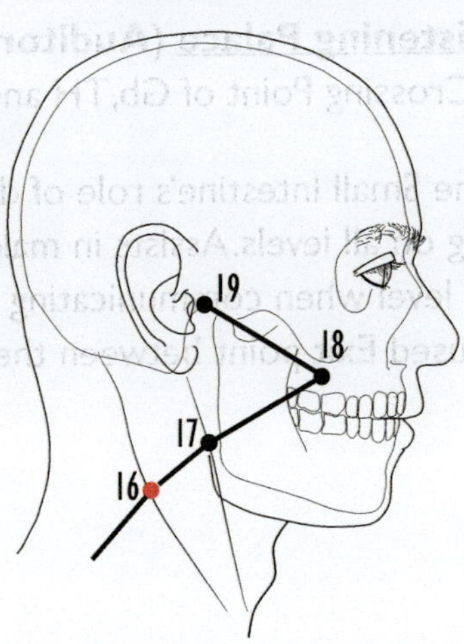
3	3-5	Lateral surface of neck Anterior border of sternocleidomastoid muscle Posterior to angle of the mandible	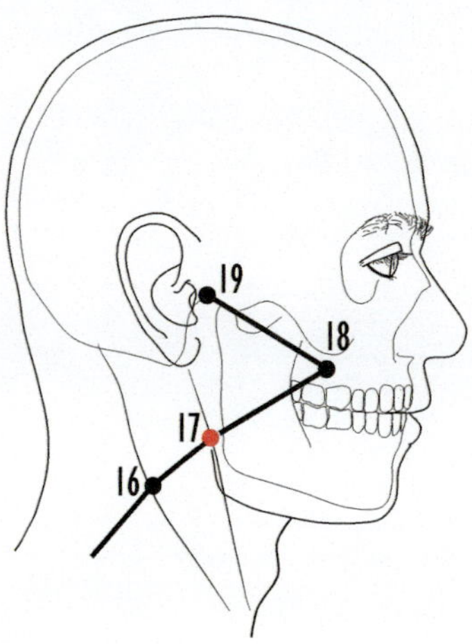
3	X	On the face — on the cheek Directly inferior to lateral canthus of the eye In the angle formed by the anterior border of the ramus of the mandible and inferior border of the zygomatic arch of the zygomatic bone	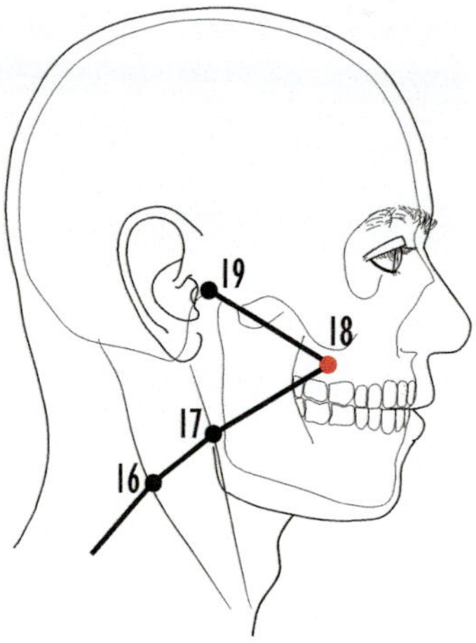

Small Intestine

SI 19 — <u>Listening Palace</u> (Auditory Palace, Temple of Understanding)
Exit Point, Crossing Point of Gb, TH and SI

Enhances the Small Intestine's role of discrimination and clear communication. Helps hearing and listening on all levels. Assists in making sense of what is being said. Helps a person to listen at a deeper level when communicating with others. Useful for tinnitus, deafness or otitis. It is a commonly used Exit point between the Small Intestine and the Bladder (connecting to Bl 1).

⊥	Δ		Location
2-3	3-5	Lateral side of face, anterior to the ear Anterior to the middle of the tragus of the ear Posterior to the condyle of the mandible bone The point lies inferior to TH 21 and superior to Gb 2 Locate with the mouth open	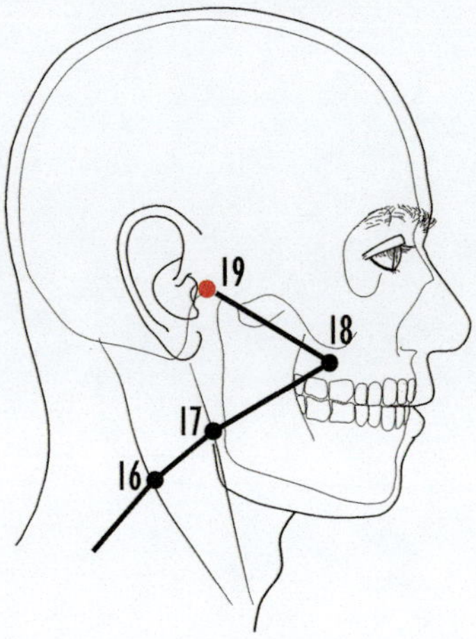

Bladder

- **The Official in Charge of Controlling the Storage of Fluids**
- **Water governs the bones, ears and hearing and the emotion Fear**

Bladder

Bl 1 — <u>Eyes Bright</u> (Eyes Clarity)
Entry Point. Crossing Point of Bl, SI, St, Gb, TH, Du Mai, Yang Qiao Mai (Heel Vessel) and Yang Wei Mai (Linking Vessel).

Helps to regulate the secretions in the Kingdom, and thus influences the hormonal system. This is a powerful point for revitalising the Spirit, Mind and Body. Can be used early on in treatment for Water CF's. It is the start of the longest meridian in the body (and the longest description of its workings in the 'Spiritual Orchid'), and connects deeply, via the Back AEP points, to the other Officials. For all eye diseases. Can help to improve eyesight. Consider for rhinitis and sinusitis. Ming in its name means 'radiance' (of the spirits) which shows in the eyes of the patient.

Bl 2 — <u>Collect Bamboo</u> (Bamboo Gathering, Beginning of Light)

This point refreshes our physical and mental faculties. Can be considered as an alternative to, or supplement for, Bl 1. For sinusitis, hay fever or eye problems. Clears the nose and head. Consider for headaches, particularly around the eyes. The eyebrow resembles a bamboo leaf, hence its name.

Bl 3 — <u>Eyebrows Rushing</u> (Eyebrow Ascension)

Rarely used, but is said to have good effects on the Spirit level of the patient. Local point for headaches, eye problems and nasal congestion.

⊥	Δ		Location
3	X	**0.1 cun** superior and medial to the medial canthus of the eye	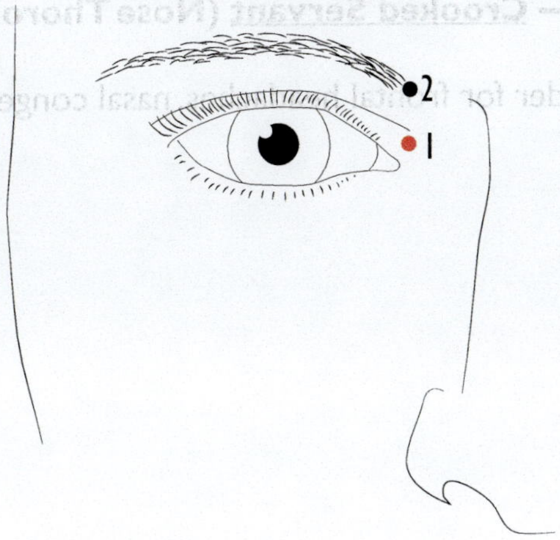
2	X	At the medial end of the eyebrow Superior to Bl 1 and the medial canthus of the eye In a depression on the superciliary arch of the frontal bone of the skull	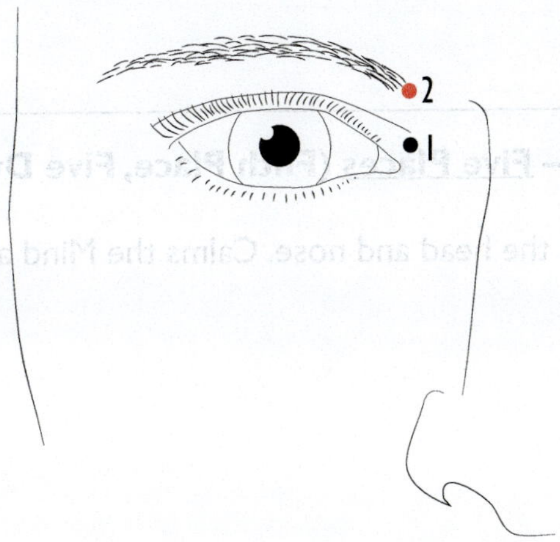
3	3	Directly superior to Bl 2 (on the medial end of the eyebrow) **0.75 cun** lateral to the anterior median line **0.5 cun** posterior to the natural anterior hairline Level with Du 24, and between Du 24 and Bl 4	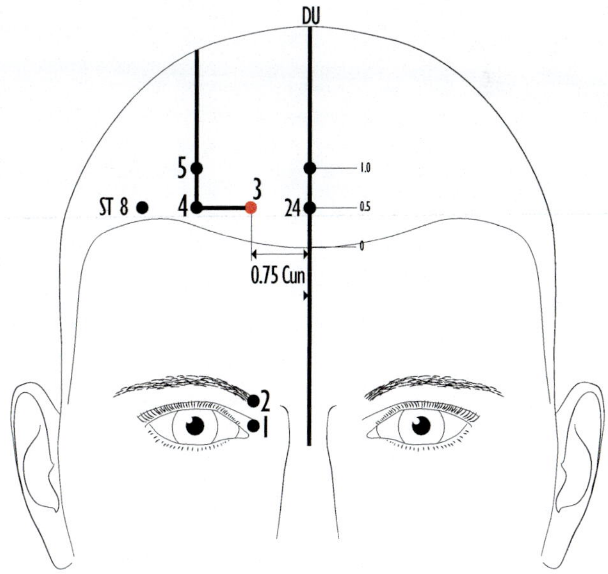

Bl 4 — Crooked Servant (Nose Thoroughfare)

Consider for frontal headaches, nasal congestion, nosebleed or nose sores.

Bl 5 — Five Places (Fifth Place, Five Dwelling)

Clears the head and nose. Calms the Mind and Spirit. Brightens the eyes.

<table>
<tr><th>⊥</th><th>Δ</th><th></th><th>Location</th></tr>
<tr><td>2</td><td>3-5</td><td>On the frontal bone
1.5 cun lateral to the anterior median line (at Du 24)
0.5 cun posterior to the natural anterior hairline
1/3 distance lateral from Du 24 to St 8</td><td>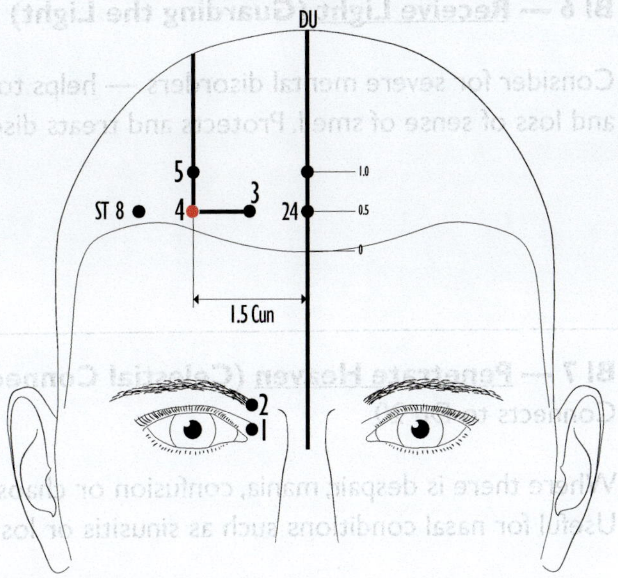
</td></tr>
<tr><td>3</td><td>X</td><td>On the frontal bone
1.5 cun lateral to the anterior median line (at Du 23)
1 cun posterior to the natural anterior hairline
0.5 cun posterior to Bl 4</td><td>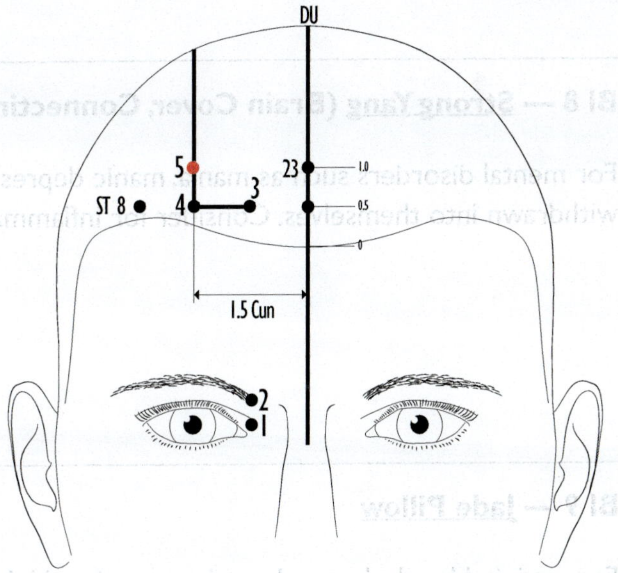
</td></tr>
</table>

Bladder

Bl 6 — Receive Light (Guarding the Light)

Consider for severe mental disorders — helps to calm the Mind and Spirit. For nasal congestion and loss of sense of smell. Protects and treats disorders of the eye. Brightens the eyes.

Bl 7 — Penetrate Heaven (Celestial Connection, Celestial White)
Connects to Du 20

Where there is despair, mania, confusion or chaos, this point brings peace and calm at a deep level. Useful for nasal conditions such as sinusitis or loss of the sense of smell.

Bl 8 — Strong Yang (Brain Cover, Connecting Cleft, Lou End)

For mental disorders such as mania, manic depression, scattered behaviour, or where a person has withdrawn into themselves. Consider for inflammation of the capillaries of the eye.

Bl 9 — Jade Pillow

For occipital headaches and nasal congestion. Helps invigorate the sense of smell and the senses in general.

⊥	△		Location
3	X	On the parietal bone **1.5 cun** lateral to the median line **2.5 cun** posterior to the natural anterior hairline **1.5 cun** posterior to Bl 5	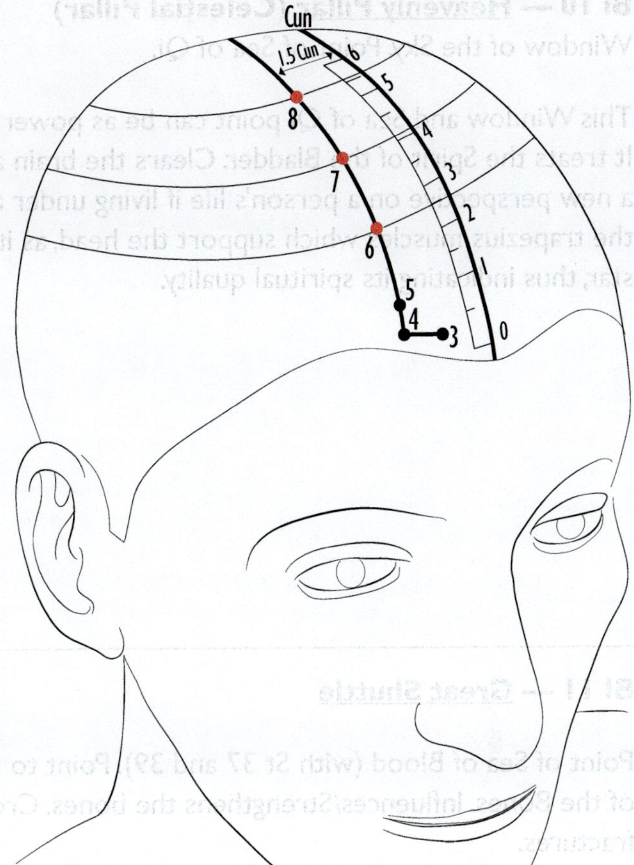
3	3-5	On the parietal bone **1.5 cun** lateral to the median line **4 cun** posterior to the natural anterior hairline **1.5 cun** posterior to Bl 6	
3	3-5	On the parietal bone **1.5 cun** lateral to the median line **5.5 cun** posterior to the natural anterior hairline **1.5 cun** posterior to Bl 7	
3-5	3-5	On the prominence of the trapezius muscle (nape of the neck) **1.3 cun** lateral to the posterior median line **2.5 cun** superior to the natural posterior hairline	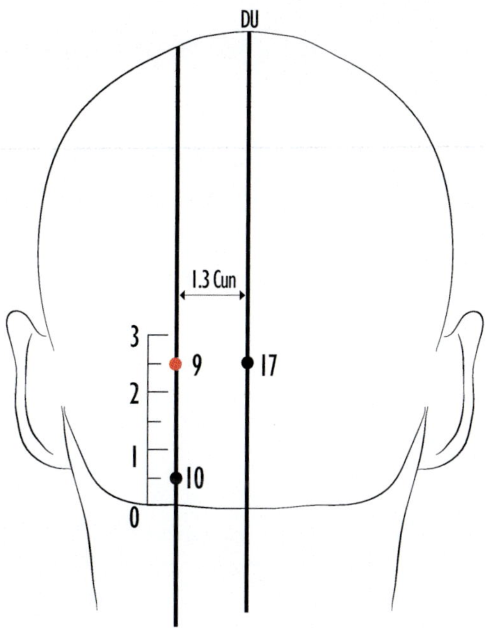

Bladder

Bl 10 — Heavenly Pillar (Celestial Pillar)
Window of the Sky. Point of Sea of Qi.

This Window and Sea of Qi point can be as powerful as the Kidney Chest Points (Kid 22-27). It treats the Spirit of the Bladder. Clears the brain and stimulates memory and concentration. Gives a new perspective on a person's life if living under a cloud of fear. Pillar in the name may refer to the trapezius muscles which support the head, as it treats disorders of the neck. Named after a star, thus indicating its spiritual quality.

Bl 11 — Great Shuttle

Point of Sea of Blood (with St 37 and 39). Point to release the External Dragons. Influential Point of the Bones. Influences/Strengthens the bones. Crossing Point of Bl, SI, Gb, TH, Du Mai. First Aid: fractures.
As a Sea of Blood, this point can be sedated for high fever or tonified for anaemia. The patient's Blood quality can be nourished and strengthened here. Helps prevent bone degeneration, particularly in the elderly. Moxa and cupping helpful here at the onset of a cold. 'Great' refers to the prominence of the 1st vertebra.

<table>
<tr><th>⊥</th><th>Δ</th><th></th><th>Location</th></tr>
<tr><td>3-5</td><td>3</td><td>On the prominence of the trapezius muscle (nape of the neck)
1.3 cun lateral to the posterior median line
0.5 cun superior to the natural posterior hairline</td><td>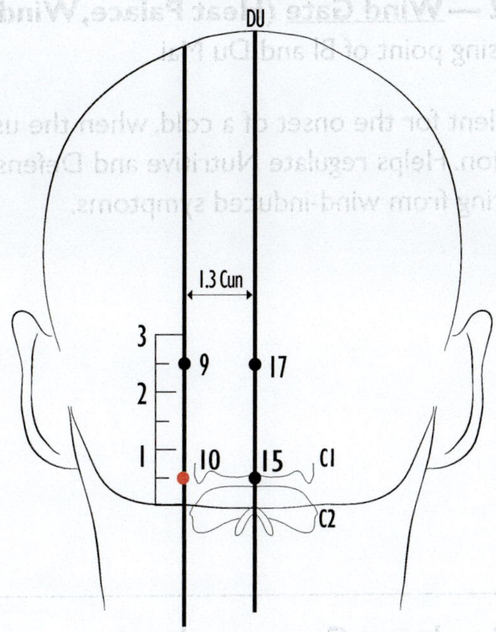
</td></tr>
<tr><td>3-7</td><td>3-7</td><td>On the inner line of the Bl Channel
1.5 cun lateral to the posterior median line
Between 1st and 2nd Thoracic vertebrae</td><td>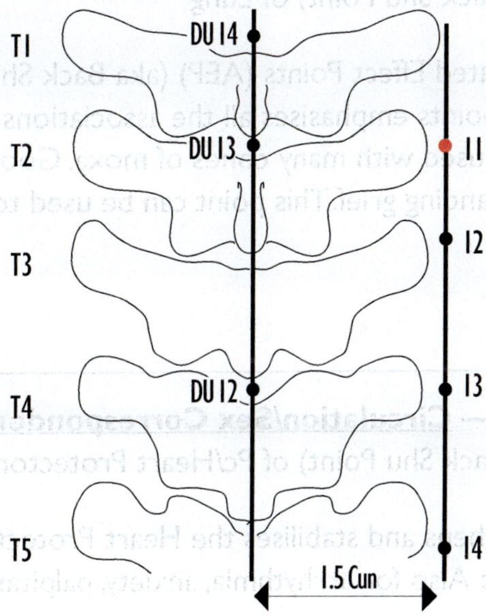
</td></tr>
</table>

Bladder

Bl 12 — Wind Gate (Heat Palace, Wind Door)
Crossing point of Bl and Du Mai

Excellent for the onset of a cold, when the use of cupping and moxa can be effective. Aids Lung function. Helps regulate Nutritive and Defensive Qi. Consider for those sensitive to the wind, or suffering from wind-induced symptoms.

Bl 13 — Lungs Correspondence
AEP (Back Shu Point) of Lung

Associated Effect Points (AEP) (aka Back Shu points) go direct to the Official, and treatment of these points emphasises all the associations of the Official and its Element. Most of these points can be used with many cones of moxa. Good for Asthma and chronic lung weakness. Consider for long-standing grief. This point can be used to drain aggressive energy, as can the other Yin AEPs.

Bl 14 — Circulation/Sex Correspondence
AEP (Back Shu Point) of Pc/Heart Protector

Strengthens and stabilises the Heart Protector. Consider for heartache, heartbreak, melancholia or sadness. Also for arrhythmia, anxiety, palpitations or shortness of breath.

<table>
<tr><th>⊥</th><th>△</th><th></th><th>Location</th></tr>
<tr><td>5</td><td>5-10</td><td>On the inner line of the Bl Channel
1.5 cun lateral to the posterior median line
Between 2nd and 3rd Thoracic vertebrae</td><td>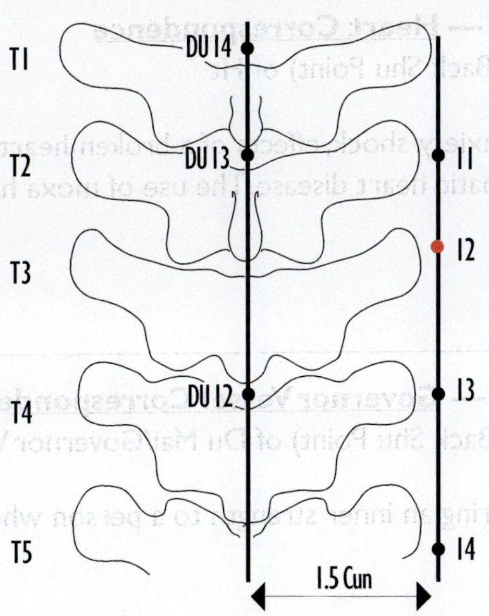
</td></tr>
<tr><td>3-5</td><td>7-20</td><td>On the inner line of the Bl Channel
1.5 cun lateral to the posterior median line
Between 3rd and 4th Thoracic vertebrae</td><td rowspan="2">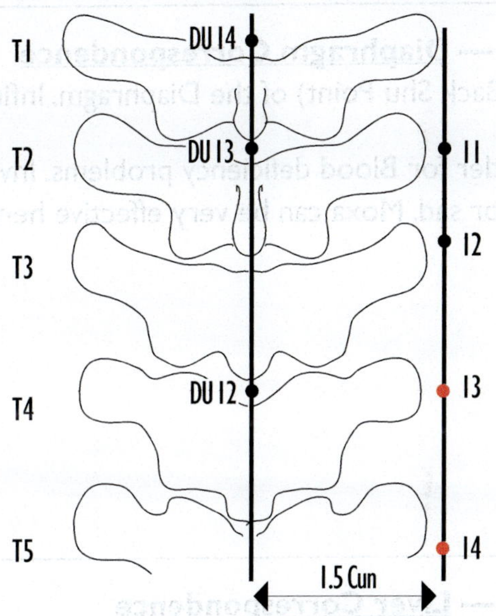
</td></tr>
<tr><td>3-5</td><td>7</td><td>On the inner line of the Bl Channel
1.5 cun lateral to the posterior median line
Between 4th and 5th Thoracic vertebrae</td></tr>
</table>

Bladder

Bl 15 — Heart Correspondence
AEP (Back Shu Point) of Ht

For anxiety, shock, effects of a broken heart, insomnia or sadness. Consider if the patient has had rheumatic heart disease. The use of moxa here, when appropriate, can give additional support.

Bl 16 — Governor Vessel Correspondence
AEP (Back Shu Point) of Du Mai/Governor Vessel

Can bring an inner strength to a person when struggling with life's trials and tribulations.

Bl 17 — Diaphragm Correspondence
AEP (Back Shu Point) of the Diaphragm. Influential Point of the Blood.

Consider for Blood deficiency problems. Invigorates the Blood. Helpful when the patient is cold, weak or sad. Moxa can be very effective here.

Bl 18 — Liver Correspondence
AEP (Back Shu Point) of Liv

For all Liver-associated conditions such as inappropriate anger, depression, lack of hope, poor vision or poor planning abilities. Can help on all levels of the BMS which are influenced by this Official.

⊥	Δ		Location
3	3	On the inner line of the Bl Channel **1.5 cun** lateral to the posterior median line Between **5th and 6th Thoracic vertebrae**	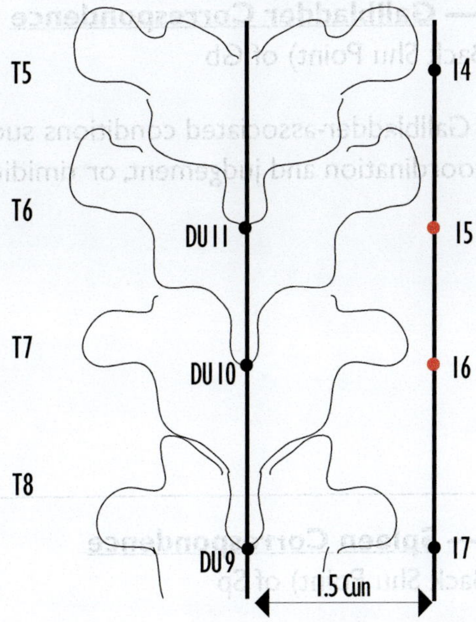
X	3	On the inner line of the Bl Channel **1.5 cun** lateral to the posterior median line Between **6th and 7th Thoracic vertebrae**	
4	7-20	On the inner line of the Bl Channel **1.5 cun** lateral to the posterior median line Between **7th and 8th Thoracic vertebrae**	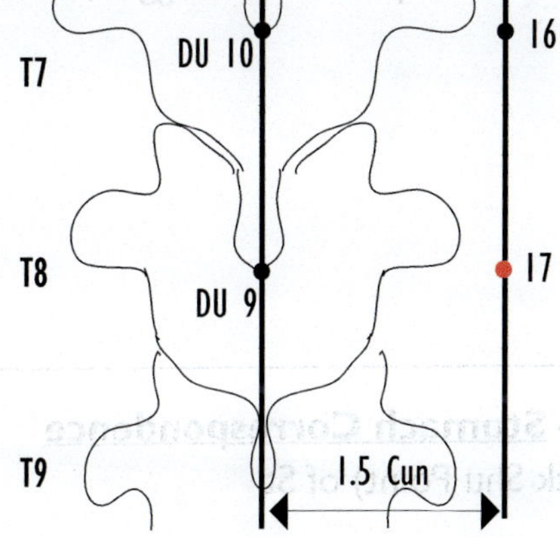
3	7-20	On the inner line of the Bl Channel **1.5 cun** lateral to the posterior median line Between **9th and 10th Thoracic vertebrae**	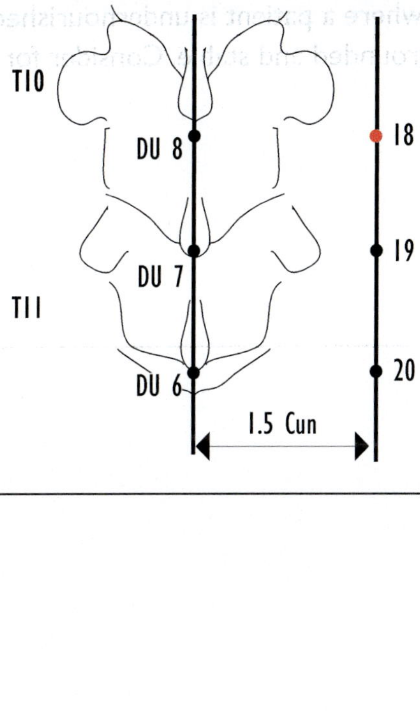

Bladder

Bl 19 — Gallbladder Correspondence
AEP (Back Shu Point) of Gb

For all Gallbladder-associated conditions such as lack of decision-making abilities and uprightness, poor coordination and judgement, or timidity. Consider using Moxa too for these deficiencies.

Bl 20 — Spleen Correspondence
AEP (Back Shu Point) of Sp

For all Spleen-associated conditions such as transformation or transportation problems, obsessive thinking patterns, lack of mental acuity, chronic exhaustion, problems with food or weight. Consider if the patient is depleted and sluggish, either physically or mentally.

Bl 21 — Stomach Correspondence
AEP (Back Shu Point) of St

For all Stomach conditions such as: poor processing abilities, poor digestion (of information or food), or where a patient is undernourished or 'stuck' in their life. Can help the patient feel more centred, grounded and stable. Consider for acid reflux problems or loss of appetite.

⊥	△		Location
3-5	3-15	On the inner line of the Bl Channel **1.5 cun** lateral to the posterior median line Between **10th and 11th Thoracic vertebrae**	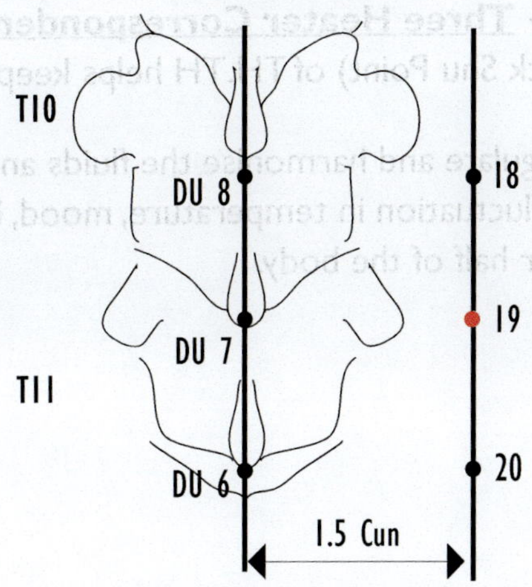
3-5	7-20	On the inner line of the Bl Channel **1.5 cun** lateral to the posterior median line Between **11th and 12th Thoracic vertebrae**	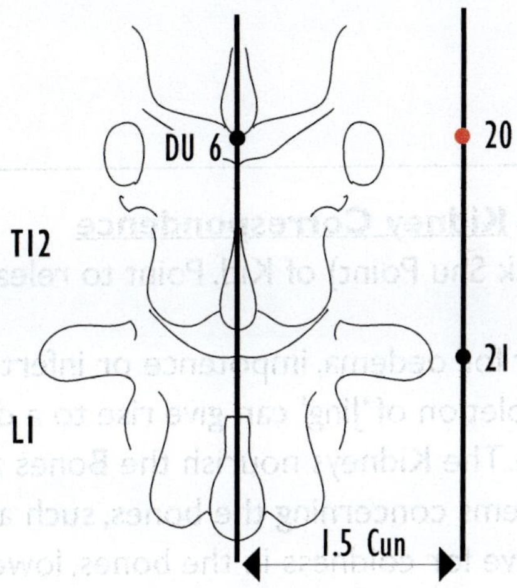
3-5	7-21	On the inner line of the Bl Channel **1.5 cun** lateral to the posterior median line Between **12th Thoracic** and **1st Lumbar vertebrae**	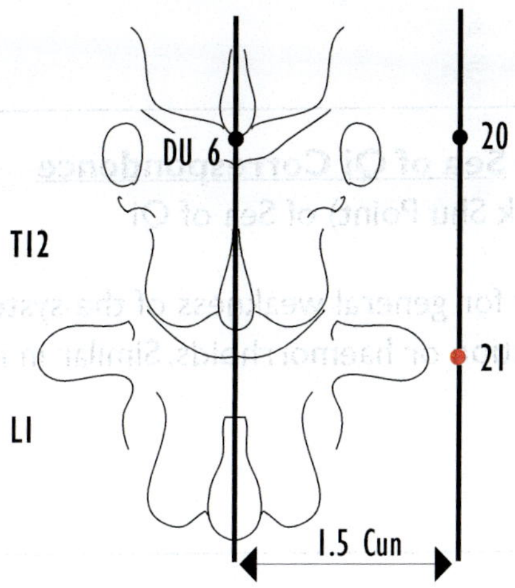

Bladder

Bl 22 — Three Heater Correspondence
AEP (Back Shu Point) of TH. TH helps keep open the Water Passages.

Helps regulate and harmonise the fluids and internal warmth within the Kingdom. Consider for a marked fluctuation in temperature, mood, behaviour or vitality. For retention of urine or swelling in the lower half of the body.

Bl 23 — Kidney Correspondence
AEP (Back Shu Point) of Kid. Point to release the External Dragons.

Consider for oedema, impotence or infertility. This point strengthens and warms the patient's 'Jing'. Depletion of 'Jing' can give rise to a depletion of energy, wisdom, determination, willpower and drive. The Kidneys nourish the Bones and Marrow, and influence hearing. Therefore consider for problems concerning the bones, such as arthritis or osteoporosis. The use of moxa here can be effective for coldness in the bones, lower back or knees.

Bl 24 — Sea of Qi Correspondence
AEP (Back Shu Point) of Sea of Qi

Consider for general weakness of the system, lower back problems, irregular or painful menstruation or haemorrhoids. Similar in its effect to Ren 6 (Sea of Qi).

⊥	Δ		Location
3-5	7-20	On the inner line of the Bl Channel **1.5 cun** lateral to the posterior median line Between **1st and 2nd Lumbar vertebrae**	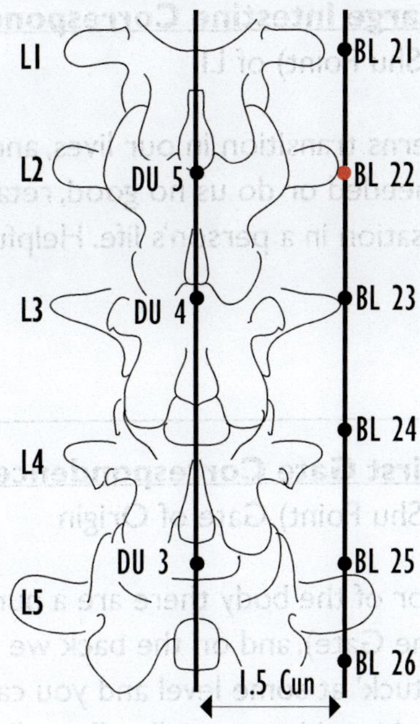
5-8	3-15	On the inner line of the Bl Channel **1.5 cun** lateral to the posterior median line Between **2nd and 3rd Lumbar vertebrae**	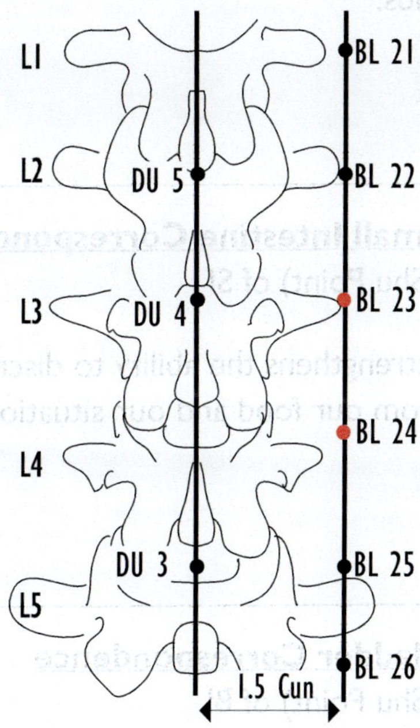
5	3-5	On the inner line of the Bl Channel **1.5 cun** lateral to the posterior median line Between **3rd and 4th Lumbar vertebrae**	

Bl 25 — <u>Large Intestine Correspondence</u>
AEP (Back Shu Point) of LI

The LI governs transition in our lives, and helps the ability to let go of things or situations that are no longer needed or do us no good, retain the worthwhile and move on. Brings quality, invigoration and revitalisation in a person's life. Helpful for constipation or diarrhoea and generalised backache.

Bl 26 — <u>First Gate Correspondence</u> (Origin Pass)
AEP (Back Shu Point) Gate of Origin

In this sector of the body there are a number of gates. On the front are Ren 4 (First Gate), and Ren 5 (Stone Gate), and on the back we have this point, above which is Du 4 (Gate of Life). Use if a patient is 'stuck' at some level and you cannot get through to their core — it opens the gate to the Officials (and is said to partially affect all the other gates in the body). For chronic lumbar pain and haemorrhoids.

Bl 27 — <u>Small Intestine Correspondence</u>
AEP (Back Shu Point) of SI

This point strengthens the ability to discriminate, separate, distinguish, sort out and extract the goodness from our food and our situations. Consider for sacral pain and stiffness.

Bl 28 — <u>Bladder Correspondence</u>
AEP (Back Shu Point) of Bl

Directly strengthens the whole of the Bladder's extensive territory and corresponding influences. For urinary problems such as retention of urine, or pain and burning on passing water. Consider for inappropriate fear. For leg and knee weakness, lower back or sacral pain and stiffness, especially if affected by cold. Consider using Moxa here.

⊥	△		Location
8-10	7-20	On the inner line of the Bl Channel **1.5 cun** lateral to the posterior median line Between **4th and 5th Lumbar vertebrae**	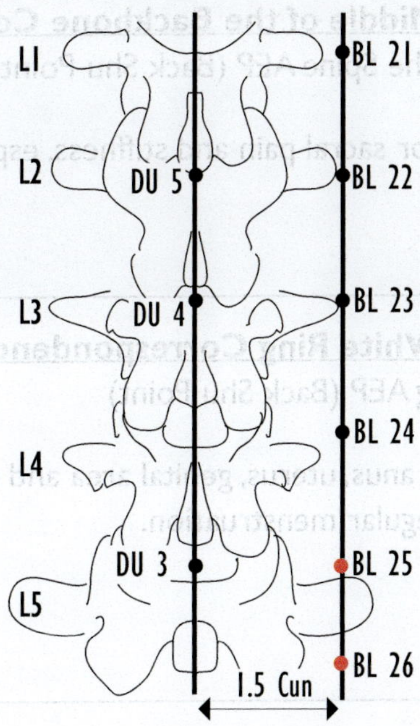
10	3	On the inner line of the Bl Channel **1.5 cun** lateral to the posterior median line Between **5th Lumbar** and **1st Sacral vertebrae**	
8-10	7-20	On the Sacrum. At the medial edge of sacroiliac joint Level with 1st sacral foramen (Bl 31) On the inner line of the Bl Channel **1.5 cun** lateral to posterior median line	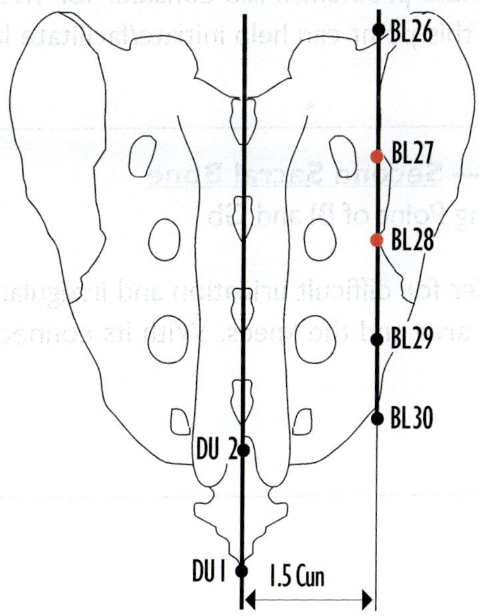
8-10	7-15	On the Sacrum. At the medial edge of sacroiliac joint At the level of the inferior and medial borders of the posterior superior iliac spine (PSIS) Level with 2nd sacral foramen (Bl 32) **1.5 cun** lateral to the posterior median line	

Bladder

Bl 29 — <u>Middle of the Backbone Correspondence</u> (Central Spine)
Middle of the Spine AEP (Back Shu Point)

For spinal or sacral pain and stiffness, especially if the pain is on both sides of the spine.

Bl 30 — <u>White Ring Correspondence</u>
White Ring AEP (Back Shu Point)

Affects the anus, uterus, genital area and sacrum. For painful defecation, haemorrhoids, lower back pain or irregular menstruation.

Bl 31-34 are all on the sacrum. They tonify the Kidneys and strengthen the lumbar area. They affect the lower jiao. Consider using Moxa. Forbidden in pregnancy.

Bl 31 — <u>Upper Sacral Bone</u>
Crossing Point of Bl and Gb

The link between Bl and Gb connects these points to the legs and knees. For infertility, impotence, or prostate problems. Also consider for weak knees and lumbar pain. With its connection to the uterus, this point can help initiate/facilitate labour.

Bl 32 — <u>Second Sacral Bone</u>
Crossing Point of Bl and Gb

Consider for difficult urination and irregular or painful periods. Strengthens the Kidneys, the lumbar area and the knees. With its connection to the uterus, this point can help initiate/facilitate labour.

⊥	△		Location
5	7-15	On the Sacrum. At the lateral edge of the body of the sacrum Level with 3rd sacral foramen (Bl 33) **1.5 cun** lateral to the posterior median line	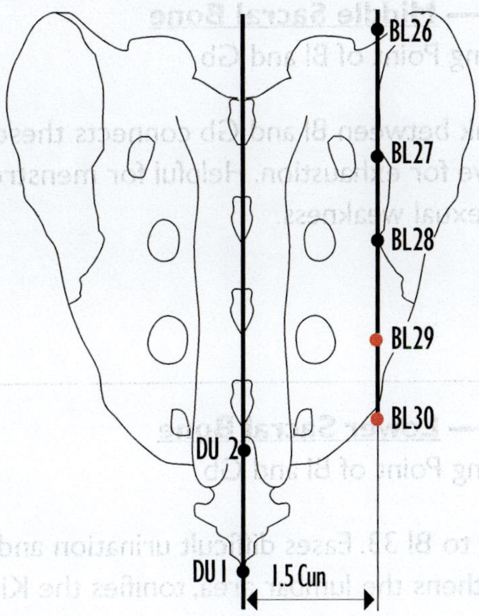
3-5	X	On the Sacrum. At the lateral edge of the body of the sacrum Level with 4th sacral foramen (Bl 34) **1.5 cun** lateral to the posterior median line	
8-10	7-15	Forbidden in pregnancy — expedites labour On the Sacrum In the 1st sacral foramen Approx at the midpoint of the posterior superior iliac spine (PSIS) and the posterior median line	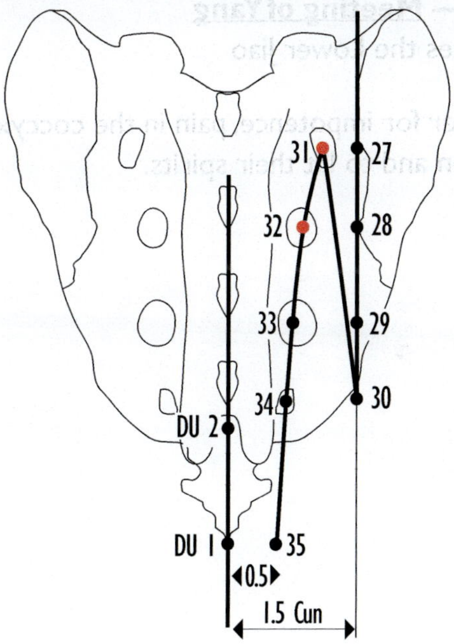
8-10	7-15	Forbidden in pregnancy — expedites labour On the Sacrum In the 2nd sacral foramen Approx at the midpoint of the posterior superior iliac spine (PSIS) and the posterior median line	

Bladder

Bl 33 — Middle Sacral Bone
Crossing Point of Bl and Gb

The link between Bl and Gb connects these points to the legs and knees. Strengthens Kid and is effective for exhaustion. Helpful for menstrual problems. Consider using Moxa here, especially for male sexual weakness.

Bl 34 — Lower Sacral Bone
Crossing Point of Bl and Gb

Similar to Bl 33. Eases difficult urination and elimination. For painful or irregular periods. Strengthens the lumbar area, tonifies the Kidneys and affects the lower jiao. Consider moxa.

Bl 35 — Meeting of Yang
Regulates the Lower Jiao

Consider for impotence, pain in the coccyx, lumbar area or legs. Moxa useful here. Said to motivate a person and to lift their spirits.

⊥	Δ		Location
8-10	7-15	On the Sacrum In the 3rd sacral foramen Level with Bl 29 Approx midway between Bl 29 and the posterior median line	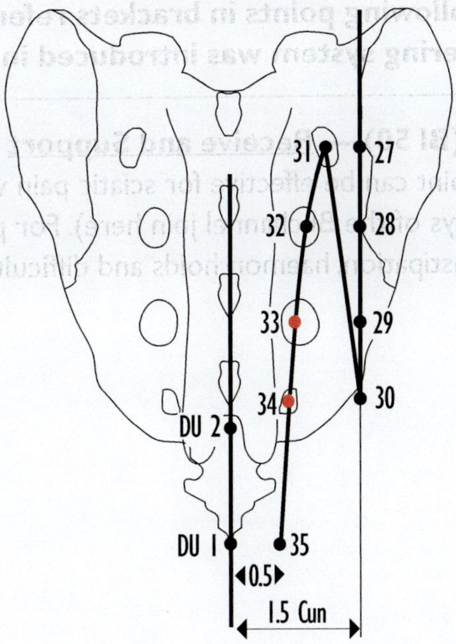
6-8	7-15	On the Sacrum In the 4th sacral foramen Level with Bl 30 Approx midway between Bl 30 and the posterior median line	
4	5	Patient is prone or in a lateral recumbent position with knees pulled towards chin Level with the tip of the coccyx (Du 1) **0.5 cun** lateral to the posterior median line (Du Mai)	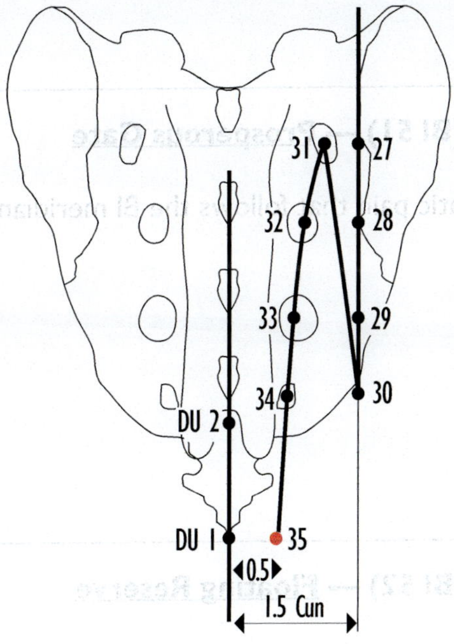

Bladder

The following points in brackets refer to the old numbering system. The new numbering system was introduced in 1985.

Bl 36 (Bl 50) — <u>Receive and Support</u> (Bearing Support, Prop Up and Hold)
This point can be effective for sciatic pain which follows the Bl meridian down the leg (the deep pathways of the Bl channel join here). For paralysis of the legs and sacral or coccyx pain. Consider for constipation, haemorrhoids and difficult urination.

Bl 37 (Bl 51) — <u>Prosperous Gate</u>

For sciatic pain that follows the Bl meridian down the leg.

Bl 38 (Bl 52) — <u>Floating Reserve</u>

Consider for constipation, difficulty urinating, or where there is a burning sensation when urinating.

⊥	Δ		Location
8	X	On the posterior surface of the Upper Thigh On the inferior border of the gluteus maximus muscle At the midpoint of the gluteal groove Between the muscles of the semitendinosus and biceps femoris	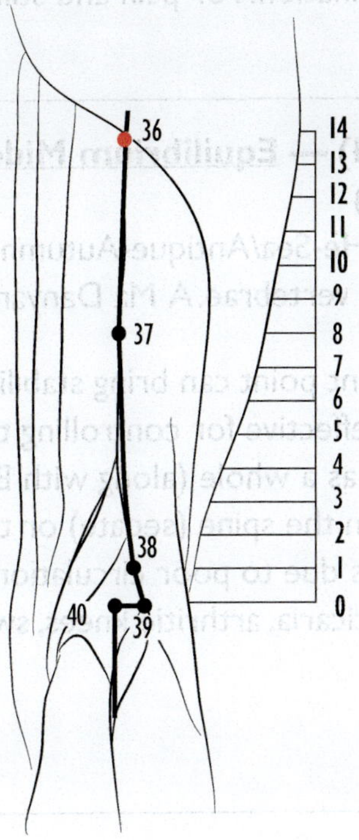
7	X	On the posterior surface of the upper thigh On a line connecting Bl 36 to Bl 40 **6 cun** inferior to Bl 36 **8 cun** proximal to the posterior aspect of the popliteal crease Between the muscles of the semitendinosus and biceps femoris	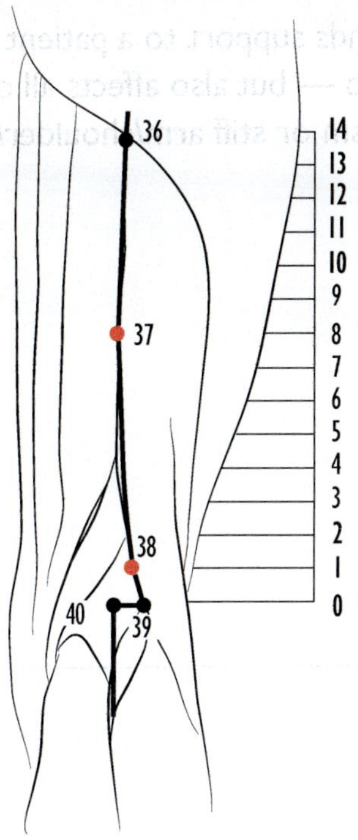
5	3-7	On the posterior surface of the lower thigh **Just** medial to the tendon of the biceps femoris muscle On a line connecting Bl 36 to Bl 40 **1 cun** proximal to the lateral end of the posterior aspect of the popliteal crease	

Bladder

Bl 39 (Bl 53) — <u>Equilibrium Yang</u>
Lower He-Sea Point of TH

Promotes urination. For pain and stiffness of the lower back, knees, legs or feet.

Bl 40 (Bl 54) — <u>Equilibrium Middle</u> (Bending Centre, Perfect Equilibrium, Supporting the Middle)
Earth Point. He-Sea/Antique-Autumn Point. Lower He-Sea Point of Bl. Greater Assembly Point of the back and vertebrae. A Ma Danyang Heavenly Star Point. Accumulation Point of Blood.

This important point can bring stability and equilibrium to an anxious, disorientated or fearful person. It is effective for controlling the Blood (along with Bl 43 (Bl 38)). Can have a direct effect on the spine as a whole (along with Bl 60) and is helpful after osteopathic manipulations; can either free rigidity in the spine (sedate) or tighten it up (tonify). For urinary troubles and night sweats. For disorders due to poor circulation (e.g. haemorrhoids). Consider for knee problems, lower backache, urticaria, arthritic knees, swollen feet or loss of head hair. Great balancer of fluids.

Bl 41 (Bl 36) — <u>Near Division</u> (Attached Branch)
Crossing point of Bl and SI

This point lends support to a patient suffering from long-term chronic illness. Good for influencing the upper jiao — but also affects all of the Triple Heater. Consider for intercostal neuralgia, arm/shoulder spasm or stiff arm/shoulder/neck. For asthma or bronchitis.

⊥	Δ		Location
7	3-5	On the posterior aspect of the popliteal crease **Just** medial to the tendon of biceps femoris muscle (in a dimple) On a line connecting Bl 36 to Bl 40	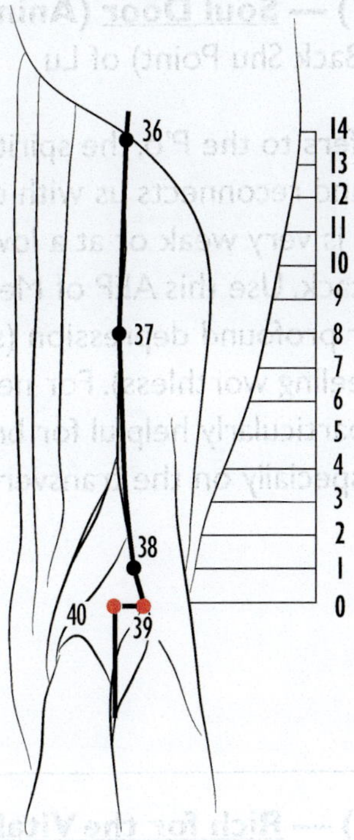
5	X	In the posterior aspect of the popliteal crease Midway between the tendons of the biceps femoris muscle and semitendinosus muscle (in a dimple) On a line connecting Bl 36 to Bl 40 and Bl 57	
4	7	On the outer line of the Bl Channel **3 cun** lateral to the posterior median line Between **2nd and 3rd Thoracic vertebrae**	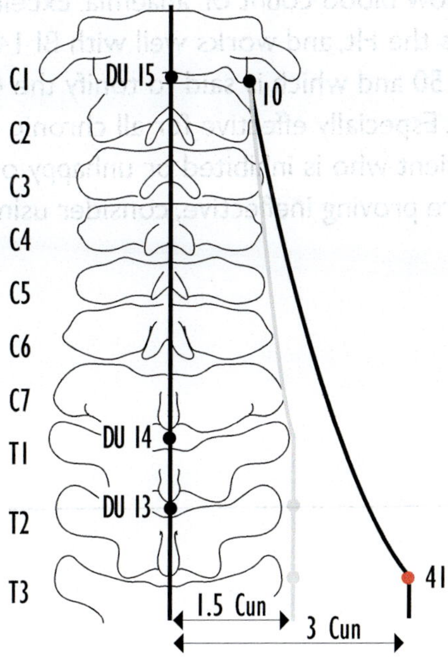

Bladder

Bl 42 (Bl 37) — Soul Door (Animal Soul Door, Door of the P'o (the Corporeal Soul)
Outer AEP (Back Shu Point) of Lu

The name refers to the P'o, the spiritual aspect of Lu, and to an important door which reinforces, strengthens and reconnects us with our authentic self. Moxa here can bring warmth directly to the Spirit if it is very weak or at a low ebb, and thus is unable to defend itself against psychic or emotional attack. Use this AEP of Metal when there is grief or lack of quality in the patient's life. For severe or profound depression (suicidal feelings, lack of physical vigour and dexterity, no sense of purpose, feeling worthless). For neuralgia affecting the arm and shoulder. The use of a Moxa stick here can be particularly helpful for bronchitis, pneumonia and general longstanding respiratory conditions, especially on the transverse line via Bl 13 and Du 12 to Bl 42 on the opposite side.

Bl 43 (Bl 38) — Rich for the Vitals (Chronic Illness Point)
Outer AEP (Back Shu Point) of Pc

A wonderful and commonly used Outer Bladder point which is effective for many blood disorders such as low blood count or anaemia. Excellent when there is a lack of vitality/warmth in the BMS. Supports the Ht, and works well with Bl 14 and Bl 15. Responds well to Moxa — sometimes as many as 50 and which is said to tonify the Qi of the whole body. Nourishes and enriches all of the Officials. Especially effective for all chronic disease, exhaustion or depression. It can be effective for a patient who is inhibited or unhappy over sex, or for low sexual energy. When the Command Points are proving ineffective, consider using this point and then return to them.

⊥	△		Location
5	7-15	On the outer line of the Bl Channel **3 cun** lateral to the posterior median line Between **3rd and 4th Thoracic vertebrae**	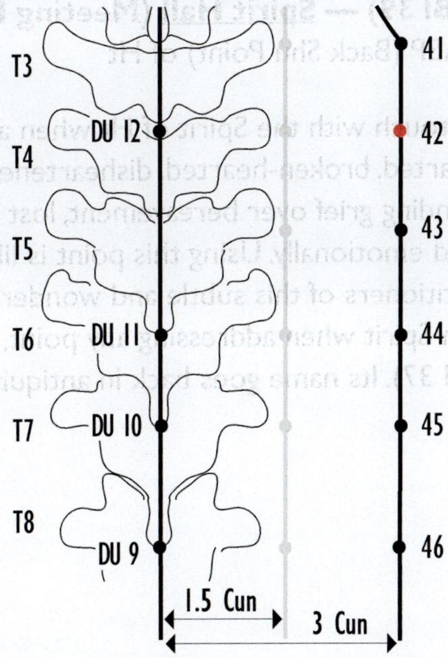
3	7-50	On the outer line of the Bl Channel **3 cun** lateral to the posterior median line Between **4th and 5th Thoracic vertebrae**	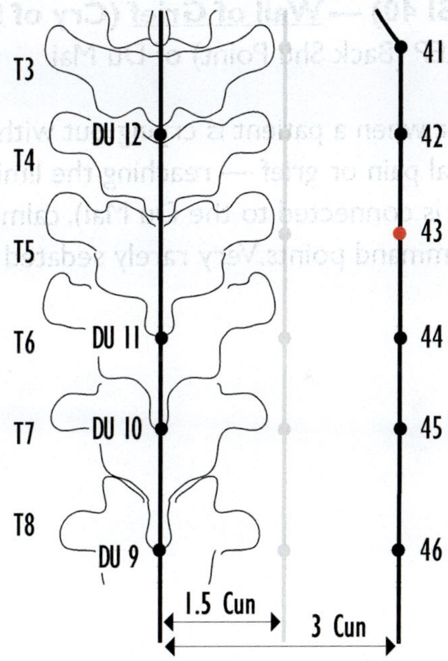

Bladder

Bl 44 (Bl 39) — Spirit Hall (Meeting Place for the Spirit)
Outer AEP (Back Shu Point) of Ht

Gets in touch with the Spirit of Ht when a person is suffering from shock, feeling downhearted, hard-hearted, broken-hearted, disheartened, lacking in joy or experiencing sadness. For long-standing grief over bereavement, lost love, broken ideals, or where the patient has been deeply wounded emotionally. Using this point is like taking the patient into a hall where the Spirit resides. As practitioners of this subtle and wonderful medicine, we need to work on being in touch with our own Spirit when addressing any point, but particularly Spirit points. Consider using alongside Bl 42 (Bl 37). Its name goes back in antiquity to the 1st century BCE.

Bl 45 (Bl 40) — Wail of Grief (Cry of Pain)
Outer AEP (Back Shu Point) of Du Mai

Consider when a patient is crying out with pain, cracked or breaking under the weight of physical or mental pain or grief — reaching the limit, having tried everything. This point strengthens the Spirit (it is connected to the Du Mai), calms everything down and lets the practitioner move on to using command points. Very rarely sedated — usually moxa'ed and/or tonified.

⊥	△		Location
3	5	On the outer line of the Bl Channel **3 cun** lateral to the posterior median line Between **5th and 6th Thoracic vertebrae**	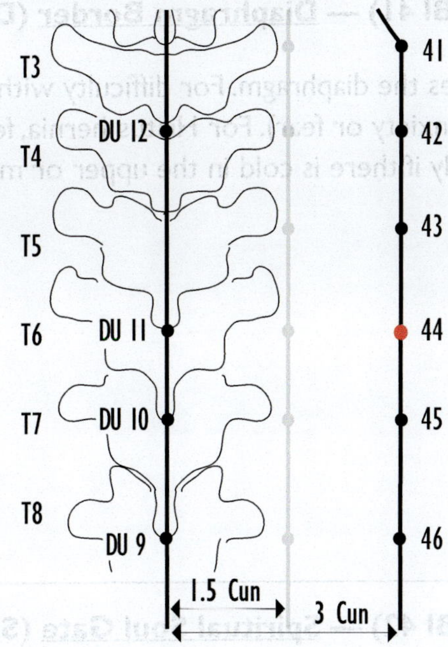
3	5-15	On the outer line of the Bl Channel **3 cun** lateral to the posterior median line Between **6th and 7th Thoracic vertebrae**	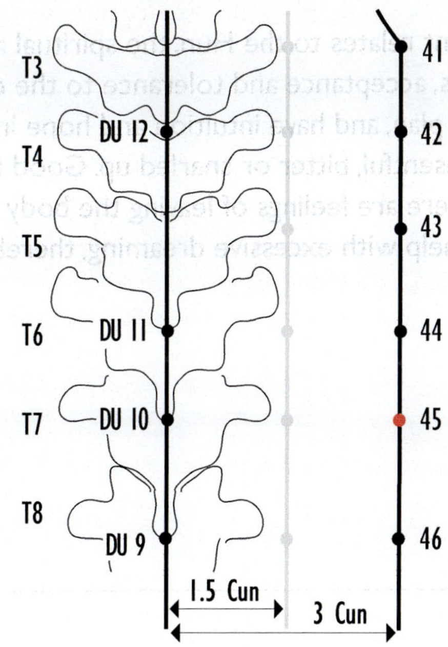

Bl 46 (Bl 41) — Diaphragm Border (Diaphragm Gate)

Regulates the diaphragm. For difficulty with breathing or digestion (especially when disturbed by shock, anxiety or fear). For Hiatus hernia, fear of the cold or the dark. Responds well to moxa, especially if there is cold in the upper or middle jiao.

Bl 47 (Bl 42) — Spiritual Soul Gate (Soul Gate, Gate of the Hun)
Outer AEP (Back Shu Point) of Liv

This point relates to the Hun, the spiritual aspect of the Liver. It roots the Ethereal Soul and brings calmness, acceptance and tolerance to the core of a person. The Hun influences our ability to imagine, plan, and have intuition and hope in our life. Use when a patient is depressed, irritable, angry, resentful, bitter or snarled up. Good for recovering alcoholics or drug addicts. Consider when there are feelings of leaving the body when going to sleep, because it 'grounds' the Hun and is said to help with excessive dreaming, thereby aiding better quality sleep.

⊥	Δ		Location
5	3-15	On the outer line of the Bl Channel **3 cun** lateral to the posterior median line Between **7th and 8th Thoracic vertebrae**	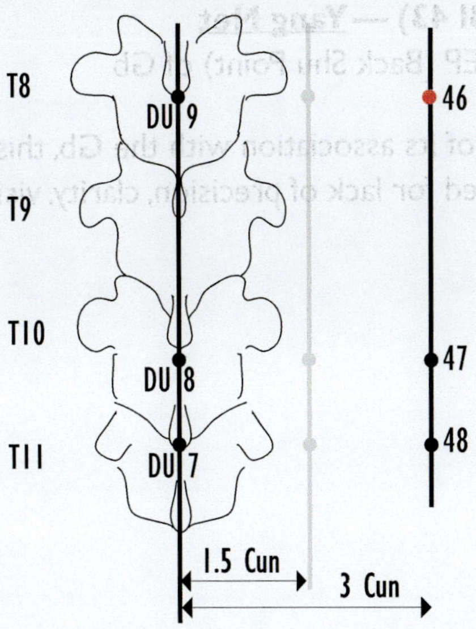
5	3-15	On the outer line of the Bl Channel **3 cun** lateral to the posterior median line Between **9th and 10th Thoracic vertebrae**	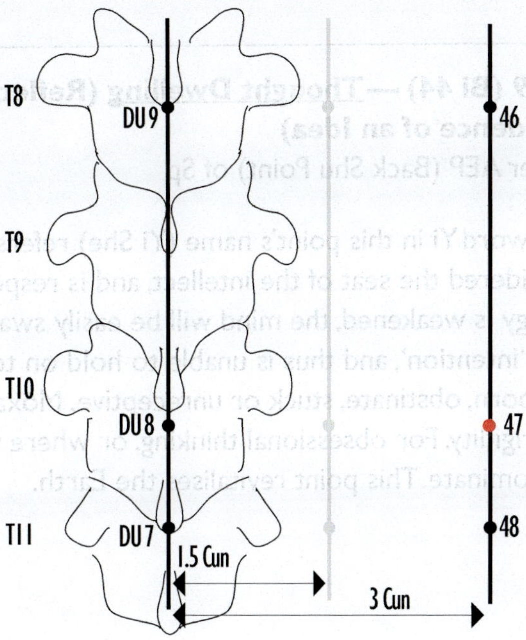

Bl 48 (Bl 43) — Yang Net
Outer AEP (Back Shu Point) of Gb

Because of its association with the Gb, this point is concerned with purity in the mind. It can be considered for lack of precision, clarity, vision, decision-making or judgement.

Bl 49 (Bl 44) — Thought Dwelling (Reflection Abode, Intelligence Lodge, Residence of an Idea)
Outer AEP (Back Shu Point) of Sp

The word Yi in this point's name (Yi She) refers to the spiritual aspect of the Spleen. Spleen is considered the seat of the intellect, and is responsible for all aspects of thinking. If the Spleen energy is weakened, the mind will be easily swayed so that a person struggles to focus and have 'intention', and thus is unable to hold on to an idea. If it is too rigid, the mind can become stubborn, obstinate, stuck or unreceptive. Moxa and tonification, when appropriate, can counteract this rigidity. For obsessional thinking, or where worry, poor memory or lack of concentration predominate. This point revitalises the Earth.

⊥	Δ		Location
5-7	5	On the outer line of the Bl Channel **3 cun** lateral to the posterior median line Between **10th and 11th Thoracic vertebrae**	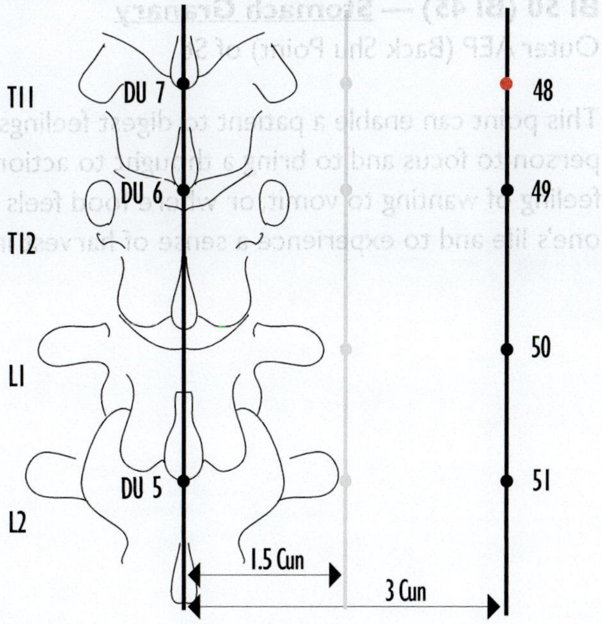
5-7	5-15	On the outer line of the Bl Channel **3 cun** lateral to the posterior median line Between **11th and 12th Thoracic vertebrae**	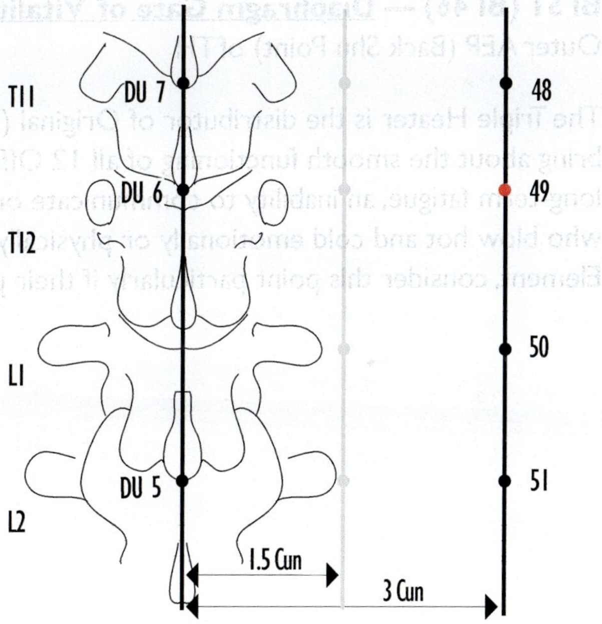

Bladder

Bl 50 (Bl 45) — <u>Stomach Granary</u>
Outer AEP (Back Shu Point) of St

This point can enable a patient to digest feelings, thoughts and ideas. Furthermore, it can help a person to focus and to bring a thought to action. Physically there may be problems digesting food, a feeling of wanting to vomit, or where food feels stuck. It is said to bestow the ability to appreciate one's life and to experience a sense of harvest in it.

Bl 51 (Bl 46) — <u>Diaphragm Gate of Vitality</u> (Vitals Gate)
Outer AEP (Back Shu Point) of TH

The Triple Heater is the distributor of Original (Yuan) Qi from the Kidneys, which in turn helps bring about the smooth functioning of all 12 Officials. Good for chronic problems such as long-term fatigue, an inability to communicate or lack of emotional control, such as among patients who blow hot and cold emotionally or physically. If the patient has an imbalance in their Fire Element, consider this point particularly if their problems are in the chest area.

⊥	Δ		Location
3-7	3-10	On the outer line of the Bl Channel **3 cun** lateral to the posterior median line Between **12th Thoracic** and **1st Lumbar vertebrae**	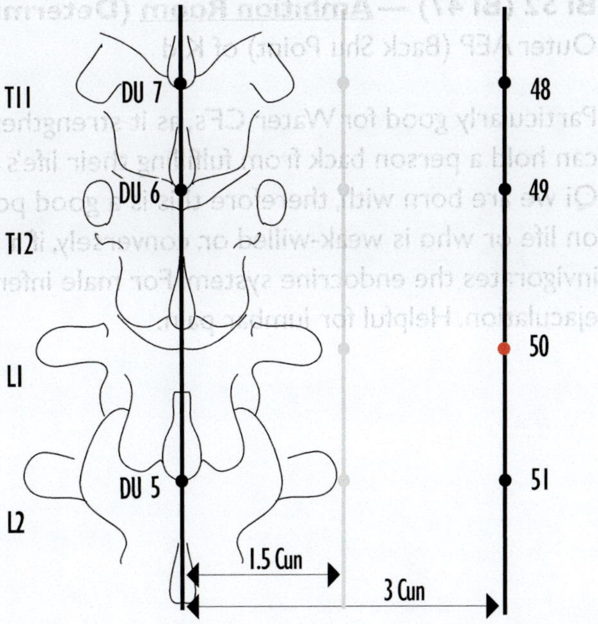
3-7	3-15	On the outer line of the Bl Channel **3 cun** lateral to the posterior median line Between **1st and 2nd Lumbar vertebrae**	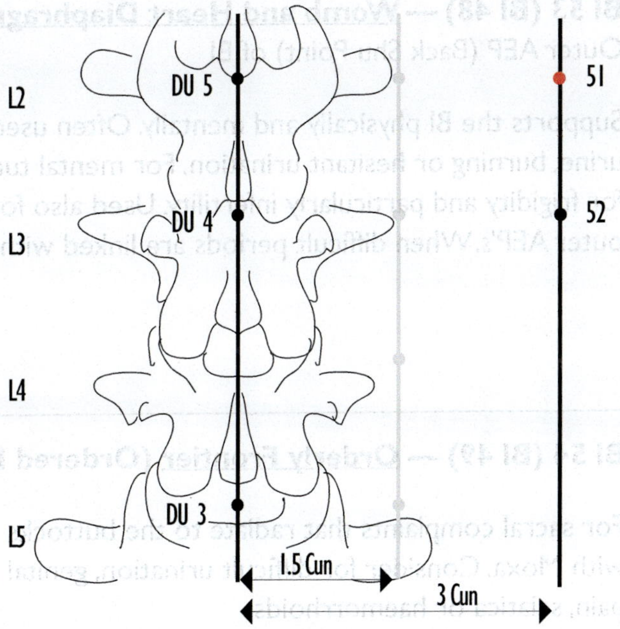

Bladder

Bl 52 (Bl 47) — Ambition Room (Determination House, Will Dwelling)
Outer AEP (Back Shu Point) of Kid

Particularly good for Water CF's, as it strengthens the Spirit of Kidney (the Zhi) which, if weakened, can hold a person back from fulfilling their life's plan. Gets directly to the Will. Kid controls the Qi we are born with, therefore this is a good point to consider for someone with a weak hold on life or who is weak-willed or, conversely, if a person is ruthlessly over-ambitious. Supports and invigorates the endocrine system. For male infertility, erectile dysfunction, impotence or premature ejaculation. Helpful for lumbar pain.

Bl 53 (Bl 48) — Womb and Heart Diaphragm (Bladder Vitals)
Outer AEP (Back Shu Point) of Bl

Supports the Bl physically and mentally. Often used for Bladder problems such as retention of urine, burning or hesitant urination. For mental turmoil, anxiety, fear or phobic behaviour. Consider for frigidity and particularly infertility. Used also for LI and SI problems since these do not have outer AEP's. When difficult periods are linked with emotional problems. Moxa is useful here.

Bl 54 (Bl 49) — Orderly Frontier (Ordered Boundary)

For sacral complaints that radiate to the buttocks and legs — often tender upon palpation. Good with Moxa. Consider for difficult urination, genital pain and swelling, menstruation problems, back pain, sciatica or haemorrhoids.

⊥	Δ		Location
5-9	3-15	On the outer line of the Bl Channel **3 cun** lateral to the posterior median line Between **2nd and 3rd Lumbar vertebrae**	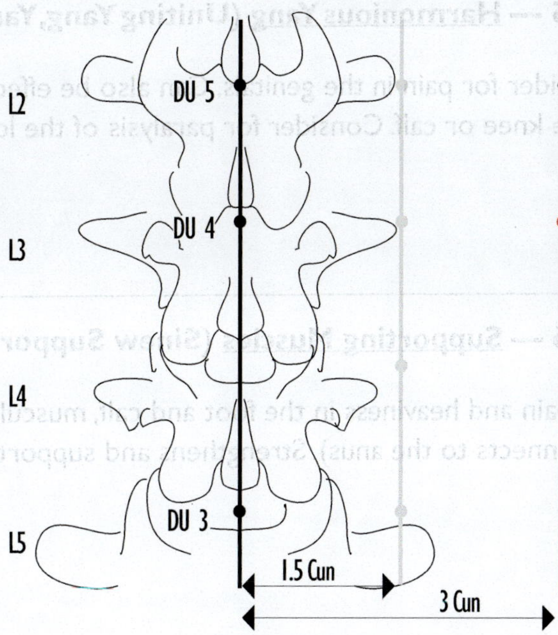
5-7	5-10	Patient is seated and upright or prone with a pillow under the pelvis On the Buttock Level with the sacrum On the outer line of the Bl Channel **3 cun** lateral to the posterior median line Level with 2nd sacral foramen	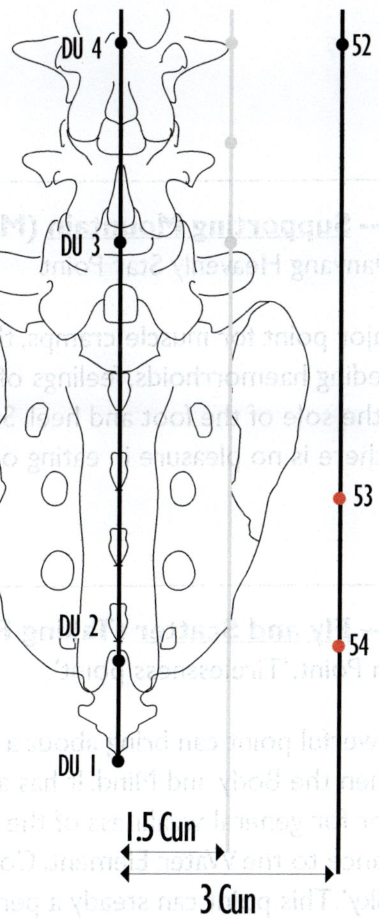
5-10	3-7	Patient is seated and upright or prone with a pillow under the pelvis On the Buttock Level with the sacrum On the outer line of the Bl Channel **3 cun** lateral to the posterior median line	

Bladder

Bl 55 — <u>Harmonious Yang</u> (Uniting Yang, Yang Union)

Consider for pain in the genitals. Can also be effective for a feeling of heaviness or muscular spasm in the knee or calf. Consider for paralysis of the lower limbs and for generalised back pain.

Bl 56 — <u>Supporting Muscles</u> (Sinew Support)

For pain and heaviness in the foot and calf, muscular cramps and all types of haemorrhoids (it connects to the anus). Strengthens and supports the muscles. Consider for sciatica.

Bl 57 — <u>Supporting Mountain</u> (Mountain Receiving)
A Ma Danyang Heavenly Star Point

As a major point for muscle cramps, this point can free up the Qi and relax the sinews. For swollen and bleeding haemorrhoids, feelings of heat in the head, lumbago, sciatica, rectal prolapse, or for pain in the sole of the foot and heel. Strengthens the legs and spine. Said to be helpful in cases where there is no pleasure in eating or, conversely, a tendency towards gluttony.

Bl 58 — <u>Fly and Scatter</u> (Taking Flight, Flying Yang)
Junction Point. 'Tirelessness point'.

This powerful point can bring about a feeling of wellbeing and greater vitality, and help to strengthen the Body and Mind. It has a direct bearing on haemorrhoids, as it connects to the anus. Consider for general weakness of the legs. Brings clarity. Often used with Kid 4 to bring harmony and balance to the Water Element. Commonly used on the mental level — almost like a 'Window of the Sky'. This point can steady a person if they are emotionally scattered because of fear.

⊥	Δ		Location
5	3-7	Between medial and lateral heads of the gastrocnemius muscle On the line connecting Bl 40 and Bl 57 **2 cun** inferior to Bl 40 **14 cun** proximal to the prominence of the lateral maleolus	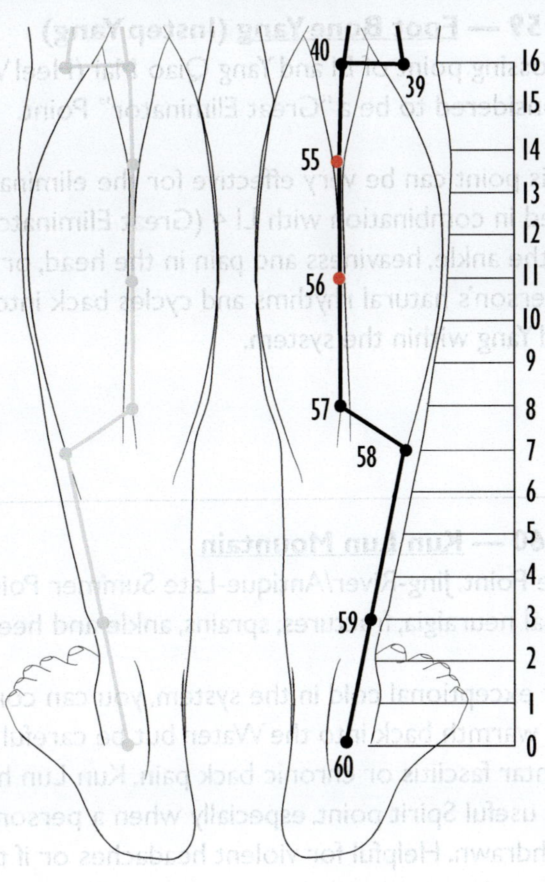
X	3-7	In the centre of the belly of the gastrocnemius muscle On the line connecting Bl 40 and Bl 57 **5 cun** inferior to Bl 40 **11 cun** proximal to the prominence of the lateral maleolus Midway between Bl 55 and Bl 57	
7	5-15	On the line connecting Bl 40 and Bl 57 At the point where the junction of the two halves of the belly of the gastrocnemius muscle meets with the tendocalcaneus (Achilles tendon) **8 cun** proximal to the prominence of the lateral maleolus	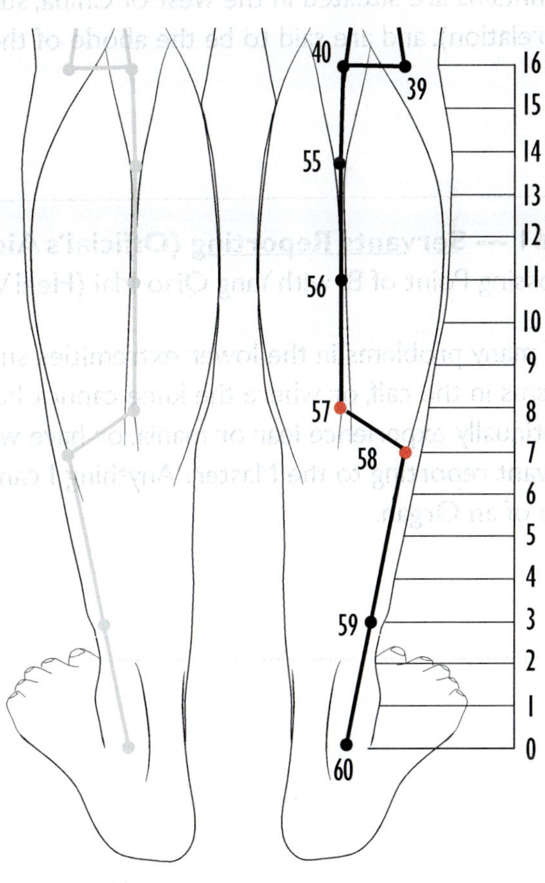
5-10	3-7	Between fibula bone and tendocalcaneus (Achilles tendon) Lateral border of tendocalcaneus Ask the patient to flex their foot against pressure to feel the border between the fibula bone and Achilles **7 cun** superior to Bl 60 (location of prominence of lateral maleolus) Approx **1 cun** lateral to Bl 57 Approx **1 cun** inferior to Bl 57	

Bladder

Bl 59 — Foot Bone Yang (Instep Yang)
Crossing point of Bl and Yang Qiao Mai (Heel Vessel). Accumulation Point of Yang Qiao Mai. Considered to be a "Great Eliminator" Point.

This point can be very effective for the elimination of toxins from the Body and Mind, and can be used in combination with LI 4 (Great Eliminator) to augment this effect. Consider for rheumatism of the ankle, heaviness and pain in the head, or an inability to raise the arms and legs. Helps to bring a person's natural rhythms and cycles back into balance because of its ability to harmonise the Yin and Yang within the system.

Bl 60 — Kun Lun Mountain
Fire Point. Jing-River/Antique-Late Summer Point. A Ma Danyang Heavenly Star Point. First Aid: facial neuralgia, fractures, sprains, ankle and heel pain.

For exceptional cold in the system, you can consider using moxa on this point along with Kid 2 to get warmth back into the Water, but be careful not to overheat. Consider for foot or ankle pain, plantar fasciitis or chronic back pain. Kun Lun has a special effect on the whole of the spine. This is a useful Spirit point, especially when a person can't communicate, has no flow, is depressed or withdrawn. Helpful for violent headaches or if there is knotting in the calf muscle. The Kun Lun Mountains are situated in the west of China, surrounded by a vermilion lake (hence the Fire point correlation), and are said to be the abode of the Immortals and to renew the Spirits.

Bl 61 — Servants Reporting (Official's Aide, Servant's Respect, Set on the Calcaneum)
Crossing Point of Bl with Yang Qiao Mai (Heel Vessel). Point to release the External Dragons.

For many problems in the lower extremities such as paralysis, pain in the knee, ankle or heel, spasms in the calf, or where the knee cannot be raised. Helps to ease the tension of those who continually experience fear or mania, or have withdrawn into themselves. An eager and willing servant reporting to the Master: 'Anything I can do to help?' is the Chinese way of describing one role of an Organ.

⊥	Δ		Location
5	5-7	Lateral aspect of the lower leg In a seam between the tendocalcaneus (Achilles tendon) and posterior border of the fibula bone **3 cun** directly superior to Bl 60 (location of prominence of lateral maleolus)	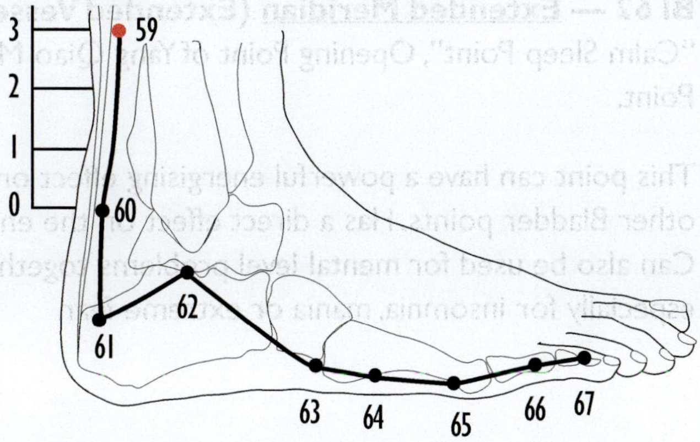
3-5	3-7	Forbidden in pregnancy Posterior to prominence of the lateral maleolus In a groove between the tendocalcaneus and the prominence of the lateral maleolus	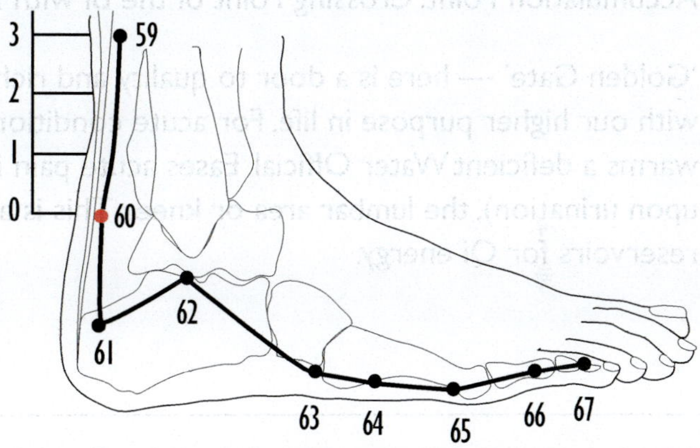
3	3-7	Lateral aspect of foot On the calcaneus itself Approx **1.5 cun** inferior to Bl 60 at the level of the prominence of the lateral maleolus At the junction of the change in skin colour and texture	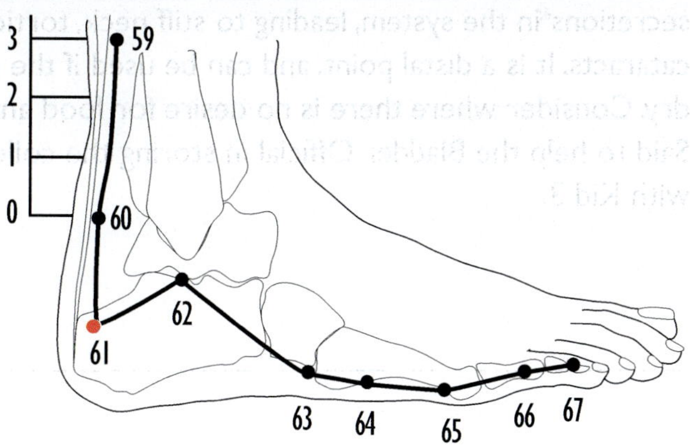

Bladder

Bl 62 — <u>Extended Meridian</u> (Extended Vessel)
"Calm Sleep Point", Opening Point of Yang Qiao Mai (Heel Vessel), Coupled Point of Du Mai. Ghost Point.

This point can have a powerful energising effect on a deficient Water Official. Use for reinforcing other Bladder points. Has a direct effect on the endocrine system. Can be sedated for pain relief. Can also be used for mental level problems together with Kid 6 (opening point of Yin Qiao Mai), especially for insomnia, mania or extreme fear.

Bl 63 — <u>Golden Gate</u>
Accumulation Point. Crossing Point of the Bl with Yang Wei Mai (Linking Vessel).

'Golden Gate' — here is a door to quality and richness which can be understood as resonating with our higher purpose in life. For acute conditions, especially fear or anxiety. Invigorates and warms a deficient Water Official. Eases acute pain in the bladder (such as a burning sensation upon urination), the lumbar area or knees. This is an under-used point. Accumulation points act as reservoirs for Qi energy.

Bl 64 — <u>Capital Bone</u> (Citadel of the Bone)
Source Point. 'Strong Tendon point'. 'Fine Appetite point'. First Aid Point for wasp or bee sting on the tongue or throat.

This point can strengthen the Bladder Official, and can be used for general stiffness or lack of secretions in the system, leading to stiff neck, torticollis, lower back pain, dimness of vision or cataracts. It is a distal point, and can be used if the inner canthus of the eye has become red and dry. Consider where there is no desire for food and drink. Helpful for sensations of cold in the legs. Said to help the Bladder Official in storing the collective memory of all the Officials. Often used with Kid 3.

⊥	△		Location
3-5	X	Lateral aspect of foot Directly inferior to prominence of lateral maleolus Approx **0.5 cun** inferior to the inferior border of the lateral maleolus	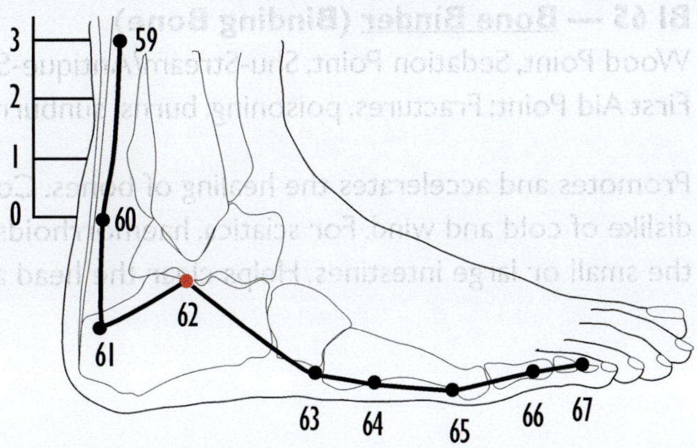
3-5	3-5	Lateral aspect of foot Proximal to tuberosity of the 5th metatarsal Inferior to the inferior border of the cuboid bone Anterior (distal) and inferior to Bl 62	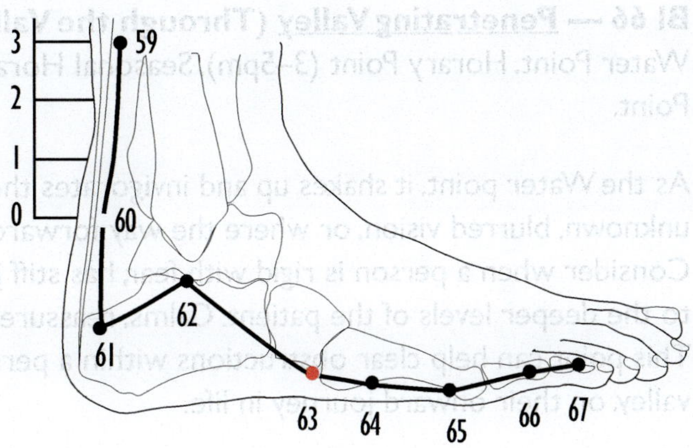
3-5	3-7	Just inferior and distal to the tuberosity of the 5th metatarsal Just distal to the flare of the base of the 5th metatarsal bone Traditionally at the junction of the change in skin colour	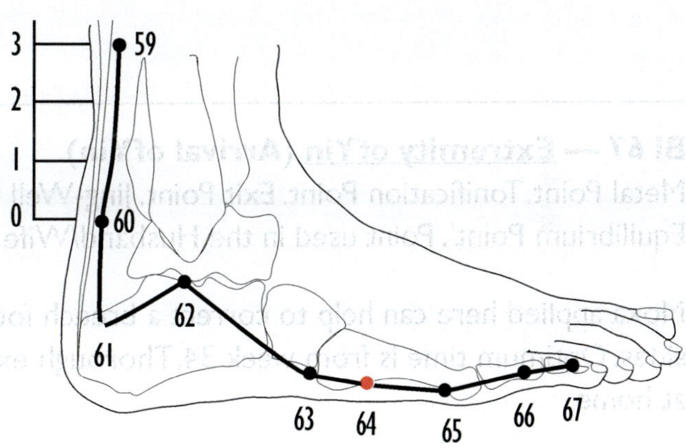

Bladder

Bl 65 — Bone Binder (Binding Bone)
Wood Point, Sedation Point, Shu-Stream/Antique-Summer Point, 'Consolation point'.
First Aid Point: Fractures, poisoning, burns, sunburn, scalds, insect bites, cystitis.

Promotes and accelerates the healing of bones. Consider in cases where there is an intense fear or dislike of cold and wind. For sciatica, haemorrhoids (it connects to the anus), cystitis or irritation in the small or large intestines. Helps clear the head and eyes (it's a distal point).

Bl 66 — Penetrating Valley (Through the Valley, Passing Valley)
Water Point. Horary Point (3–5pm). Seasonal Horary Point — Winter. Ying-Spring/Antique-Spring Point.

As the Water point, it shakes up and invigorates the Bladder Official. Consider for fear of the unknown, blurred vision, or where the way forward is not clear. Refreshes the Mind and Spirit. Consider when a person is rigid with fear, has stiff joints and is unable to flow. Useful for reaching to the deeper levels of the patient. Calms, reassures and captures the essence of the Water Official. This point can help clear obstructions within a person as they progress, via the protection of this valley, on their onward journey in life.

Bl 67 — Extremity of Yin (Arrival of Yin)
Metal Point. Tonification Point. Exit Point. Jing-Well Point/Antique-Winter Point. 'General Equilibrium Point'. Point used in the Husband/Wife treatment Protocol.

Moxa applied here can help to correct a breech foetal presentation — 10 minutes each day, both sides. Optimum time is from week 34. Thorough explanation needed for safe use of the moxa stick at home.

Consider for fear, anxiety and depression — when a patient has reached the limits of their endurance. When used with Bl 1 it can enhance the body's hormonal secretions, as it influences the endocrine and lymphatic systems. Consider for eye troubles, especially where there is excessive lacrimation or if pain is present. Metal within Water brings quality, purity and sparkling clarity to this Official, and helps in maintaining internal rhythms and processes. Connects to the uterus and is said to help with a difficult labour.

⊥	△		Location
3-5	3-5	Proximal and inferior to the flare of the head of the 5th metatarsal bone Proximal and inferior to the metatarso-phalangeal joint of 5th digit Traditionally at the junction of the change in skin colour	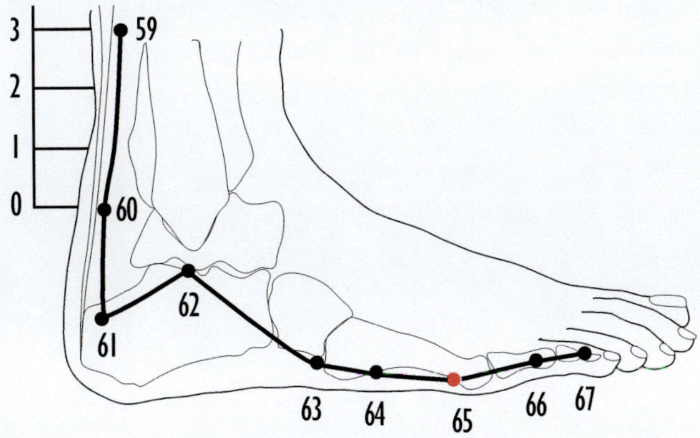
2	3-5	Distal and inferior to the flare of the base of the 5th proximal phalanx Distal and inferior to the metatarso-phalangeal joint of 5th digit Traditionally at the junction of the change in skin colour	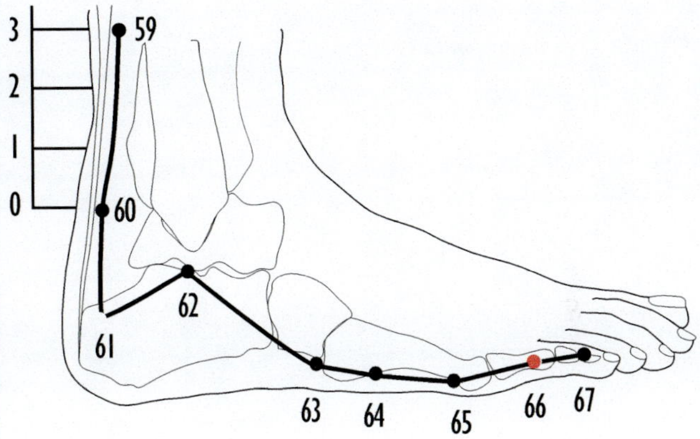
2	3	Forbidden to needle or moxa during pregnancy — except to turn Breech Baby Lateral nail point of the 5th digit Approx **0.1 cun** proximal to corner of nail. Distal to the flare of the distal phalanx	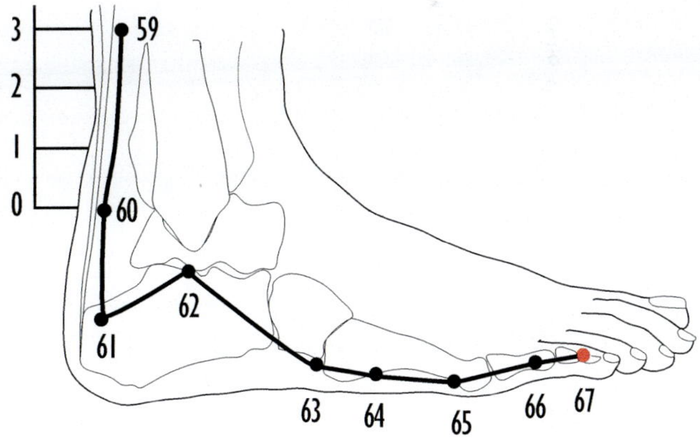

Kidney

- **Controls all the fluids within the Kingdom**
- **It is the Seat of the Will (the Zhi) and a Storehouse of the Vital Essence, our Jing**
- **Masters the bones and marrow. Ability, skill and cleverness stem from them**

Kidney

Kid 1 — Bubbling Spring (Fountain of Life, Earth Surge)

Entry Point. Wood Point. Sedation Point. Jing-Well/Antique-Winter Point. 'Courage Point'. 'Taoist Yoga Power Point.' 'Corpse Reviver'. One of the nine needles for returning Yang (used in cases of extreme Yang deficiency). Emergency point for high blood pressure.

This is the only acupuncture point on the sole of the foot; it connects us with the Earth. Kidney stores our Jing — the ancestral energy. It is the Seat of Will, "creates power within the Kingdom", and is what enables us to do things. Here is where vital Qi energy comes into the meridian. As long as the spring is bubbling, we have pure, revitalised Qi from the source. If there is a deficiency in the Kid, where energy is blocked from entering, this can manifest as stagnant energy levels, stiffness in the bones, or hot and dry feet. If there is excess energy, the feet can be hot and wet, the face can appear very red, or there can be excessive sweating. Oedema, memory loss and insomnia can also result from an imbalance here. If the patient is fearful or agitated, this point can help Earth and stabilise them, bringing a sense of calm because of its grounding effect. It can also revitalise and invigorate the system. Consider for infertility (Wood and growth).

Kid 2 — Blazing Valley (Dragon Spring)

Fire Point. Ying-Spring/Antique-Spring Point. Secondary Sedation point. First Aid after kick to the testicles (with strong thumb pressure bilaterally).

Water is transformed and regulated by Fire. Without it we may get anxious, become relentlessly driven or, conversely, exhausted, lose expansiveness, become disinterested in sex or constantly fearful. This point deals with rigidity, lack of movement or painful articulation (especially spinal pain). If Fire is in excess: a person can be very hot, suffer from night sweats, or have hot, sweaty feet, polyuria or dehydration (treatment is usually sedation). If deficient: a person can be cold and lethargic, have no moisture on their feet, rarely perspire, or suffer from oedema, especially around the ankles (treatment is usually tonification). If you find one ankle swollen, or that one foot is hot and the other is cold, then consider an Akabane test. Helpful for genital itching.

⊥	Δ		Location
5	3-7	Forbidden from 8th month of pregnancy One third down from top of foot (excluding toes) In line with middle phalanx Between 2nd and 3rd metatarsal bones, just distal to where the bases flare. Flex the foot and curl the toes under; depression forms in the foot at the point of Kid 1	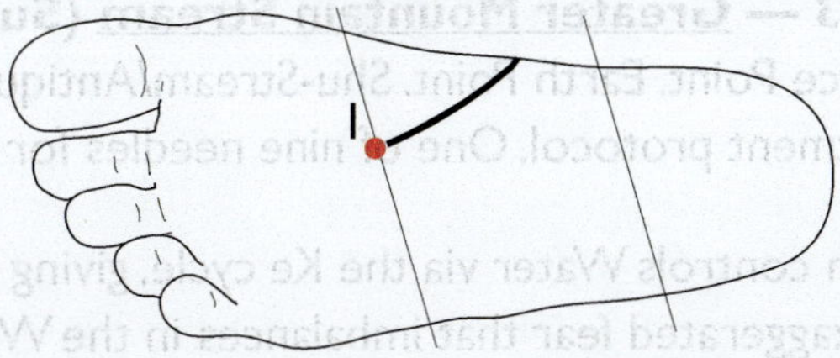
5	3-5	Forbidden from 8th month of pregnancy Inferior to the distal corner of the tuberosity of the navicular Traditionally at change of skin colour	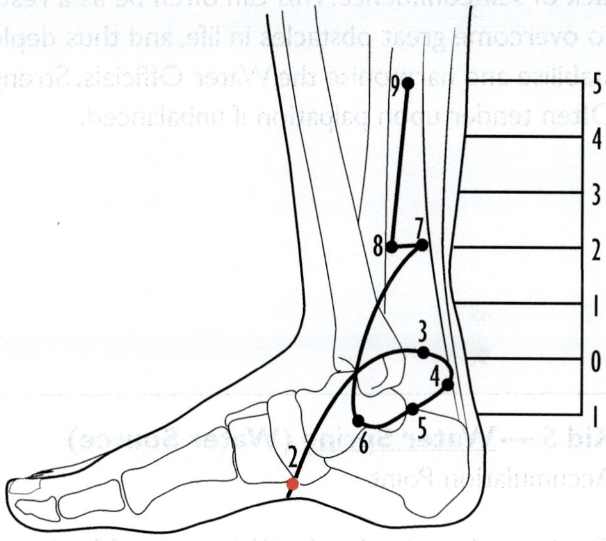

Kidney

Kid 3 — <u>Greater Mountain Stream</u> (Supreme Stream, Reflecting Sea, Great Torrent)
Source Point. Earth Point. Shu-Stream/Antique Summer Point. Point used in the Husband/Wife treatment protocol. One of nine needles for returning Yang.

Earth controls Water via the Ke cycle, giving it stability and steadying it. This point calms the type of exaggerated fear that imbalances in the Water Element can sometimes produce. If the Earth within the Kidney is deficient, a person can also experience sore throat, insomnia, inertia, cystitis, a feeling of heaviness and weariness in the four limbs, or irregular menstruation. This Shu-Stream point regulates the function of the uterus and the water pathways. Kid 3 has a strong connection to the Original (Yuan) Qi. Consider for lack of Will, for those who are 'excessively driven', or for hypertension. Often tender upon palpation if unbalanced.

Kid 4 — <u>Great Bell</u> (Big Bell Clock, Great Cup)
Junction Point

This point can have a powerful effect on calming a person's emotions, particularly fear or for a lack of self-confidence. This can often be as a result of working too relentlessly, forcing their Will to overcome great obstacles in life, and thus depleting their reserves, their Jing. It helps to balance, stabilise and harmonise the Water Officials. Strengthens the back. Stores our reserves of energy. Often tender upon palpation if unbalanced.

Kid 5 — <u>Water Spring</u> (Water Source)
Accumulation Point

The image here is of a plentiful supply of fresh, pure water which can be used for the general support of the Kidney, especially in acute conditions. Consider when fear and depression are both present, or when a person is held back in life, creating a prison around themselves leading to agoraphobia, a fear of leaving the house — "something might happen to me". Consider with Bl 59 for a cleansing, freeing, energising action. For irregular menstruation, cystitis or excessive urination.

⊥	Δ		Location
3	3-5	Level with the prominence of the Medial Maleolus In the groove midway between prominence and the posterior median line of the Achilles tendon	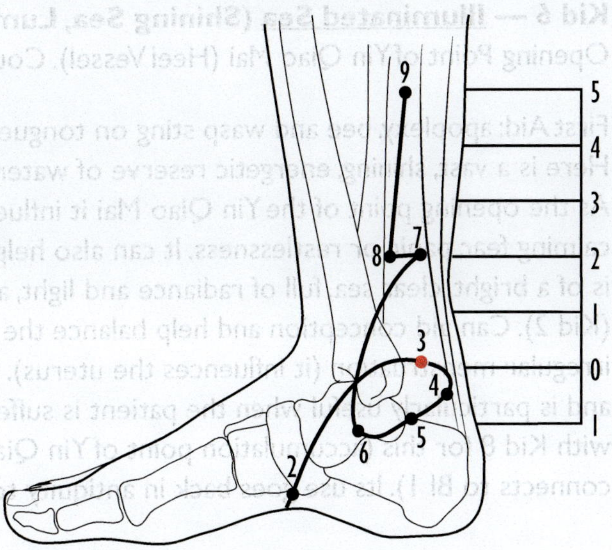
3	3-7	Forbidden from 3rd month of pregnancy **0.5 cun** inferior and slightly posterior to Kid 3 in the depression medial to the attachment of the Achilles tendon	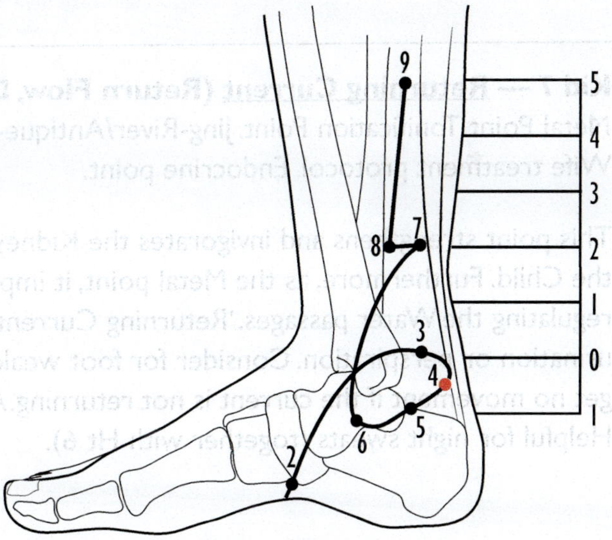
4	5	**1 cun** directly inferior to Kid 3. Anterior to tuberosity of the Calcaneus	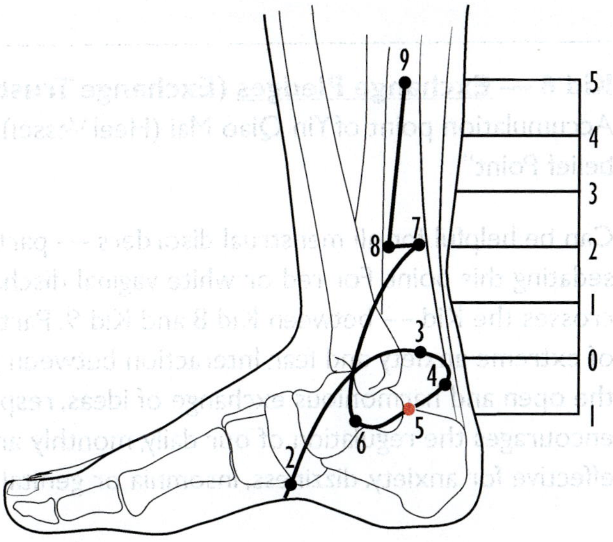

Kidney

Kid 6 — <u>Illuminated Sea</u> (Shining Sea, Luminous Sea)
Opening Point of Yin Qiao Mai (Heel Vessel). Coupled Point of Ren Mai. "Joyous Sleep point".

First Aid: apoplexy, bee and wasp sting on tongue or throat, snake bite, concussion.
Here is a vast, shining, energetic reserve of water which has a resonance with Ren 6 (Sea of Qi). As the opening point of the Yin Qiao Mai it influences and nourishes the Yin, steadying the mind, calming fear, panic or restlessness. It can also help in treating a dry, sore throat. The image here is of a bright, clear sea, full of radiance and light, and is said to reflect this from the Blazing Valley (Kid 2). Can aid conception and help balance the hormones in cases of menopausal problems or irregular menstruation (it influences the uterus). It can be effective in regulating the body's cycles, and is particularly useful when the patient is suffering from insomnia when it is often used together with Kid 8 for this (accumulation point of Yin Qiao Mai). Consider for eye problems (Yin Qiao Mai connects to Bl 1). Its use goes back in antiquity to the 1st century BCE.

Kid 7 — <u>Returning Current</u> (Return Flow, Deeply White, Bearing White)
Metal Point. Tonification Point. Jing-River/Antique-Late Summer point. Point used in the Husband/Wife treatment protocol. Endocrine point.

This point strengthens and invigorates the Kidney meridian, bringing energy from the Mother to the Child. Furthermore, as the Metal point, it imparts quality and structure to this Official, thus regulating the Water passages. 'Returning Current' — it regulates the body's rhythms, e.g. sleep, urination or perspiration. Consider for foot weakness and paralysis (especially in children) — you get no movement if the current is not returning. Also for male infertility, e.g. low sperm count. Helpful for night sweats (together with Ht 6).

Kid 8 — <u>Exchange Pledges</u> (Exchange Trust, Faith Intersection)
Accumulation point of Yin Qiao Mai (Heel Vessel). "Strengthener and Calmer Point". "Communicate belief Point".

Can be helpful for all menstrual disorders — particularly heavy periods where you may consider sedating this point. For red or white vaginal discharges. This intersection is where the Sp meridian crosses the Kid — between Kid 8 and Kid 9. Particularly good on a mental level, especially in cases of extreme anxiety and fear. Interaction between groups, people and officials are dependent upon the open and harmonious exchange of ideas, responsibilities and knowledge. Affects fluidity, and encourages the regulation of our daily, monthly and seasonal rhythms. Good with moxa. Can be effective for anxiety, dizziness, insomnia or genital itching.

⊥	Δ		Location
3	3-5	**1 cun** inferior to prominence of Medial Maleolus Flex foot (invert and evert) to feel bones of the foot In depression immediately inferior to the talus bone and superior to the sustentaculum tali of the calcaneus bone, i.e. between these two bones	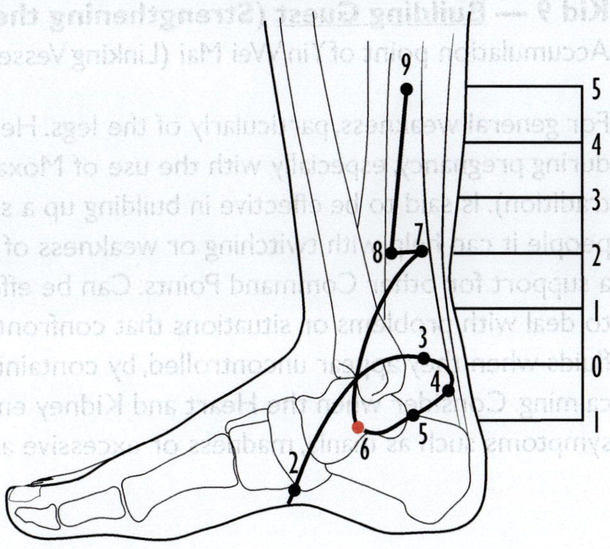
4	3-7	Forbidden from 8th month of pregnancy **2 cun** superior to Kid 3 on the anterior border of the Achilles tendon	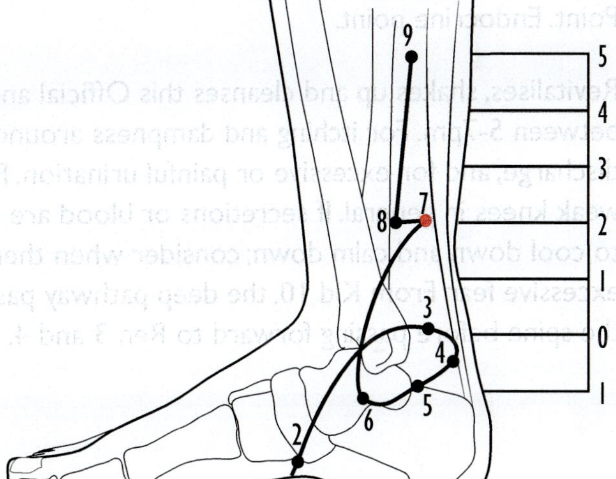
3	5	**2 cun** superior to Kid 3 **0.5 cun** anterior to Kid 7	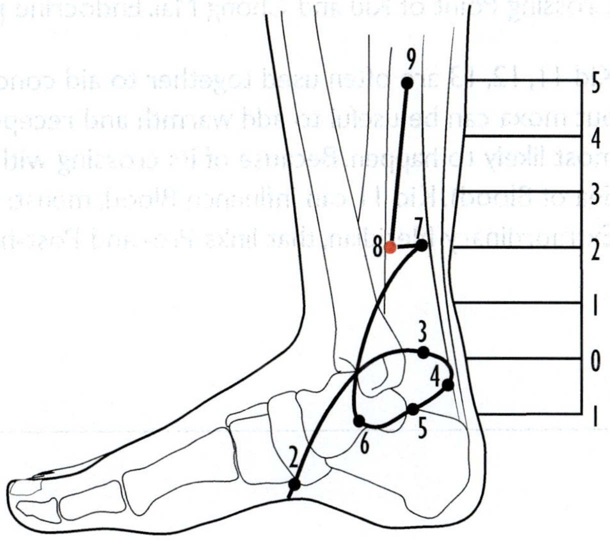

Kidney

Kid 9 — <u>Building Guest</u> (Strengthening the River Bank, Guest House)
Accumulation point of Yin Wei Mai (Linking Vessel, which connects all the Yin meridians)

For general weakness, particularly of the legs. Helps strengthen the Mother (and thus the child) during pregnancy, especially with the use of Moxa at the 3rd, 6th and 9th month (in the Japanese tradition). Is said to be effective in building up a supply of breastmilk for the mother. In older people it can help with twitching or weakness of the legs, occurring most often at night. Acts as a support for other Command Points. Can be effective in supporting the patient as they strive to deal with problems or situations that confront them in life. Kid 9 can help regulate and settle fluids when they appear uncontrolled, by containing them between the river banks. Profoundly calming. Consider when the Heart and Kidney energies are not harmonised, and for psychological symptoms such as mania, madness or excessive anger.

Kid 10 — <u>Yin Valley</u>
Water Point. Horary Point (5–7pm). Seasonal Horary Point — Winter. He-Sea/Antique Autumn Point. Endocrine point.

Revitalises, shakes up and cleanses this Official and thus the fluid secretions, especially when used between 5-7pm. For itching and dampness around the scrotum or vagina. For all types of vaginal discharge, and for excessive or painful urination. Excellent for knee trouble and injury. Strengthens weak knees in general. If secretions or blood are overheating, they can be taken through this valley to cool down and calm down; consider when there is blood in the urine. Calms the raging seas of excessive fear. From Kid 10, the deep pathway passes through to the coccyx and Du 1, and then up the spine before passing forward to Ren 3 and 4. Connects to the root of the tongue.

Kid 11 — <u>Transverse Bone</u>
Crossing Point of Kid and Chong Mai. Endocrine point.

Kid 11, 12, 13 are often used together to aid conception. This point is usually forbidden to needle, but moxa can be useful to add warmth and receptivity at the time just before conception is most likely to happen. Because of its crossing with the Chong Mai (alternatively known as the Sea of Blood), Kid 11 can influence Blood, menstruation and conception. The Chong Mai is an Extraordinary Meridian, that links Pre- and Post-heavenly Essence. Can help sperm production.

⊥	Δ		Location
5	3-7	**5 cun** superior to Kid 3 Medial border of gastrocnemius muscle Not always in the seam of the muscle; crucial to feel for this point and its energy Mark the position of Kid 10 to verify the position of Kid 9	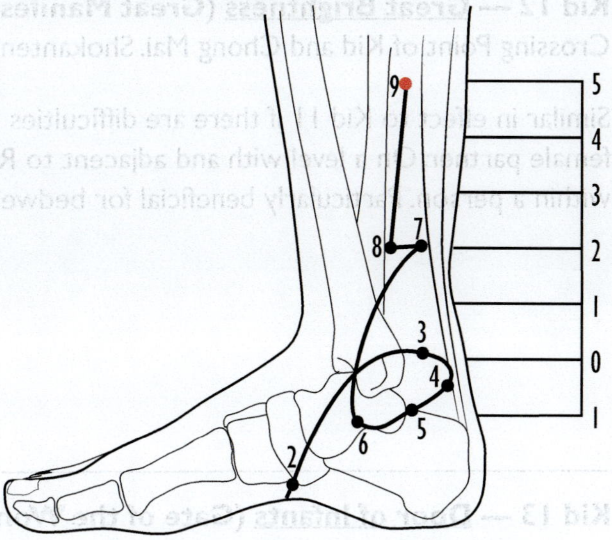
4	3	Medial end of popliteal crease between tendons of semitendinosus (ST) and semimembranosus (SM) muscles with knee semi-flexed The first tendon you will feel is the ST, which feels like a tight guitar string; roll over this tendon medially to the surface of the SM tendon. The point is needled on the SM tendon	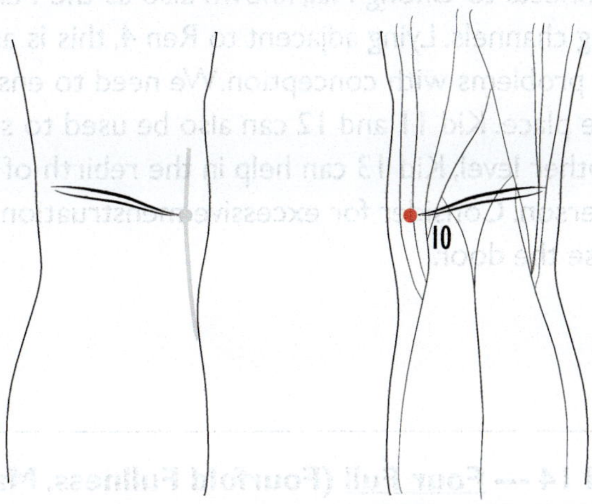
X	5-15	**0.5 cun** lateral to anterior median line (Ren Mai) On the superior border of symphysis pubis **5 cun** inferior to the level with the centre of the umbilicus Level with Ren 2	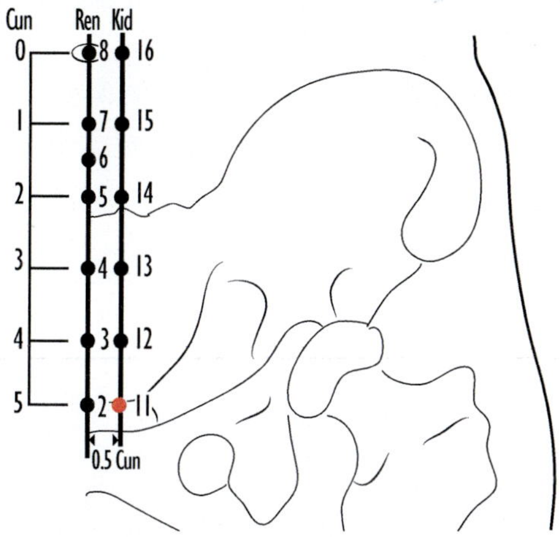

Kidney

Kid 12 — <u>Great Brightness</u> (Great Manifestation, Yin Gate)
Crossing Point of Kid and Chong Mai. Shokanten Point.

Similar in effect to Kid 11 if there are difficulties with conception — particularly helpful for the female partner. On a level with and adjacent to Ren 3. Can also lift the Spirits and help calm fear within a person. Particularly beneficial for bedwetting in children.

Kid 13 — <u>Door of Infants</u> (Gate of the Womb, Qi Cave)
Crossing Point of Kid and Chong Mai

Connects to Chong Mai, known also as the Penetrating Vessel and the Sea of the 5 yin and 6 yang channels. Lying adjacent to Ren 4, this is another wonderful point to consider when there are problems with conception. We need to ensure that this door opens freely for conception to take place. Kid 11 and 12 can also be used to supplement the effect of Kid 13 in this respect. On another level, Kid 13 can help in the rebirth of the Spirit and the development of new ideas within a person. Consider for excessive menstruation, urination, or vomiting — here we may have to close the door.

Kid 14 — <u>Four Full</u> (Fourfold Fullness, Marrow Mansion)
Crossing Point of Kid and Chong Mai

For warmth on the Mental level; can use many moxa cones here. 'Four' relates to the fullness of Blood, Food, Qi and Water. Consider for irregular or heavy periods, abdominal pain or distension.

⊥	Δ		Location
5-10	5-10	**0.5 cun** lateral to anterior median line (Ren Mai) **1 cun** superior to superior border of symphysis pubis **1 cun** superior to Kid 11 **4 cun** inferior to the level with the centre of the umbilicus Level with Ren 3	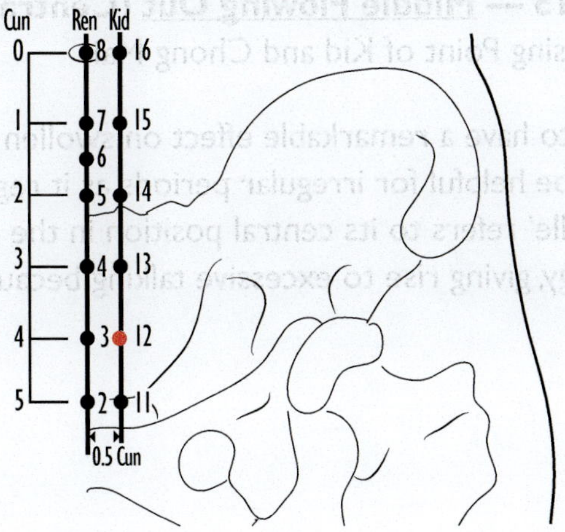
5-10	5-10	**0.5 cun** lateral to anterior median line (Ren Mai) **2 cun** superior to superior border of symphysis pubis **2 cun** superior to Kid 11 **3 cun** inferior to the level with the centre of the umbilicus Level with Ren 4	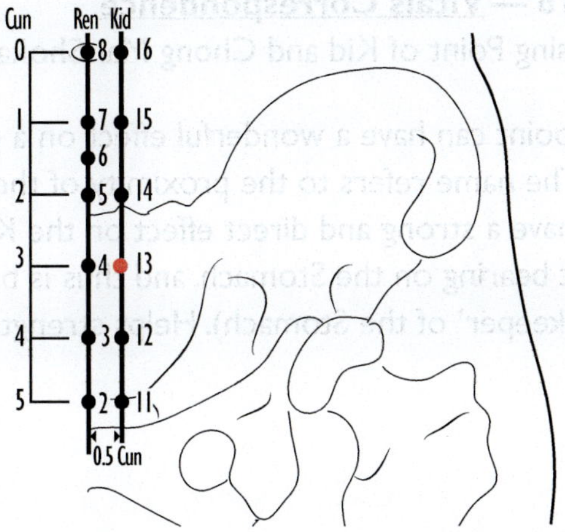
7-10	5-30	**0.5 cun** lateral to anterior median line (Ren Mai) **3 cun** superior to superior border of symphysis pubis **2 cun** inferior to the level with the centre of the umbilicus Level with Ren 5	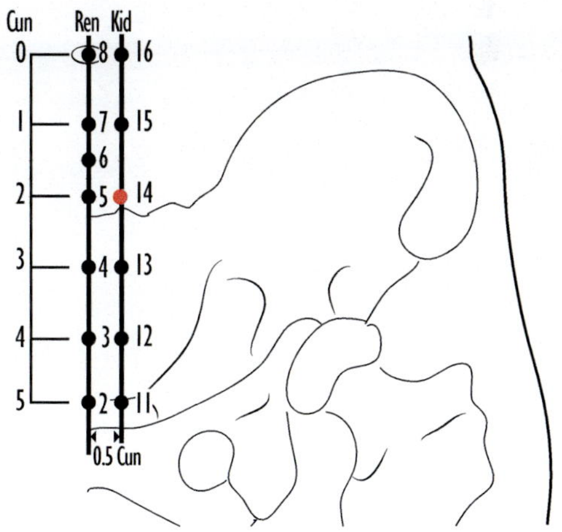

Kidney

Kid 15 — Middle Flowing Out (Central Flow)
Crossing Point of Kid and Chong Mai

Said to have a remarkable effect on swollen hands, as well as for arthritis of the hands and fingers. Can be helpful for irregular periods as it regulates and balances the flow of fluids within the body. 'Middle' refers to its central position in the body. Consider when there is a great depletion of energy, giving rise to excessive talking because of feelings of intense Fear.

Kid 16 — Vitals Correspondence
Crossing Point of Kid and Chong Mai. Shokanten Point.

This point can have a wonderful effect on a person worn down by overwork, illness or chronic fear. The name refers to the proximity of the Kid meridian's pathway to the Heart and diaphragm. Can have a strong and direct effect on the Kid, and help restore order to this Official. Has a direct bearing on the Stomach, and thus is beneficial for many stomach complaints (Kidney is the 'Gatekeeper' of the Stomach). Helps strengthen the Zhi, our Will. On a level with Ren 8.

⊥	△		Location
7-10	5-15	**0.5 cun** lateral to anterior median line (Ren Mai) **4 cun** superior to superior border of symphysis pubis **1 cun** inferior to the level with the centre of the umbilicus Level with Ren 7	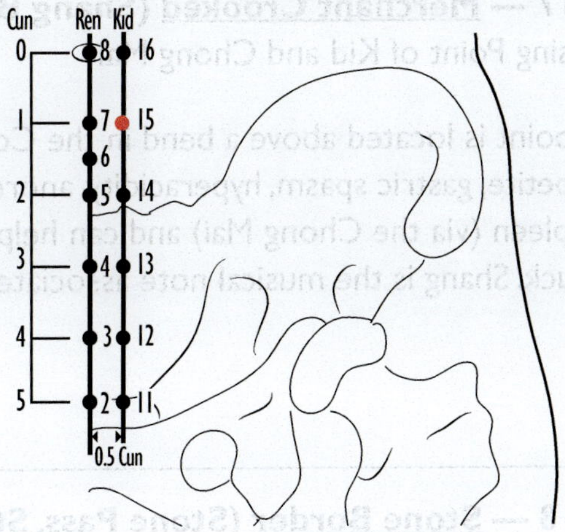
10	7	**0.5 cun** lateral to anterior median line (Ren Mai) **5 cun** superior to superior border of symphysis pubis Level with the centre of the umbilicus Level with Ren 8	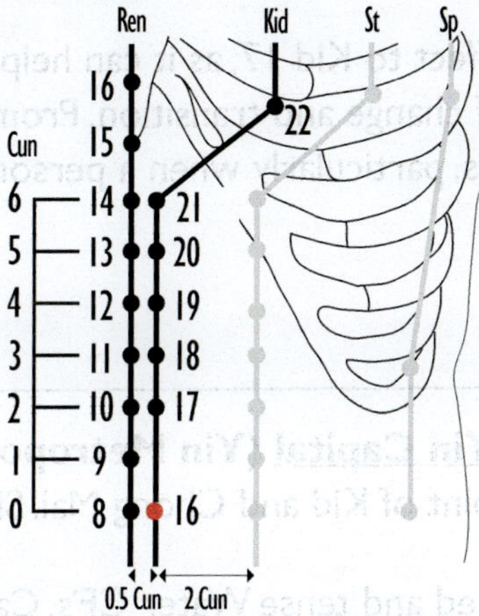

Kidney

Kid 17 — <u>Merchant Crooked</u> (Shang Bend)
Crossing Point of Kid and Chong Mai

This point is located above a bend in the Colon. It influences the intestines, and is helpful for lack of appetite, gastric spasm, hyperacidity, anorexia or where there is no pleasure in eating. Fortifies the Spleen (via the Chong Mai) and can help a person move on in life if they are tired of living, sad or stuck. Shang is the musical note associated with the Metal element.

Kid 18 — <u>Stone Border</u> (Stone Pass, Stone Gate)
Crossing Point of Kid and Chong Mai

Similar in effect to Kid 17, as it can help the patient remove a barrier and move on in life; this is a point of change and transition. Promotes fluidity and helps the BMS find a way through obstructions, particularly when a person is afraid and wary of change. Consider for infertility.

Kid 19 —<u>Yin Capital</u> (Yin Metropolis)
Crossing Point of Kid and Chong Mai. Shokanten Point.

For distressed and tense Water CF's. Can steady and settle a scattered or fearful person and bring them back to their centre. A 'capital' or 'metropolis' is where information and ideas are exchanged or processed. Strongly affects the Yin aspect of a person, enabling them to reflect and receive. Consider for infertility. Fortifies the Spleen.

⊥	Δ		Location
10	7	**0.5 cun** lateral to anterior median line (Ren Mai) **2 cun** superior to the level of the centre of the umbilicus Level with Ren 10	
7-10	7	**0.5 cun** lateral to anterior median line (Ren Mai) **3 cun** superior to the level with the centre of the umbilicus Level with Ren 11	
7-10	7-10	**0.5 cun** lateral to anterior median line (Ren Mai) **4 cun** superior to the level with the centre of the umbilicus Level with Ren 12	

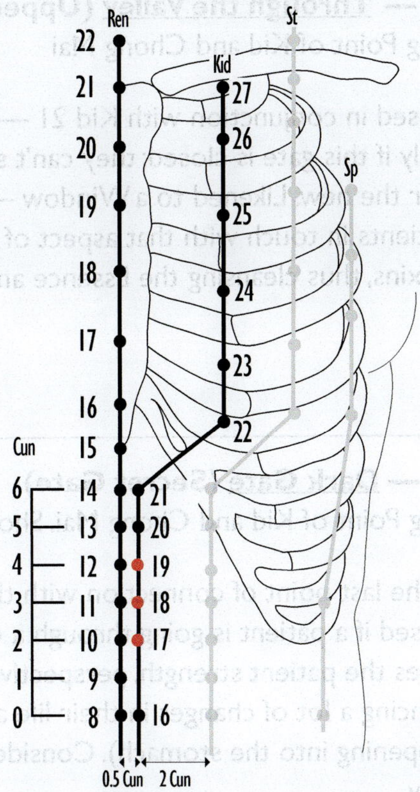

Kidney

Kid 20 — Through the Valley (Upper Gate)
Crossing Point of Kid and Chong Mai

Often used in conjunction with Kid 21 — a person may be stuck, lonely, fearful or suicidal, especially if this gate is closed; they can't see a way forward. Helps to let go of the old and brings hope for the new. Likened to a Window — gives the ability to see. Concerned with the Spirit — puts patients in touch with that aspect of themselves. Enhances the quality of Water by clearing away toxins, thus cleansing the Essence and allowing them to move forward in life more freely.

Kid 21 — Dark Gate (Secret Gate)
Crossing Point of Kid and Chong Mai. Shokanten Point.

This is the last point of connection with the Chong Mai. If this gate is closed, everything looks black. Used if a patient is going through a dark, negative time — suffering from phobias or extreme fear. Gives the patient strength, perspective and the will to face their fears, especially if they are experiencing a lot of changes in their life at this time. It affects the stomach (it is located adjacent to the opening into the stomach). Consider for morning sickness or where breastmilk doesn't flow correctly.

Kid 22 — Walking on the Verandah (Corridor Walk)
Exit point

Kid 22 to Kid 27 are important points to treat the Spirit (said to have been forbidden to use during the Cultural Revolution in China). A verandah is a safe place for aiding convalescence. Gives a sense of new horizons, and helps the patient to face the outside world once again from a position of safety and confidence. Frees the chest area. Consider for patients who can't raise their arms.

Kid 23 — Spirit Seal (Spirit's Altar, Altar Mound)

This point is like a personal seal which stamps the uniqueness and authority of an individual, bestowing a sense of identity upon a person, reconnecting them with their true self. It is often used after Kid 24. We are dealing here with the (Shen) Spirit — bright-eyed, vivacious, extrovert — the perpetuator of good in a person. Great for fragmented Water CF's experiencing intense emotion, shock or sadness, as this point also supports the Heart and its Protector. Affects the will to live. Lies on a level with Ren 17. Helps with breathing problems and frees the chest.

⊥	Δ		Location
5	7-10	**0.5 cun** lateral to anterior median line (Ren Mai) **5 cun** superior to the level with the centre of the umbilicus Level with Ren 13	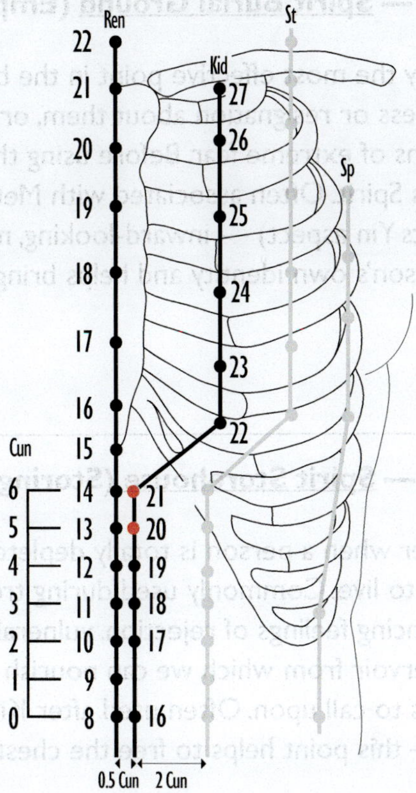
5	7-10	**0.5 cun** lateral to anterior median line (Ren Mai) **6 cun** superior to the level with the centre of the umbilicus Level with Ren 14	
3	5	In the **5th IC Space** **2 cun** lateral to anterior median line (Ren Mai) Level with Ren 16 Level with Xiphisternal Joint	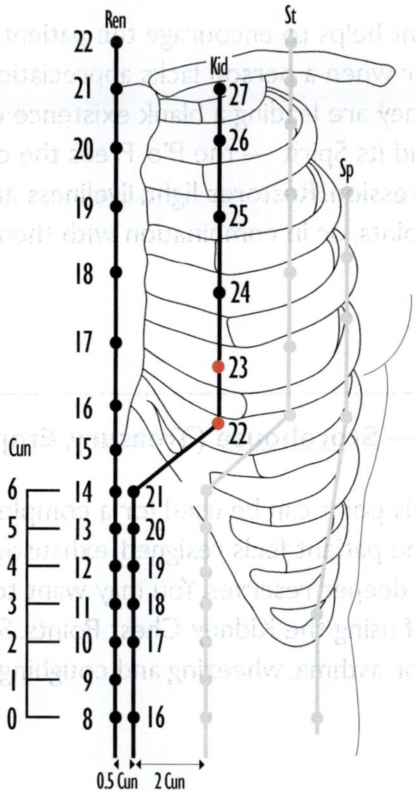
3	5	In the **4th IC Space** **2 cun** lateral to anterior median line (Ren Mai) Level with Ren 17	

Kidney

Kid 24 — <u>Spirit Burial Ground</u> (Empty Spirit, Spirit Ruins)

Probably the most effective point in the body to resurrect the (Ling) Spirit. The patient may have a deadness or resignation about them, or they may experience dreams of wildernesses, ghosts or situations of extreme fear. Before using the Internal Dragons, consider the need to resurrect the patient's Spirit. Often associated with Metal and Water CF's. We are dealing here with the Ling Spirit (its Yin aspect) — inward-looking, mysterious, receptive, serene, hidden. Gives a strong sense of a person's own identity and helps bring purpose, meaning and direction back in their life.

Kid 25 — <u>Spirit Storehouse</u> (Storing the Spirit)

Consider when a person is totally depleted on the Spirit level — in this case the Shen Spirit. Affects the will to live. Commonly used during treatment of Ht and Pc CF's. Excellent if the patient is experiencing feelings of rejection, vulnerability or loneliness. For lack of spiritual reserves — here is a reservoir from which we can nourish and support the Spirit when the patient has no more reserves to call upon. Often used after Kid 24. For chest disorders where the chest can't expand easily — this point helps to free the chest area. Consider for insomnia due to worry.

Kid 26 — <u>Amidst Elegance</u> (Elegant Centre, Lively Centre)

This point helps to encourage the patient back into the midst of peace, serenity and beauty. Consider when a person lacks appreciation or respect for their own Spirit or for that of others; where they are leading a blank existence or just 'going through the motions'. Lies in the area of the Lungs and its Spirit — the P'o. Frees the chest, and is helpful for asthma, cough, congestion, grief and depression. Restores light, liveliness and elegance to the Spirit. Often used after other Kidney Chest Points, or in combination with them.

Kid 27 — <u>Storehouse</u> (Treasury, Empty Treasury)

Again, this point can be used for a complete lack of Spiritual reserves — when the storehouse is empty, the patient feels resigned, exhausted and hopeless. Here we can support and enhance the patient's deeper reserves. You may want to use Kid 27 before Kid 25 in order to gauge the possible effects of using the Kidney Chest Points. Strengthens Ancestral Qi, frees the chest, and can be helpful for asthma, wheezing and coughing.

⊥	△		Location
3	5	In the 3rd **IC Space** **2 cun** lateral to anterior median line (Ren Mai) Level with Ren 18	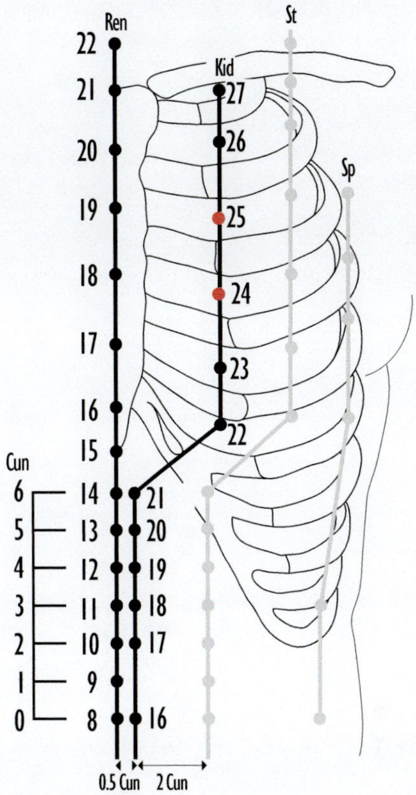
3	5	In the 2nd **IC Space** **2 cun** lateral to anterior median line (Ren Mai) Level with Ren 19	
3	5	In the 1st **IC Space** **2 cun** lateral to anterior median line (Ren Mai) Level with Ren 20	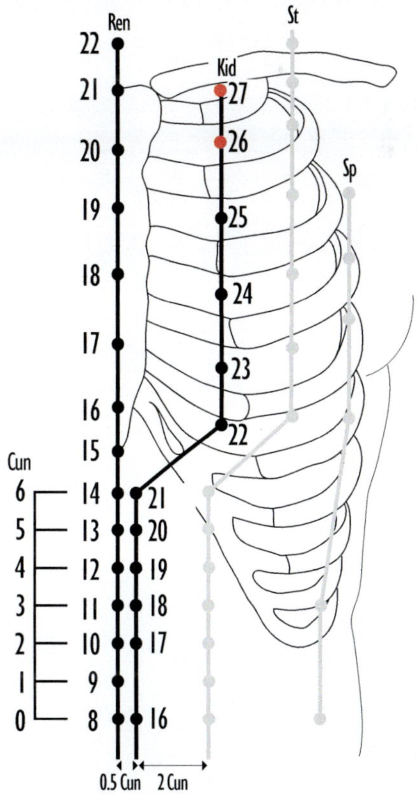
3	5	In the depression between the lower border of the sternal end of the clavicle and the upper border of the 1st rib **2 cun** lateral to anterior median line (Ren Mai) Level with Ren 21	

Pericardium. Heart Protector. Circulation Sex. Tan Zhong

- **Ambassador, Servant and Protector of the Heart**
- **Fire governs the blood vessels, the emotion joy, and produces the scorched odour**

Pericardium. Heart Protector. Circulation Sex. Tan Zhong

Pc 1 — Heavenly Pond (Celestial Pool)
Entry Point (Men). Window of the Sky (Men). Crossing Point Pc, Liv, Gb, TH. Forbidden on Women.

This is a powerful point — it can reach to the depths of a person's Spirit. It can be effective in cases of sadness or a broken heart, and helps facilitate the process of regaining appropriate relationships with other people without feeling too vulnerable. Heavenly Pond bathes the Spirit. The Pericardium connects to our Ancestral Chest energy. Pc protects the Ht (particularly from emotional turmoil or excessive heat) and thus guards the Spirits. Pc 1 and 2 work well together (on men). Pc 1 puts patients in touch with themselves; Pc 2 allows them to do something with it.

Pc 2 — Heavenly Spring (Celestial Source, Heavenly Fountain)
Entry Point (Women). Window of the Sky (Women).

This point is named after a star, which is an indication of its heavenly quality. It invigorates and enlivens the vital energy in the meridian. Soothes and cleanses the Official at the Spirit level, but is also helpful for emotional problems, especially profound hurt. For nursing mothers who don't have enough milk. Classic point for fear of wind and cold. Has a major effect on the chest when combined with Command Points, e.g. palpitations, cardiac pain, or arrhythmia.

Pc 3 — Crooked Marsh (Marsh at the Bend)
Water Point. He-Sea Point/Antique-Autumn Point.

A marsh is a fertile place (at least in rice-cultivating communities). This Water point can calm and cool the Fire if it is raging out of control, where the patient is hot, anxious, restless, agitated or manic. As the Water point it can be used for transferring Qi across the K'e cycle from the Kidneys. Consider for fear of meeting people. Local point for muscular pain in the arm or elbow.

⊥	Δ		Location
Male 3 Female X	Male 3-5 Female X	On the anterior torso — chest **1 cun** lateral to centre of the nipple In the **4th IC Space**	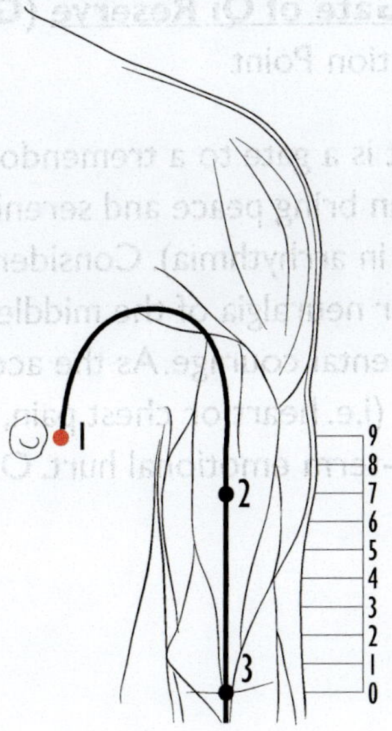
5	3	Anterior surface of upper arm Between two muscle bellies of biceps brachii muscle **7 cun** proximal to the flexure of the elbow (transverse cubital crease) **2 cun** distal to the axillary fold	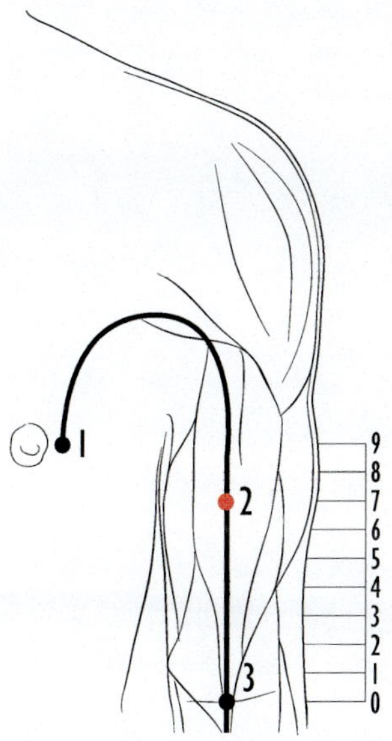
3	3-5	On flexure of the elbow Medial to the tendon of the biceps brachii Arm slightly flexed Midpoint of the transverse cubital crease	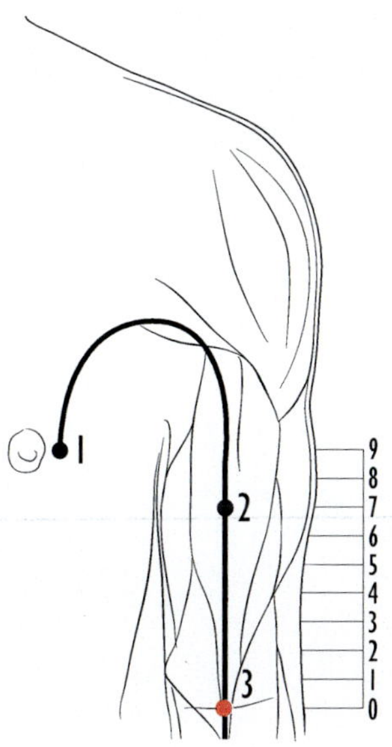

Pc 4 — Gate of Qi Reserve (Gate of the Meridian, Cleft Gate, Accumulation Door)
Accumulation Point

This point is a gate to a tremendous reserve of energy. One of the strongest points on the body, it can bring peace and serenity to a troubled heart. It can help regulate the rhythm of the Heart (as in arrhythmia). Consider this point for generalised apprehension and fear of strangers. Helpful for neuralgia of the middle forearm, hand or fingers. It is said to strengthen the mind and bestow mental courage. As the accumulation point it strengthens the meridian, especially in acute situations (i.e. heart or chest pain, or as a result of shock). Helps calm Pc-type disturbances arising from long-term emotional hurt. Often used with TH 7.

⊥	Δ		Location
4	5	**5 cun** proximal to Pc 7 Between the tendons of the Palmaris Longus and Flexor Carpi Radialis Between ulna (medial) and Radius (lateral) if muscles and tendons cannot be felt	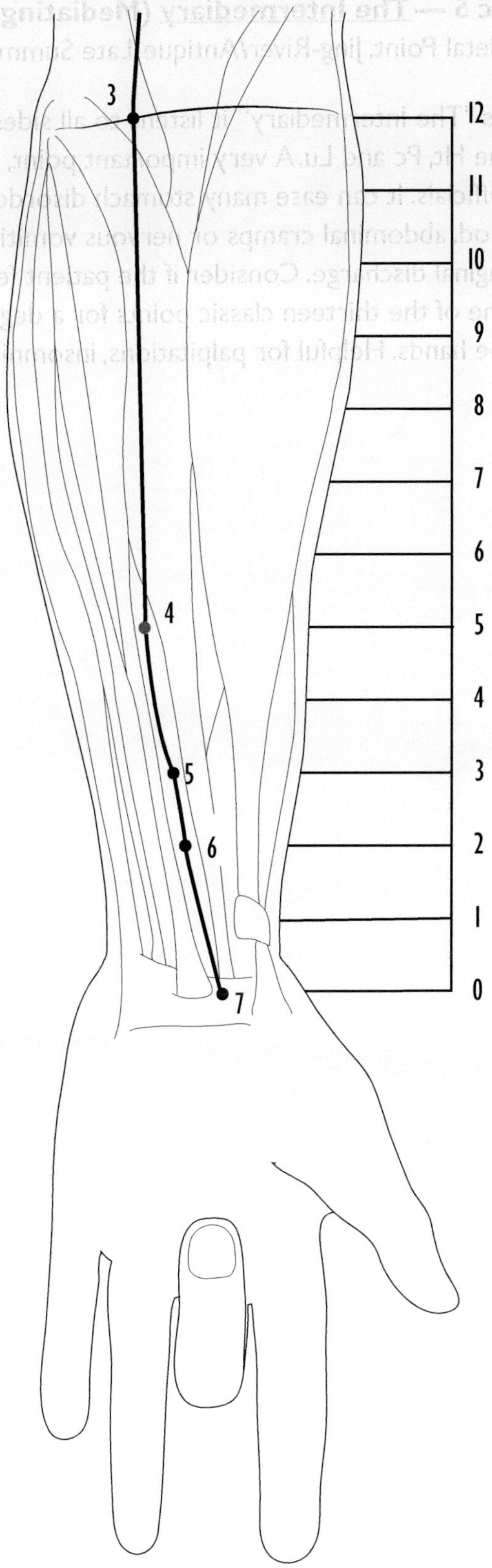

Pericardium. Heart Protector. Circulation Sex. Tan Zhong

Pc 5 — The Intermediary (Mediating Messenger, Intermediate Emissary)
Metal Point. Jing-River/Antique-Late Summer Point. Crossing Point of Ht, Pc, Lu. Ghost Point.

As "The Intermediary" it listens to all sides and brings harmony. This point mediates between the Ht, Pc and Lu. A very important point, assisting the Ht in its communication with the other Officials. It can ease many stomach disorders (Fire is the Mother of Earth), e.g. inability to digest food, abdominal cramps or nervous vomiting. Beneficial for cardiac pains, irregular periods or vaginal discharge. Consider if the patient feels as though they are possessed by the devil — this is one of the thirteen classic points for a degree of possession. For a sensation of heat in the palms of the hands. Helpful for palpitations, insomnia, hysteria or manic depression.

⊥	△		Location
3-7	3-5	**3 cun** proximal to Pc 7 Between the tendons of the Palmaris Longus and Flexor Carpi Radialis Between ulna (medial) and Radius (lateral) if muscles and tendons cannot be felt	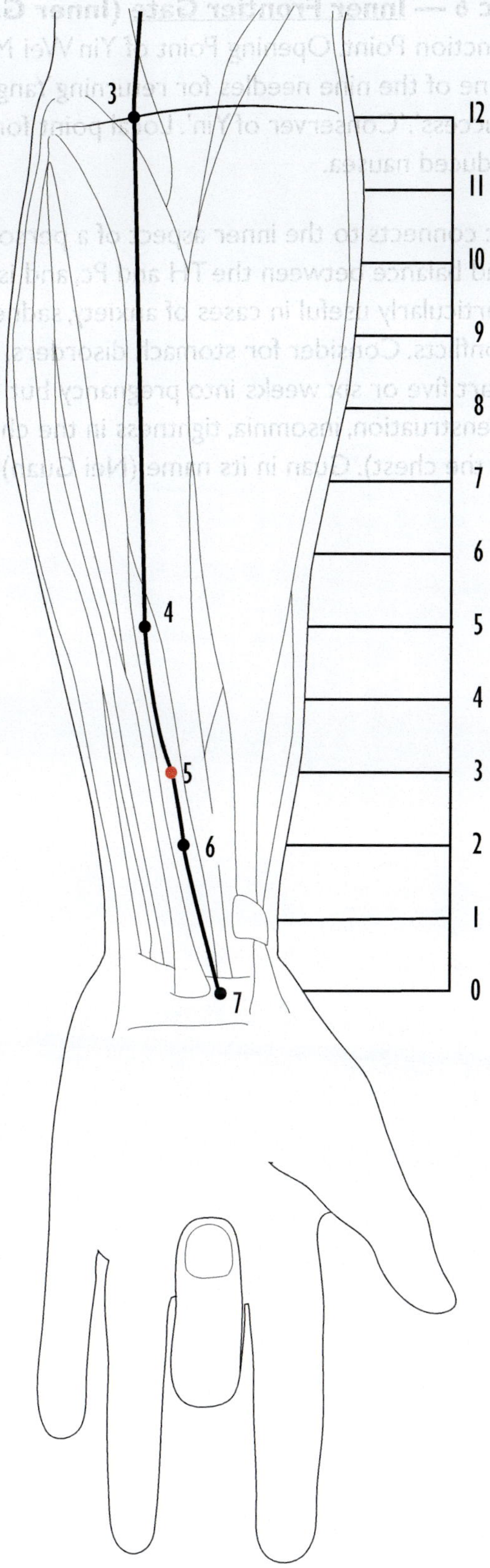

Pericardium. Heart Protector. Circulation Sex. Tan Zhong

Pc 6 — <u>Inner Frontier Gate</u> (Inner Gate, Inner Pass)
Junction Point. Opening Point of Yin Wei Mai. Coupled Point of Chong Mai. General Junction Point. One of the nine needles for returning Yang, 'Perfect Love Point'. 'Broken Heart Gate'. 'Gate to Success'. 'Conserver of Yin'. Local point for travel sickness, morning sickness or chemotherapy-induced nausea.

Pc connects to the inner aspect of a person, TH to the outer. This potent point restores harmony and balance between the TH and Pc, and is often used with TH 5 (Outer Frontier Gate). Particularly useful in cases of anxiety, sadness or lack of joy, perhaps as a result of relationship conflicts. Consider for stomach disorders, especially nausea, and morning sickness which may start five or six weeks into pregnancy but is often gone by the 14th week. For irregular or painful menstruation, insomnia, tightness in the chest, heavy-heartedness or palpitations (Pc and TH meet in the chest). Guan in its name (Nei Guan) indicates the importance of this gate.

⊥	Δ		Location
3	5	Forbidden from 4th month of pregnancy **2 cun** proximal to Pc 7 Between the tendons of the Palmaris Longus and Flexor Carpi Radialis Between ulna (medial) and Radius (lateral) if muscles and tendons cannot be felt	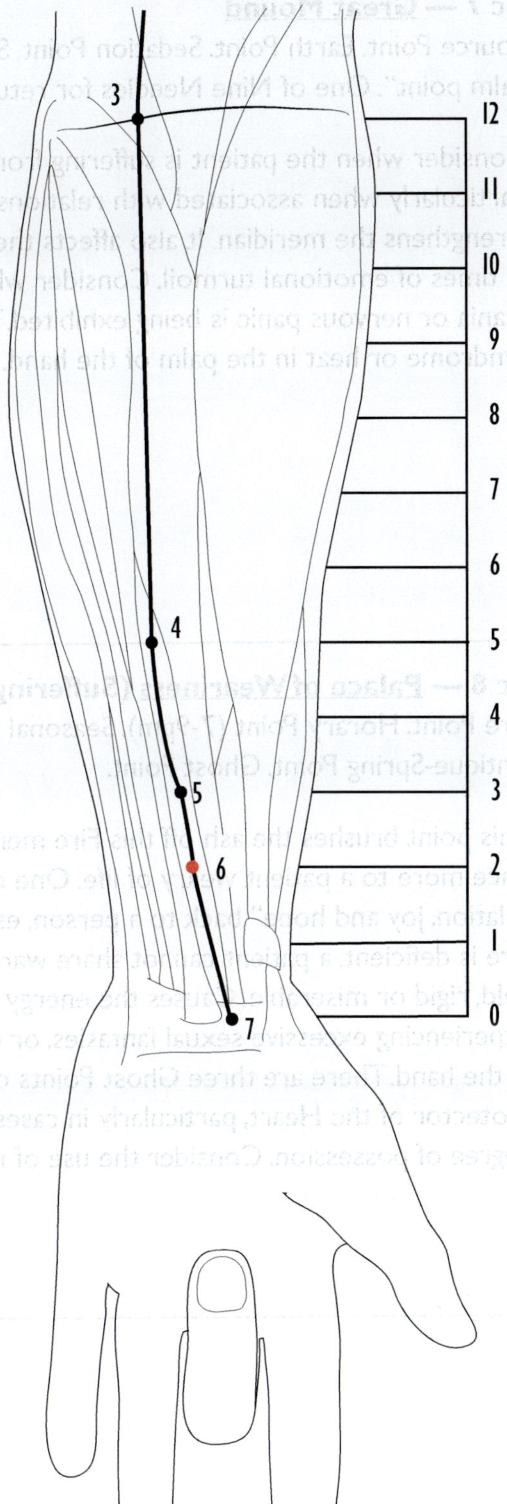

Pc 7 — Great Mound
Source Point. Earth Point. Sedation Point. Shu-Stream/Antique-Summer Point. Ghost Point. "Sexual calm point". One of Nine Needles for returning Yang.

Consider when the patient is suffering from insecurity, vulnerability, sadness, rejection or lack of joy, particularly when associated with relationship difficulties. As the Earth point it calms, stabilises and strengthens the meridian. It also affects the Heart in this way, protecting and steadying it especially in times of emotional turmoil. Consider when there is hysterical laughter or crying, or where mania or nervous panic is being exhibited. This point can be effective in cases of carpal tunnel syndrome or heat in the palm of the hand.

Pc 8 — Palace of Weariness (Suffering Palace, Labour Palace, Temple of Hard Work)
Fire Point. Horary Point (7-9pm). Seasonal Horary Point — Summer. Exit Point. Ying-Spring/Antique-Spring Point. Ghost Point.

This point brushes the ash off this Fire meridian, allowing joy, love, vitality and vigour to emerge once more to a patient weary of life. One of the most powerful points on the body, bringing "elation, joy and hope" back to a person, especially if depressed or when very low in spirit. If the Fire is deficient, a patient cannot share warmth or affection — this may result in their becoming cold, rigid or miserable. Causes the energy of the Heart to leap up. Helpful where a patient is experiencing excessive sexual fantasies, or conversely, impotence. Local point for pain and stiffness in the hand. There are three Ghost Points on this meridian, which further illustrates its role as protector of the Heart, particularly in cases such as "out of control" behaviour, mania or some degree of possession. Consider the use of moxa here, but take care not to overheat.

⊥	Δ		Location
3	X	Proximal ulnar corner of the scaphoid bone Between the tendons of the flexor carpi radialis and the palmaris longus muscles.	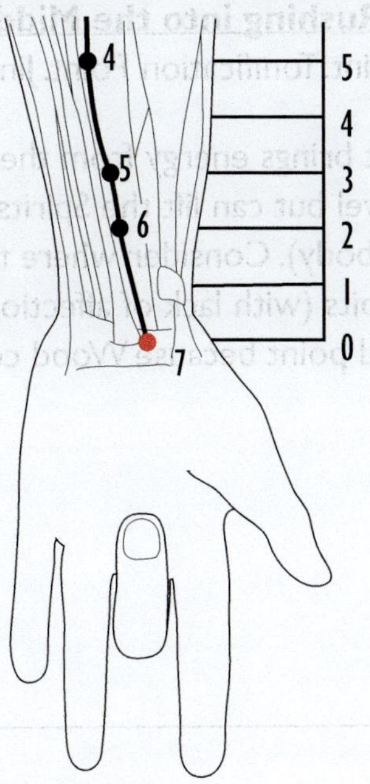
2-3	3	Forbidden from 3rd month of Pregnancy Palmar surface of the hand Between 2nd and 3rd metacarpal bones (closer to 3rd) Proximal to head of the 3rd metacarpal bone Normally lies just proximal to the proximal transverse crease	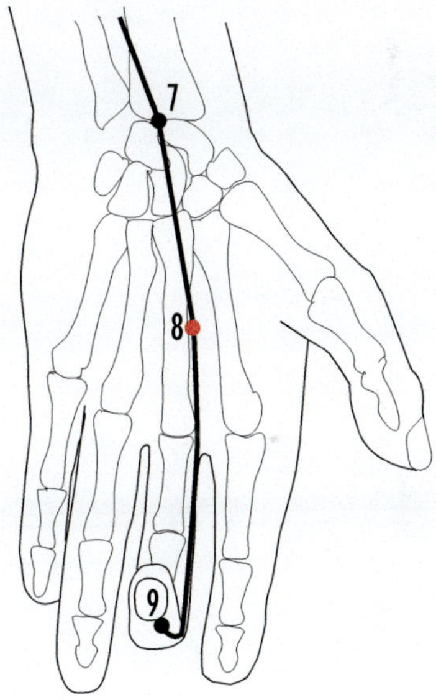

Pc 9 — <u>Rushing into the Middle</u> (Central Surge)
Wood Point. Tonification Point. Jing-Well/Antique-Winter Point. "Balanced Friendliness Point".

This point brings energy from the Mother to the Child via the Sheng cycle. Works directly on the Mental level but can lift the Spirits too. For unconsciousness or fainting (cutting off of the mind from the body). Consider where the hands are hot or cold. May be beneficial for uncontrollable sexual habits (with lack of affection), or for people who have difficulty expressing themselves. An often used point because Wood commonly has more available energy in it than Fire.

⊥	△		Location
I	3	Radial nail point of the 3rd digit Distal to the flare of the distal phalanx Pc 9 alternative location, historically at the tip of the 3rd digit	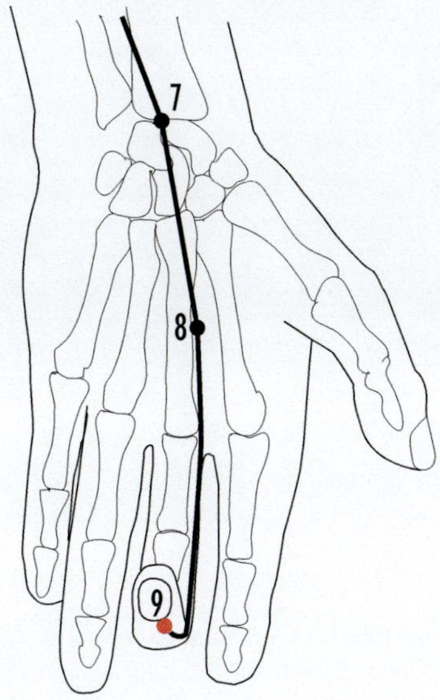

Triple Heater. Three Heater. Triple Burner. San Jiao

- As the "Official of balance and harmony" it plays a key role in the regulation and diplomatic communication amongst all of the Officials. It pervades the entire Kingdom
- Opens and irrigates the Water passages
- Regulates the fluids — the 'ye' — Governs the distribution of Yuan Qi
- Maintains correct heat balance in the system, both physically and emotionally

Triple Heater. Three Heater. Triple Burner. San Jiao

TH 1 — <u>Rushing the Frontier Gate</u> (Thoroughfare Gate, Passage Hub)
Metal Point. Entry Point. Jing-Well/Antique-Winter Point.

With Guan in its name (Guan Chong), this Point is thus defined as a major, important gate. It is also the Metal point which brings quality and rhythmic order to the Official. This frontier gate must be allowed to function correctly as it opens and irrigates the Water passages of the Kingdom, which is its Yin aspect. This point also has an influence on the regulation of heat within the body, its Yang aspect. If the gate is closed, the system can become cold, rigid, numb with articulation problems and poor communication amongst the Officials. The throat area may become numb, affecting speech. As a distal point it influences the shoulder, ear, eye, head, throat and tongue.

TH 2 — <u>Fluid Secretion Gate</u> (Door of fluids)
Water Point. Ying-Spring/Antique-Spring Point.

This next gate controls and balances Water within the Fire. It regulates heat in the body which, for a human being, lies within a narrow bandwidth of only 3.4°C (6.1°F). It has a special effect on the ears. This is a gate that controls secretions within the Kingdom — we need to be fluid, knowing when to yield and when to take a stand. Consider using this point for all your patients. When stimulated it can, over time, increase fluid secretions (the ye) in the spine, joints, bone marrow and brain. Consider for arthritis of the fingers, or paralysis or swelling of the hands and fingers. Can be helpful when there are fluctuations of the emotions, or when the hands and feet feel very cold or very hot. When using TH 2, consider adding TH 10 (Earth point) to control and contain Water.

⊥	△		Location
1	3	Ulnar nail point of the 4th digit Distal to the flare of the distal phalanx	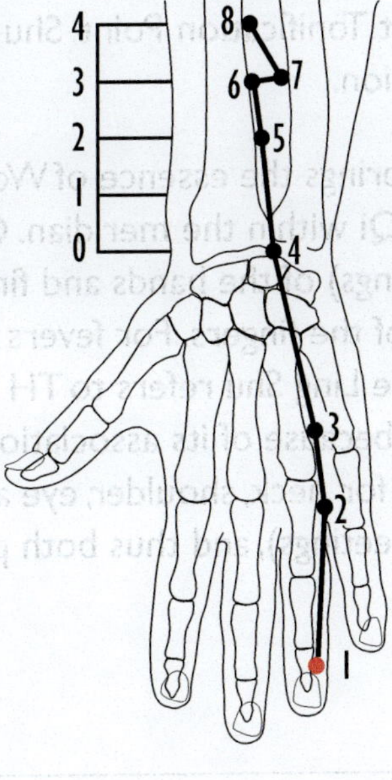
1	3	Distal to metacarpo-phalangeal joint Distal to flare of base of proximal phalanx of 4th digit Proximal to web margin when digits are spread out	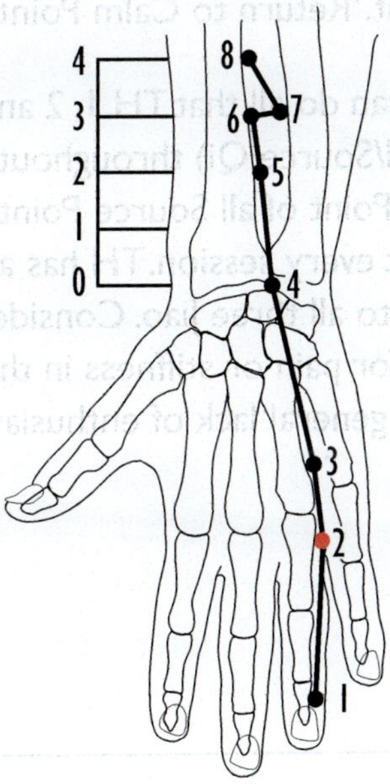

Triple Heater. Three Heater. Triple Burner. San Jiao

TH 3 — Middle Islet (Central Islet, Middle of the Pond)
Wood Point. Tonification Point. Shu-Stream/Antique-Summer Point. 'Warm Joy Point'. First Aid point for Exhaustion.

This point brings the essence of Wood to the Fire. As the Mother point, it has the natural ability to control Qi within the meridian. Can be helpful for lack of articulation (and thus a lack of ability to grasp things) of the hands and fingers; to a lesser extent, the wrists and elbows. Consider for numbness of the fingers. For fevers and emotions that rage and then subside (lack of balance and control). The Ling Shu refers to TH as 'the central river that protects the Spirits from perverse influences', because of its association with defensive 'Wei Qi'. As a distal point it can be used to good effect for neck, shoulder, eye and ear disorders. Has a connection to the area of Du 20 (One Hundred Meetings), and thus both points can be considered for raising the Spirits.

TH 4 — Yang Pond (Accumulation of Yang)
Source Point. 'Return to Calm Point'.

This point can do all that TH 1, 2 and 3 can do, but to a lesser degree. TH evenly distributes Yuan Qi (Original/Source Qi) throughout the entire system. TH 4 is a potent point, and can be seen as the Source Point of all Source Points. Some schools, mainly Japanese, recommend treatment of this point at every session. TH has a strong analogy with Water, warmth and communication, as it connects to all three Jiao. Consider for an inability to grasp things or to raise the arm, or as a local point for pain or stiffness in the wrist, arm and shoulder. For hearing problems (e.g. tinnitus, deafness), a general lack of enthusiasm or emotional instability.

⊥	△		Location
3	3-5	Proximal to metacarpo-phalangeal joint Proximal to flare of the head of the 4th metacarpal bone when a loose fist is made	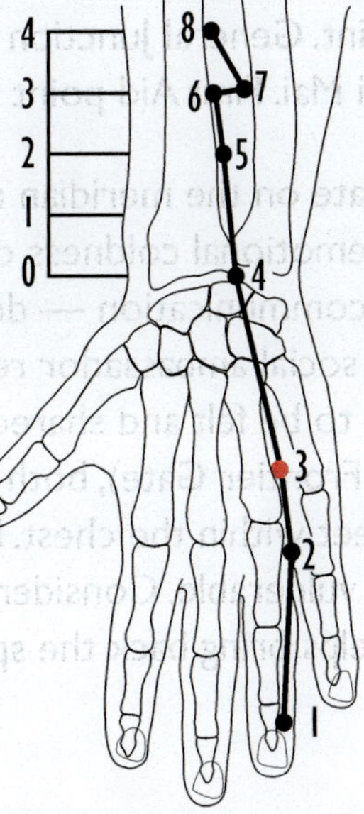
3	Moxa generally forbidden	Forbidden from 3rd month of pregnancy At flexure of wrist on a continuum of the border of the 4th metacarpal bone In the depression between ulna and radius Between tendons of extensor digitorum communis and extensor digiti minimi Feel for space between triquetral and lunate bones	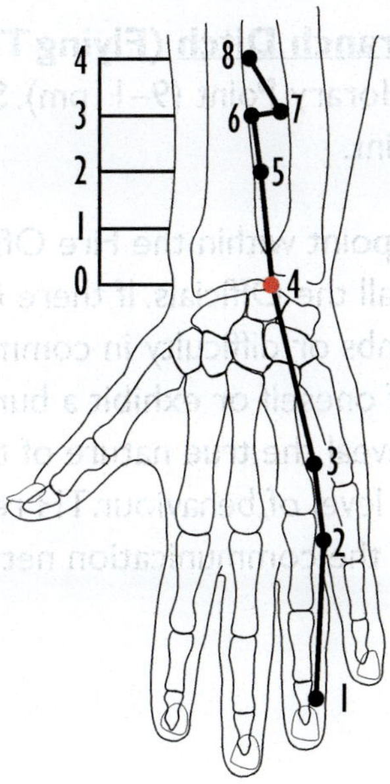

Triple Heater. Three Heater. Triple Burner. San Jiao

TH 5 — <u>Outer Frontier Gate</u> (External Gate, Conserver of Yang)
Junction Point. General Junction Point. Opening Point of Yang Wei Mai (Linking Vessel). Coupling Point of Dai Mai. First Aid point for Fever.

This third gate on the meridian regulates the balance of heat within a person, which can manifest as physical or emotional coldness or, conversely, as excessive openness. Perhaps the patient is shutting the gate of communication — doesn't want to hear, see or know. Perhaps it is wedged open.
TH is like a social ambassador reaching out into the world, giving a wider perspective on things. Allows love to be felt and shared between the two worlds — inner and outer. Often paired with Pc 5 (Inner Frontier Gate), both of which have Guan in their names indicating major gates. Both channels meet within the chest. Helps with relationship difficulties, especially if a person is feeling insecure or vulnerable. Consider for deafness, tinnitus, trigeminal neuralgia, throbbing headache or migraine. Helps bring back the sparkle in a person's life, particularly after a severe fever.

TH 6 — <u>Branch Ditch</u> (Flying Tiger)
Fire Point. Horary Point (9–11pm). Seasonal Horary Point — Summer. Jing-River/Antique-Late Summer Point.

As the Fire point within the Fire Official, TH 6 enlivens the meridian and regulates heat in all 3 Jiao and thus in all the Officials. If there is too little Fire, Water can flow unchecked, resulting in swollen and puffy limbs or difficulty in communicating with others. If the Fire is excessive, one can be brash, full of oneself or exhibit a burning ego. It can also result in urticaria, psoriasis or angina. This point can reveal the true nature of the Official, and help return the patient to a more mature and appropriate level of behaviour. TH regulates the 'ditches, sluices and waterways', which are the vital pathways of the communication network within the Kingdom.

⊥	△		Location
5	3-7	Posterior median line of forearm **2 cun** proximal to wrist flexure Between ulna and radius Between extensor digitorum communis and extensor pollicis	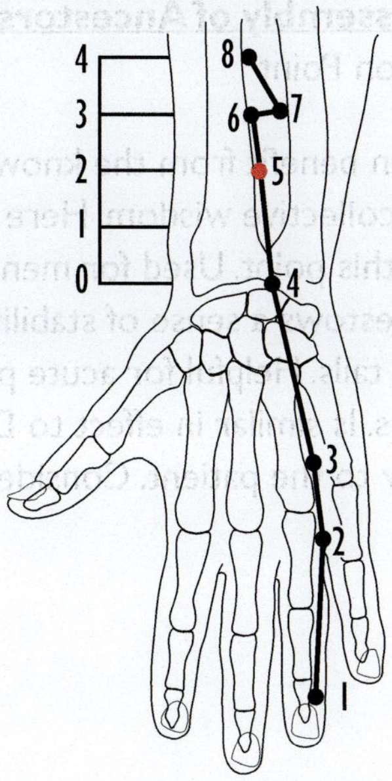
5	5	As for TH 5, but **3 cun** proximal to wrist flexure	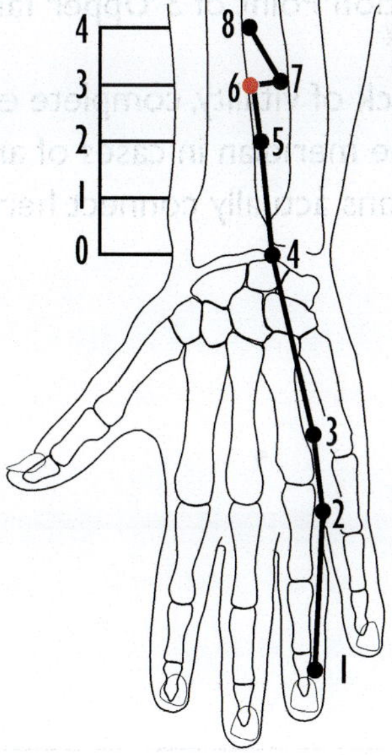

Triple Heater. Three Heater. Triple Burner. San Jiao

TH 7 — Assembly of Ancestors (Ancestral Cooperation)
Accumulation Point

Here we can benefit from the knowledge, authority and experience of our ancestors; we can draw upon their collective wisdom. Here our ancestors have assembled for our benefit — we can turn to them at this point. Used for mental and emotional disorders when moods alternate wildly; this point bestows a sense of stability and calm. Use when the Qi gets snarled up and we end up chasing our tails. Helpful for acute problems — painful skin conditions, pain in the arm, ear, temples or eyebrows. Is similar in effect to Du 20 (One Hundred Meetings), in that it brings clarity, peace and serenity to the patient. Consider combining with TH 6, which lies on the same level.

TH 8 — Three Yang Junction (Three Yang Connection)
Group Junction Point of 3 Upper Yang Meridians (SI, TH, LI)

Good for lack of vitality, complete exhaustion or inertia. Consider for deafness or loss of voice. Activates the meridian in cases of arm or shoulder pain. Texts are not clear as to whether the 3 Yang meridians actually connect here, or whether their function and proximity are merely similar.

⊥	Δ		Location
3	5-7	**3 cun** proximal to wrist flexure Level with and one finger width medial to TH 6 Between extensor Carpi ulnaris and extensor digiti minimi muscles Between the radius and ulna	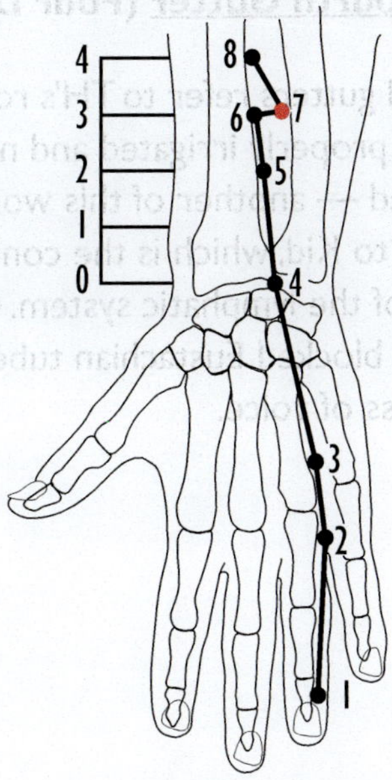
X	7	**4 cun** proximal to wrist flexure between radius and ulna Between extensor digitorum and abductor pollicis longus	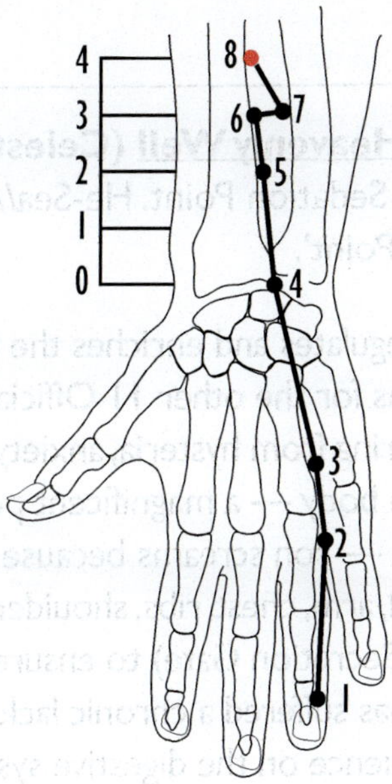

TH 9 — Fourth Gutter (Four Ditches, Four Rivers)

Ditches and gutters refer to TH's role in distributing and regulating the fluids around the system so that it is properly irrigated and not clogged up. Thus, communication amongst all the Officials is maintained — another of this wonderful, but mysterious, Official's roles. The TH has a close connection to Kid, which is the controller of the fluids. Some think of the TH as the oriental equivalent of the lymphatic system. Consider for ear disorders, especially tinnitus. Also for deafness caused by a blocked Eustachian tube. Useful for physical problems in the forearm and elbow, or for a sudden loss of voice.

TH 10 — Heavenly Well (Celestial Well)

Earth Point. Sedation Point. He-Sea/Antique-Autumn Point. Upper Meeting Point. 'Serene Tranquillity Point'.

This point regulates and enriches the Earth within the Fire. Heavenly Well can have far-reaching repercussions for the other 11 Officials, bringing stability, strength and serenity to a volatile patient who may be suffering from hysteria, anxiety, sadness or depression. This is one of the most neglected points of the whole body — a magnificent point. No negative actions emanate from this 'Well'. Deals with all types of pain — son screams because Mother is sick; Mother screams because son is sick. For pain in the jaw, hand, arm, chest, ribs, shoulder, elbow or behind the ear. Consider adding this point when using TH 2 (Fluid Secretion Gate) to ensure the Earth is not dried out. Said to be supportive in cases where the patient has suffered a chronic lack of love during childhood, and to be effective for lack of appetite as it has an influence on the digestive system via the sheng cycle.

⊥	△		Location
6	3-7	**7 cun** proximal to wrist flexure between radius and ulna Between extensor digitorum and extensor carpi ulnaris	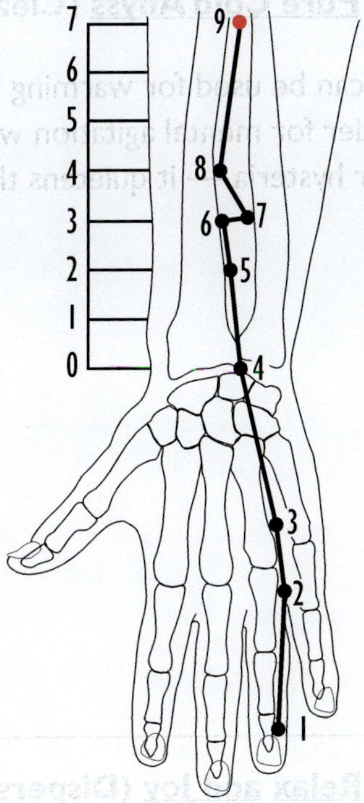
3-5	3-5	Forbidden from 4th month of pregnancy Approx **1 cun** proximal to the tip of the olecranon of the ulna Superior to the superior border of the olecranon In depression in the tendon of triceps brachii For TH 10 to TH 14 the patient is seated with arms at 90° angle with palmar surface upwards.	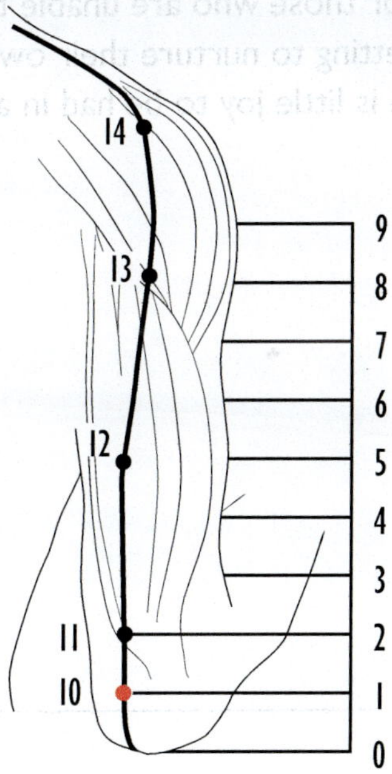

Triple Heater. Three Heater. Triple Burner. San Jiao

TH 11 — Pure Cold Abyss (Clear Cold Abyss)

This point can be used for warming the TH if it is too cold, or for cooling or calming it if it is too hot. Consider for mental agitation within the patient if the Fire is out of control, perhaps causing madness or hysteria — it quietens the mind. For problems in the arm, elbow or shoulder.

TH 12 — Relax and Joy (Dispersing Brilliance)

Consider for those who are unable to relax, who are running around seeing to the needs of others whilst forgetting to nurture their own need to relax and be joyful. A very comforting point. Helpful when there is little joy to be had in a person's life.

⊥	Δ		Location
3	3-7	Posterior midline of upper arm Superior to superior border of the olecranon process Approx **2 cun** proximal to the tip of the olecranon of the ulna bone In a depression in the tendon of the triceps brachii muscle in the midline **1 cun** superior to TH 10	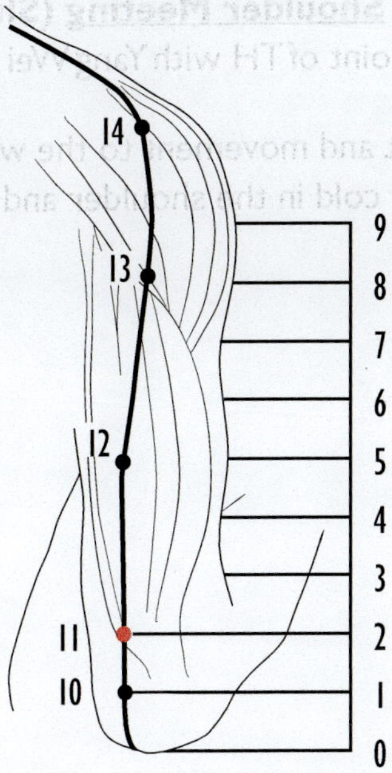
5	3-7	Posterior midline of upper arm On the triceps brachii muscle Approx **5 cun** prox to the tip of the olecranon of the ulna bone. Midway between TH 11 and TH 13	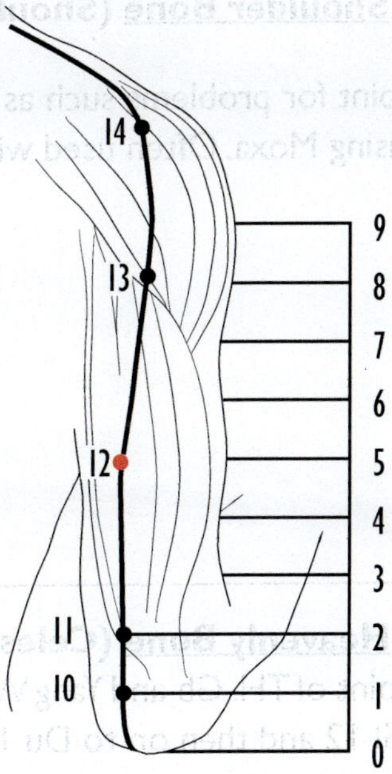

Triple Heater. Three Heater. Triple Burner. San Jiao

TH 13 — <u>Shoulder Meeting</u> (Shoulder Convergence)
Crossing point of TH with Yang Wei Mai (Linking Vessel — which links all Yang meridians)

Brings heat and movement to the whole shoulder region. Excellent for shoulder paralysis. Consider for pain or cold in the shoulder and shoulder blade. Good with Moxa or Moxa roll.

TH 14 — <u>Shoulder Bone</u> (Shoulder Opening)

A classic point for problems such as pain, fibrositis, arthritis or paralysis of the arms and shoulders. Consider using Moxa. Often used with LI 15 and LI 16.

TH 15 — <u>Heavenly Bone</u> (Celestial Hearing, Heavenly Foramen)
Crossing Point of TH, Gb and Yang Wei Mai (Linking Vessel). From TH 14, a deep pathway travels to TH 15 via SI 12 and then on to Du 14 before passing over to Gb 21 and St 12.

For shoulder, arm and neck stiffness and pain. For feelings of oppression in the area of the Upper Jiao. The channel's connection with Gb (both pass through and around the ear) accounts for TH 15's effect on hearing and ear pain, and for its alternative name of Celestial Hearing. Consider Moxa or cupping here for chills and fevers.

⊥	△		Location
3-7	5-15	Posterior midline of upper arm Inferior border of the deltoid muscle Approx **3 cun** inferior to the acromial angle and TH 14	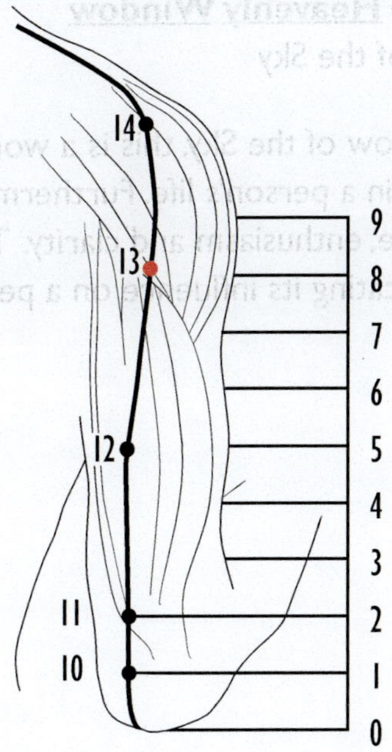
7	5-7	Patient is seated with arms at 90° Palmar surface upwards At the infero-lateral corner of Acromion process of scapula At the acromial angle Approx **1 cun** posterior to LI 15 when arm is abducted	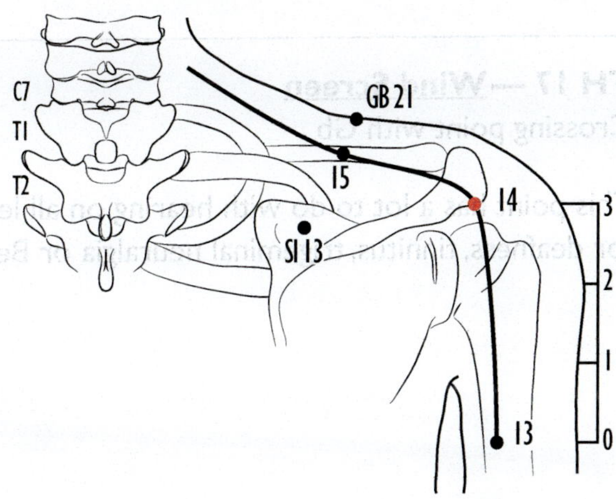
3-8	5-7	On the trapezius muscle At the transverse midpoint between Du 14 (on posterior midline) and the lateral tip of the Acromion of the scapula Midway between SI 13 and Gb 21 On a vertical line from SI 13 to TH 15 ending at Gb 21	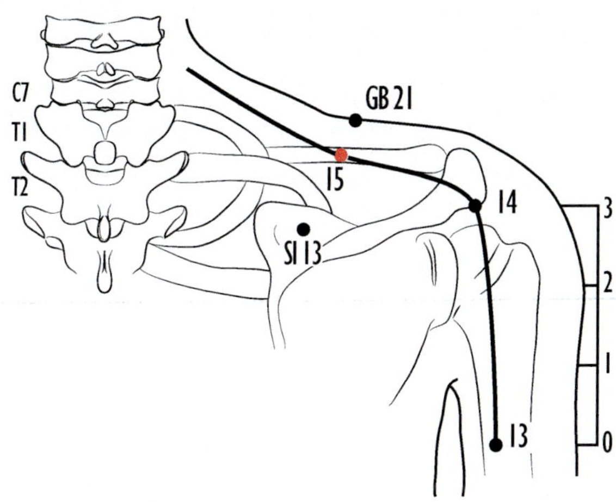

Triple Heater. Three Heater. Triple Burner. San Jiao

TH 16 — <u>Heavenly Window</u>
Window of the Sky

As a Window of the Sky, this is a wonderful point for lifting the spirits if sadness or lack of joy is present in a person's life. Furthermore, it can help bring back to them a sense of purpose, perspective, enthusiasm and clarity. This is the third point on the TH meridian with Heavenly in its name, indicating its influence on a person's relationship with their higher self.

TH 17 — <u>Wind Screen</u>
Crossing point with Gb

This point has a lot to do with hearing on all levels (both TH and Gb connect to the ear). Consider for deafness, tinnitus, trigeminal neuralgia or Bell's Palsy. Take care when needling.

<table>
<tr><th>⊥</th><th>Δ</th><th></th><th>Location</th></tr>
<tr><td>3-5</td><td>X</td><td>On the posterior border of the sternocleidomastoid muscle
Posterior and inferior to the mastoid process of the temporal bone
Inferior to the inferior border of the medial aspect of the temporal bone
Approx 1 cun inferior to Gb 12
Level with angle of mandible (SI 17)
Approx level with Bl 10</td><td>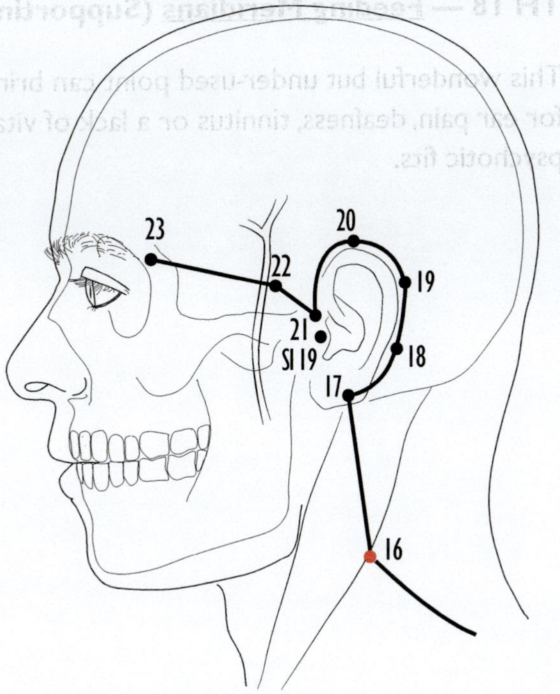
</td></tr>
<tr><td>3</td><td>3-7</td><td>In the depression halfway between the ramus of the mandible and the mastoid process of the temporal bone posterior to the ear lobe
Open the mouth to expose the hollow</td><td>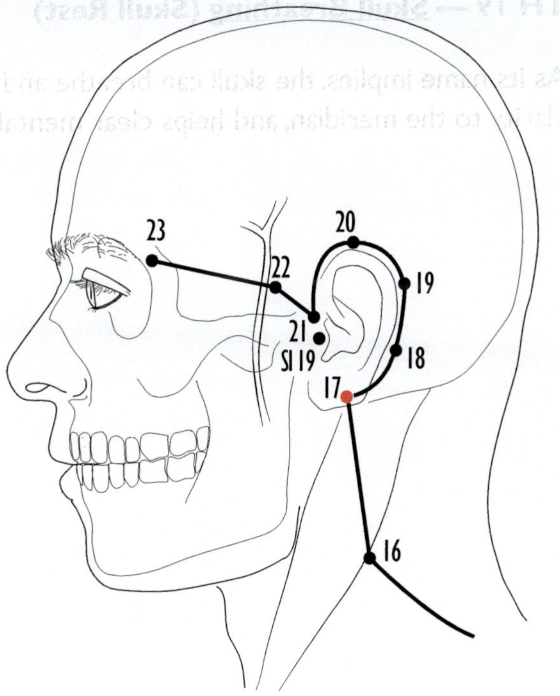
</td></tr>
</table>

TH 18 — Feeding Meridians (Supporting Vessel)

This wonderful but under-used point can bring vitality, clarity and warmth to a person. Consider for ear pain, deafness, tinnitus or a lack of vitality. It is said to be effective for treating epileptic or psychotic fits.

TH 19 — Skull Breathing (Skull Rest)

As its name implies, the skull can breathe and move; this point aids in bringing a freshness and clarity to the meridian, and helps clear mental congestion. Useful for ear problems.

⊥	△		Location
I	X	On the mastoid bone directly posterior to the helix of the ear when this is flattened against the skull One third of the distance from TH 17 to TH 20	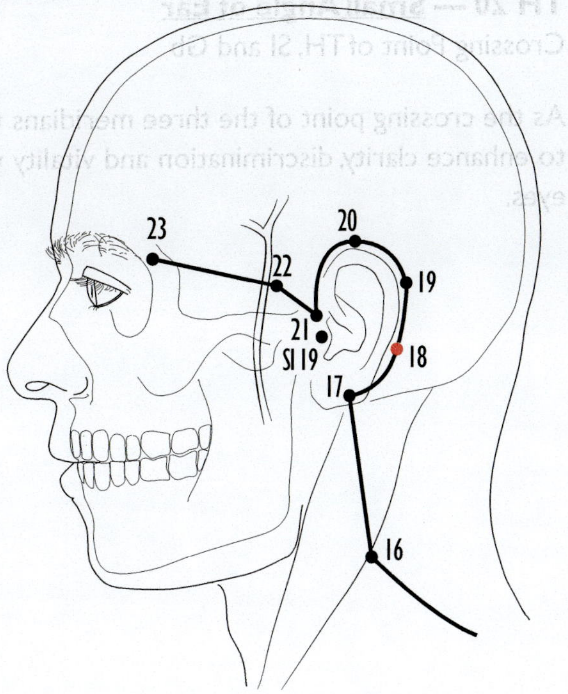
X	3-7	On the mastoid bone directly posterior to the helix of the ear when this is flattened against the skull Two thirds of the distance from TH 17 to TH 20	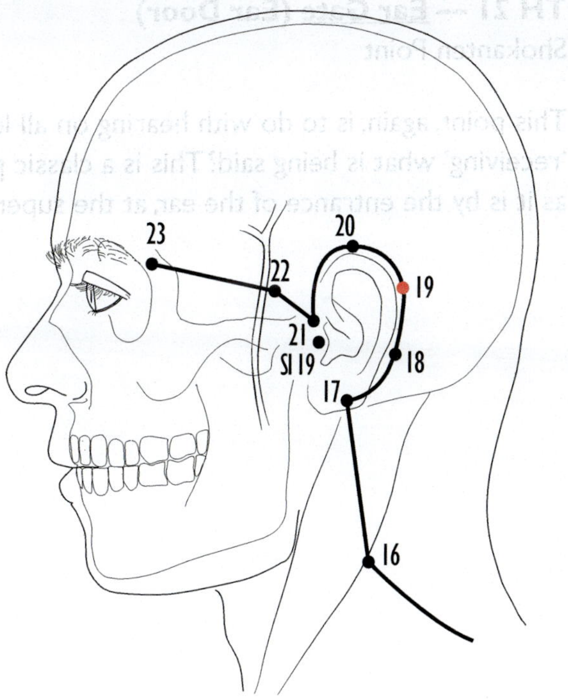

Triple Heater. Three Heater. Triple Burner. San Jiao

TH 20 — Small Angle of Ear
Crossing Point of TH, SI and Gb

As the crossing point of the three meridians that connect to the ear, this is one of the main points to enhance clarity, discrimination and vitality within this Organ. Connects with the face, mouth and eyes.

TH 21 — Ear Gate (Ear Door)
Shokanten Point

This point, again, is to do with hearing on all levels of the Body, Mind and Spirit. Is the patient 'receiving' what is being said? This is a classic point for deafness and restoration of hearing, located as it is by the entrance of the ear, at the superior edge of the tragus.

⊥	△	Location	
X	3-7	On the temporal bone, directly superior to the apex of the pinna	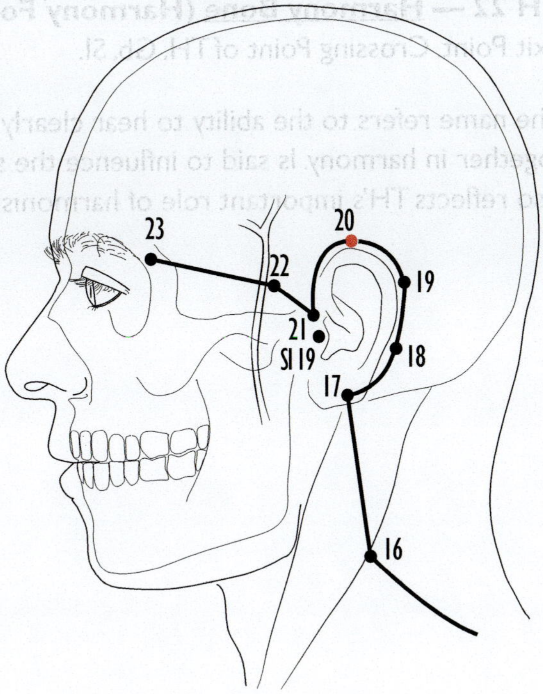
3	3-7	When the mouth is open the point lies anterior to the superior edge of the tragus In the depression at the posterior border of the condyle of the mandible (superior to SI 19)	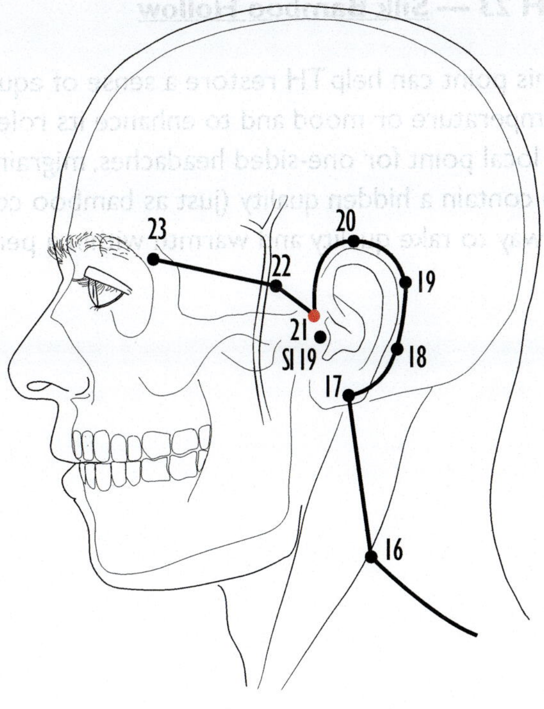

Triple Heater. Three Heater. Triple Burner. San Jiao

TH 22 — Harmony Bone (Harmony Foramen)
Exit Point. Crossing Point of TH, Gb, SI.

The name refers to the ability to hear clearly the five tones, and for the system to bring them together in harmony. Is said to influence the state of the Kidneys which govern the ears. The name also reflects TH's important role of harmonising the workings of all Tweleve Officials.

TH 23 — Silk Bamboo Hollow

This point can help TH restore a sense of equilibrium to a person in cases of unbalanced temperature or mood and to enhance its role of 'guarding the Spirits against perverse influences'. A local point for one-sided headaches, migraines, facial paralysis and many eye disorders. It is said to contain a hidden quality (just as bamboo contains its flower within it), and the connotation is of a 'way to take quality and warmth within a person'.

⊥	△		Location
3-7	3-5	On the lateral aspect of the head **0.5 — 1.5 cun** anterior to the superior root of the pinna of the ear Just posterior to the superficial temporal artery At the midpoint between Gb 7 and Gb 3	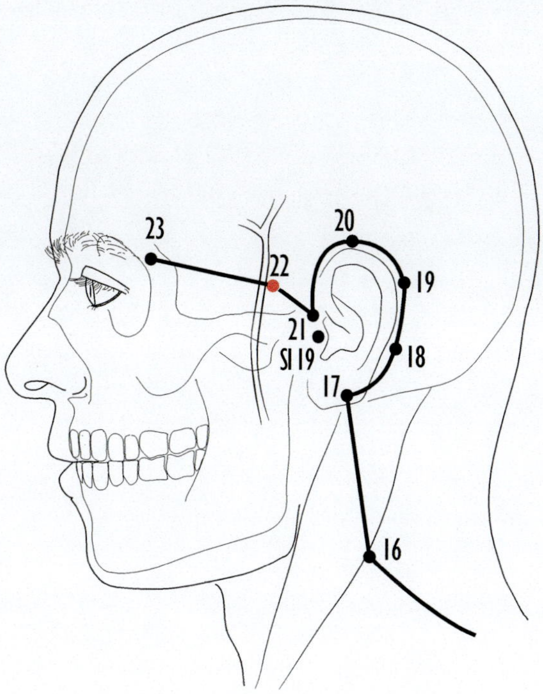
3	X	At the lateral extremity of the eyebrow Just posterior to the supraorbital ridge	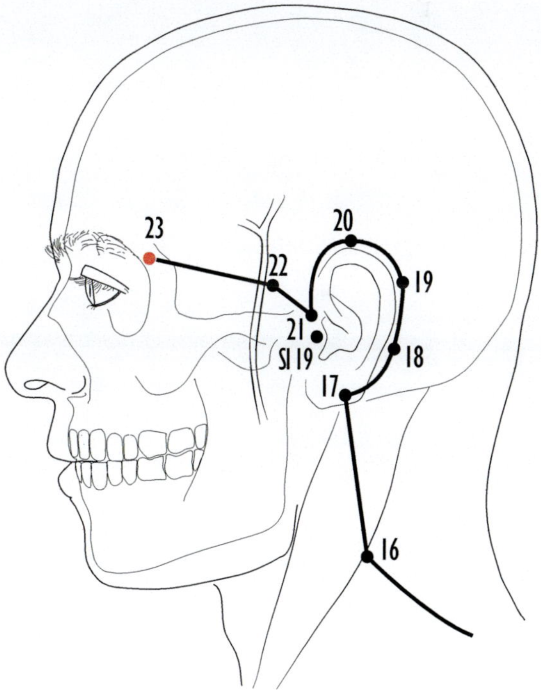

Gallbladder

- **The upright Official of Decision-Making and Judgement**
- **Responsible for what is just and exact. Influences clarity and purity**
- **Wood governs the sinews, tendons, nails, tears and eyes**

Gallbladder

Gb 1 — <u>Orbit Bone</u> (Pupil Crevice, Pupil Foramen)
Entry point. A branch from the primary meridian makes connections with St 5, St 6, St 12 and SI 18, and in doing so it crosses the TH meridian.

Consider this point for many types of eye disorders, early stages of glaucoma, conjunctivitis, photophobia and also facial paralysis. Helps with clarity, vision and decision-making of the Body, Mind and Spirit, strengthening resolve and self-assertion if timidity is present within a person.

Gb 2 — <u>Hearing Assembly</u> (Auditory Convergence)
Needle with the mouth open

This point can be used to good effect for hearing disorders such as deafness, tinnitus, hearing loss or discharge from the ear (the meridian passes around and within the ear). Often used with TH 17 to supplement its treatment of ear problems. Local point for trigeminal neuralgia.

⊥	Δ		Location
3	5	On the temporal region of the head Just lateral to the orbital ridge of the zygomatic bone Approx **0.5 cun** lateral and level to the lateral canthus of the eye In the depression on the lateral aspect of the orbit bone.	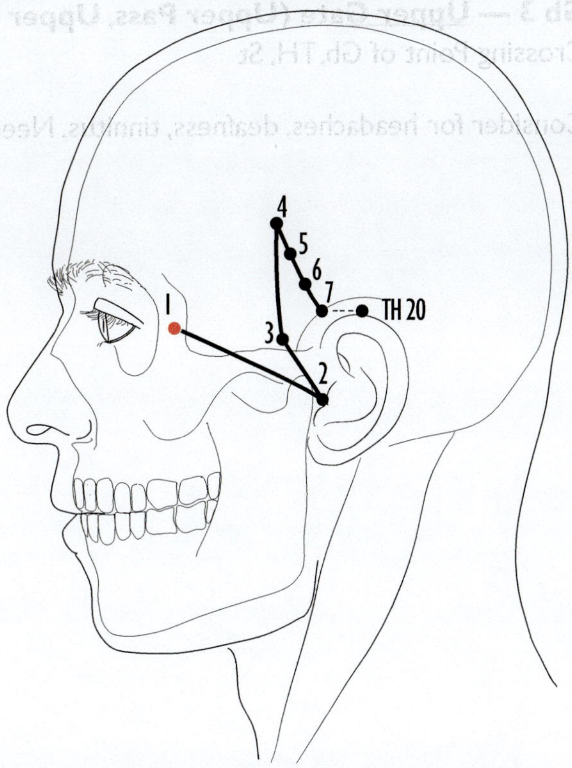
5	5	Forbidden from 1st month of pregnancy On the posterior border of the condyle of the mandible bone Anterior and just inferior to the inferior border of the tragus of the ear Inferior to SI 1	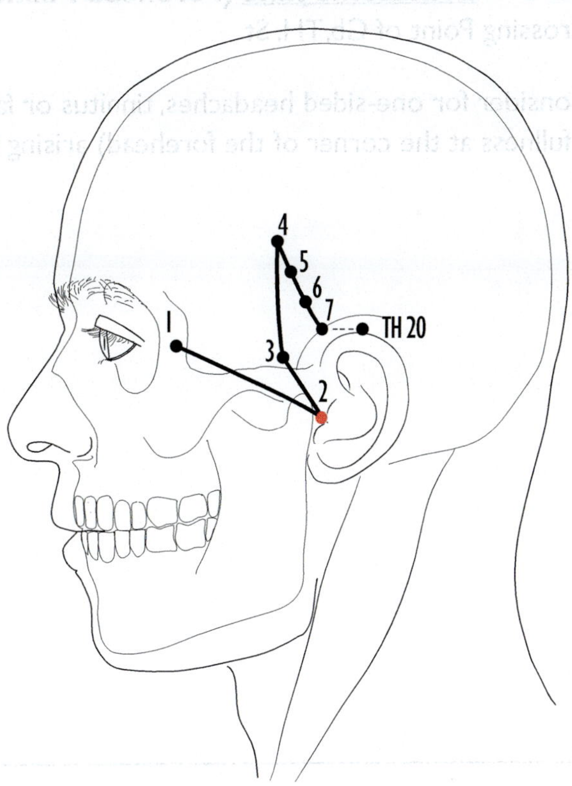

Gallbladder

Gb 3 — Upper Gate (Upper Pass, Upper Fortified Gate)
Crossing Point of Gb, TH, St

Consider for headaches, deafness, tinnitus. Needling usually forbidden, unless it is shallow.

Gb 4 — Loathsome Jaws (Forehead Fullness)
Crossing Point of Gb, TH, St

Consider for one-sided headaches, tinnitus or facial paralysis. Beneficial for tension in the jaws (and a fullness at the corner of the forehead) arising from frustration, anger or impatience.

⊥	Δ		Location
X	3-5	Anterior to the ear On the upper border of the zygomatic arch of the temporal bone Superior to the anterior border of the condyle of the mandible Directly superior to St 7, superior to Gb 2 and SI 19	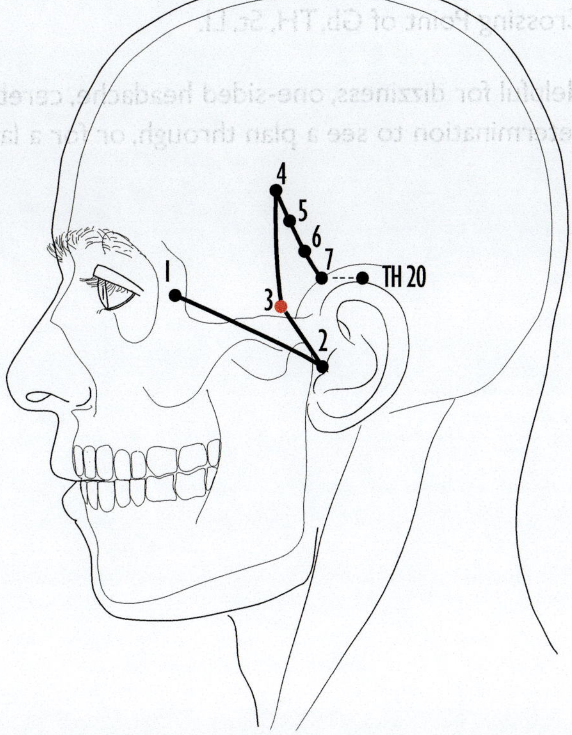
2	3	Posterior to the natural hairline on temporal region of the head Approx **1 cun** inferior to St 8 ¼ of the distance between St 8 and Gb 7	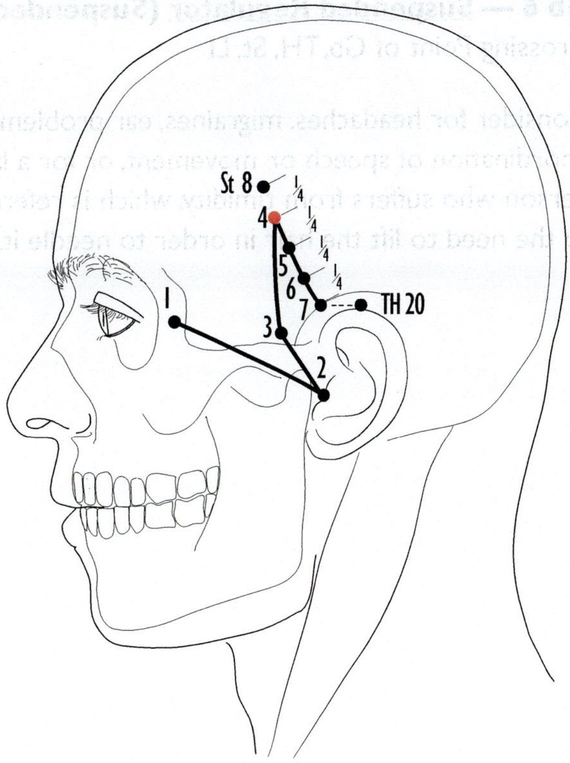

Gallbladder

Gb 5 — <u>Suspended Skull</u>
Crossing Point of Gb, TH, St, LI.

Helpful for dizziness, one-sided headache, cerebral weakness and congestion. Consider for a lack of determination to see a plan through, or for a lack of coordinated movement or speech.

Gb 6 — <u>Suspended Regulator</u> (Suspended Tuft)
Crossing Point of Gb, TH, St, LI

Consider for headaches, migraines, ear problems or cerebral weakness. For difficulties with coordination of speech or movement, or for a lack of penetrative thought. Can be effective for a person who suffers from timidity, which is referred to as 'small Gallbladder'. The point name refers to the need to lift the hair in order to needle it.

⊥	Δ		Location
3	3	Posterior to the natural hairline on temporal region of the head ½ of the distance between St 8 and Gb 7	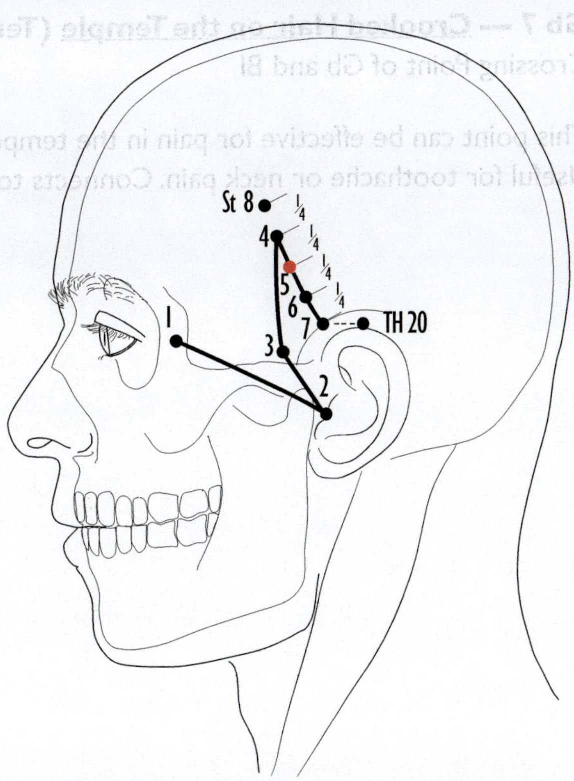
2	3	Temporal region of the head Posterior to the hairline ¾ of the distance between St 8 and Gb 7	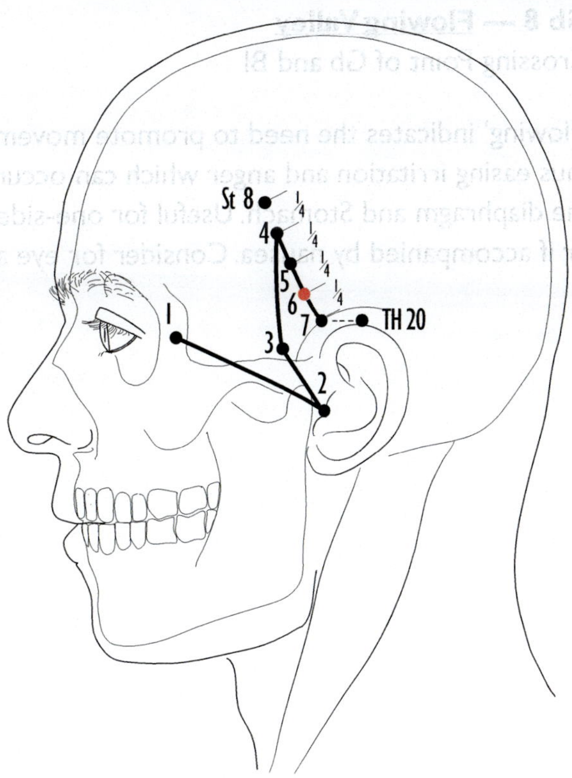

Gb 7 — Crooked Hair on the Temple (Temporal Hairline Curve)
Crossing Point of Gb and Bl

This point can be effective for pain in the temporal areas. Promotes clarity of Mind and Spirit. Useful for toothache or neck pain. Connects to the mouth and jaw.

Gb 8 — Flowing Valley
Crossing Point of Gb and Bl

'Flowing' indicates the need to promote movement (rather than blockage) within the meridian, thus easing irritation and anger which can occur if the Gb energy is thwarted. Said to harmonise the diaphragm and Stomach. Useful for one-sided headaches or migraine, particularly if it is tender or if accompanied by nausea. Consider for eye and ear disorders.

⊥	Δ		Location
3	3-5	On the temporal bone, posterior to the hairline On a transverse level with TH 20 and the apex of the pinna of the ear Approx 1 finger width anterior to TH 20	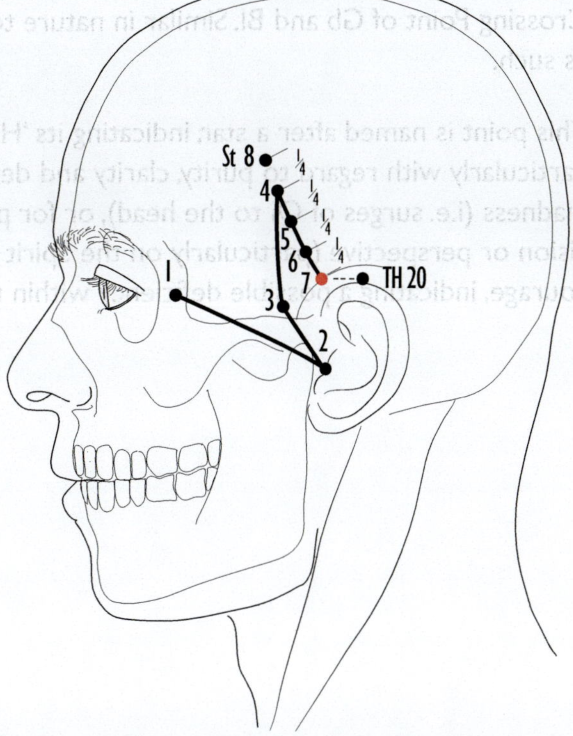
3	3-5	Lateral aspect of the head On the parietal bone **1 — 1.5 cun** superior to the apex of the pinna of the ear Directly superior to TH 20 (which is at the apex of the pinna of ear)	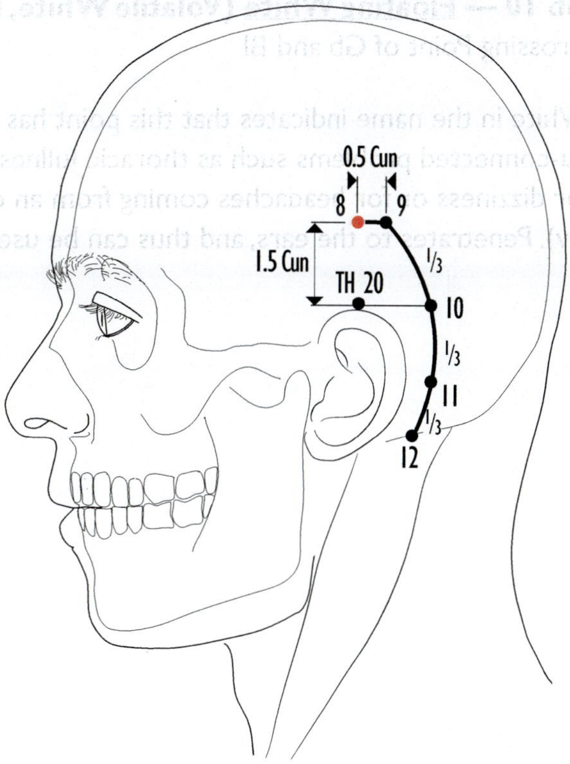

Gallbladder

Gb 9 — <u>Heaven Rushing</u> (Penetrating Heaven, Celestial Crossroads, Celestial Surge)
Crossing Point of Gb and Bl. Similar in nature to a Window of the Sky, and is listed in the Classics as such.

This point is named after a star, indicating its 'Heavenly' aspect and its effect upon the Spirit, particularly with regard to purity, clarity and decision-making. Consider for headaches, epilepsy, madness (i.e. surges of Qi to the head), or for poor coordination. It can be beneficial for lack of vision or perspective (particularly on the Spirit level). Useful if a patient is timid and lacking in courage, indicating a possible deficiency within this Official.

Gb 10 — <u>Floating White</u> (Volatile White, Rising White)
Crossing Point of Gb and Bl

White in the name indicates that this point has a Metal association, and as such can be helpful with Lu-connected problems such as thoracic fullness, cough or shortness of breath. Can be considered for dizziness or for headaches coming from an overactive Wood Official (heat rising up from Gb or Liv). Penetrates to the ears, and thus can be useful for some ear problems.

⊥	Δ		Location
3	3-5	Forbidden from 4th month of pregnancy Lateral aspect of the head on the parietal bone **0.5 cun** posterior to Gb 8 Directly superior to the posterior border of the root of the pinna Approx **2 cun** superior to the natural hairline	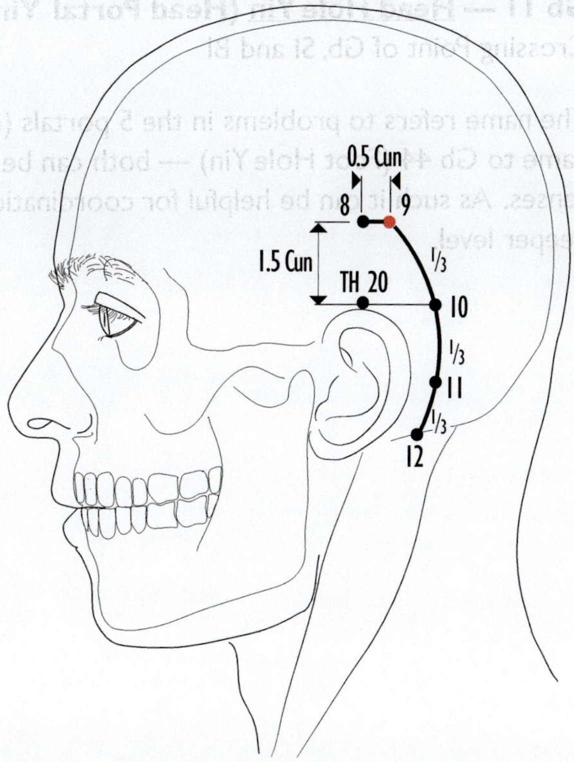
3	3-5	Posterior and superior to the mastoid process Approximately level with the superior root of the pinna Approx **1 cun** posterior to the lateral natural hairline On the curvature of the Gb channel halfway between Gb 9 and Gb 11 TH channel is anterior to the GB channel at this point	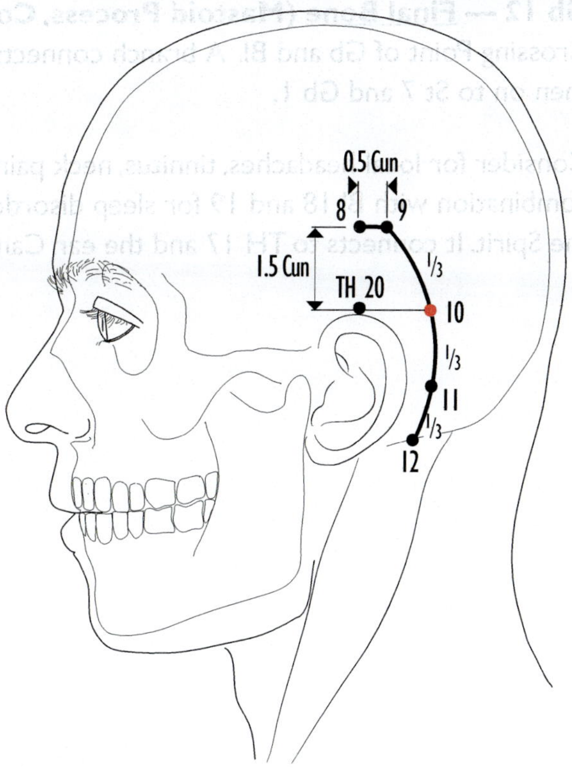

Gallbladder

Gb 11 — <u>Head Hole Yin</u> (Head Portal Yin, Penetration of Yin)
Crossing Point of Gb, SI and Bl

The name refers to problems in the 5 portals (eyes, ears, mouth, nose, tongue). It has a similar name to Gb 44 (Foot Hole Yin) — both can be used together to enhance, brighten and purify the senses. As such it can be helpful for coordination, judgement and decision-making, particularly at a deeper level.

Gb 12 — <u>Final Bone</u> (Mastoid Process, Completed Bone)
Crossing Point of Gb and Bl. A branch connects to TH 17, passes through the ear to SI 19 and then on to St 7 and Gb 1.

Consider for local headaches, tinnitus, neck pain, psychosis, mania or insomnia (often used in combination with Bl 18 and 19 for sleep disorders or violent dream disturbance). This point calms the Spirit. It connects to TH 17 and the ear. Can be effective for facial paralysis.

<table>
<tr><th>⊥</th><th>Δ</th><th></th><th>Location</th></tr>
<tr><td>3</td><td>3-7</td><td>In a depression posterior and superior to the mastoid process
On the curvature of the Gb channel halfway between Gb 10 and Gb 12
TH channel is anterior to the GB channel at this point</td><td>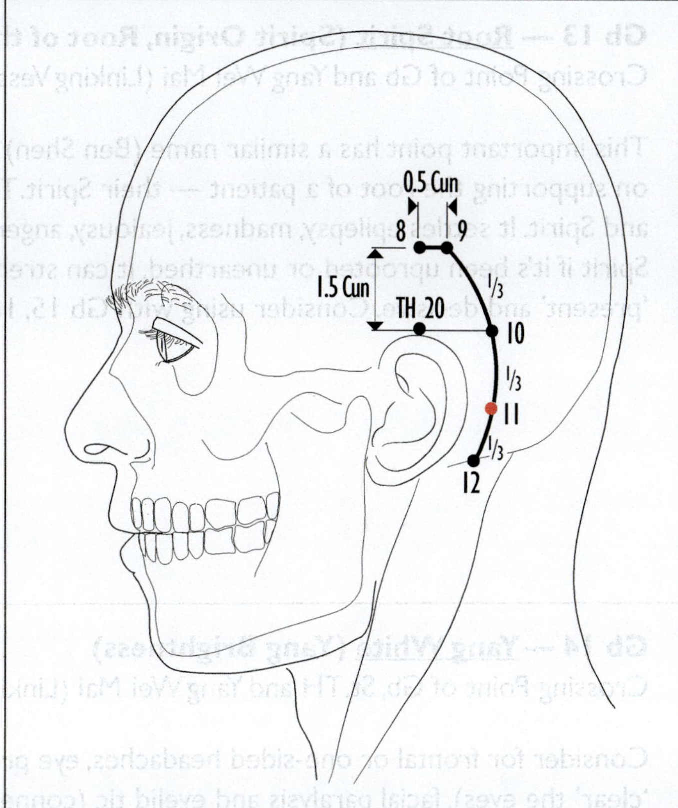
</td></tr>
<tr><td>5</td><td>3-7</td><td>In a depression just posterior and inferior to the mastoid process
Level with the prominence of the mastoid process in the articulation between the occipital bone and the mastoid process of the temporal bone
Approx 1 cun superior to TH 16</td><td>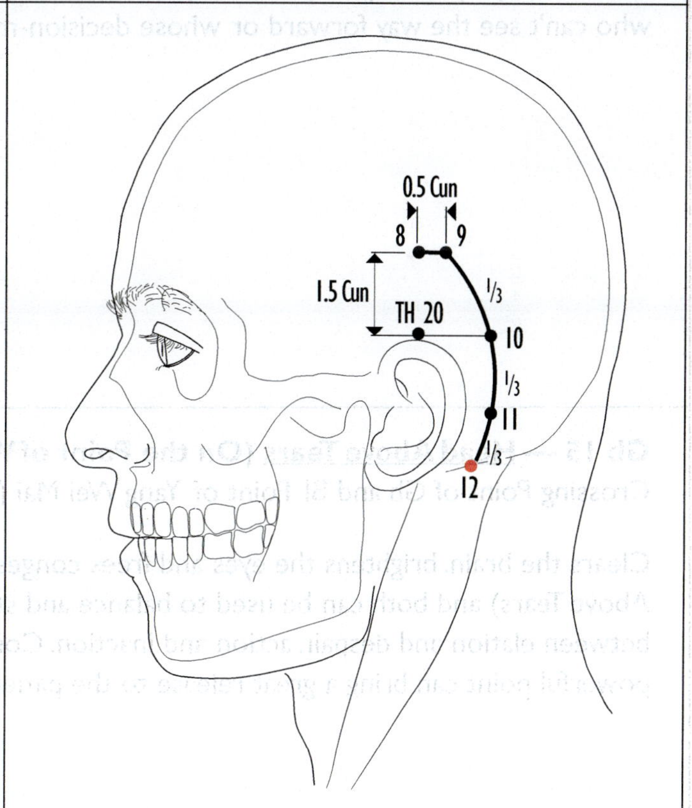
</td></tr>
</table>

Gallbladder

Gb 13 — <u>Root Spirit</u> (Spirit Origin, Root of the Spirit)
Crossing Point of Gb and Yang Wei Mai (Linking Vessel)

This important point has a similar name (Ben Shen) to Chapter 8 of the Ling Shu which focusses on supporting the root of a patient — their Spirit. This point is used for disorders of the Mind and Spirit. It settles epilepsy, madness, jealousy, anger, obsessive thinking and suspicion. It calms the Spirit if it's been uprooted or unearthed. It can strengthen a person's ability to be more assertive, 'present' and decisive. Consider using with Gb 15, 16, 38, Ht 5, Ren 4 or Du 24.

Gb 14 — <u>Yang White</u> (Yang Brightness)
Crossing Point of Gb, St, TH and Yang Wei Mai (Linking Vessel)

Consider for frontal or one-sided headaches, eye problems, blurred vision (it can brighten and 'clear' the eyes), facial paralysis and eyelid tic (connects to Bl 1). Helpful for confused Wood CF's who can't see the way forward or whose decision-making processes need to be firmed up.

Gb 15 — <u>Head Above Tears</u> (On the Point of Weeping)
Crossing Point of Gb and Bl. Point of Yang Wei Mai (Linking Vessel)

Clears the brain, brightens the eyes and frees congestion in the nose. Related to Gb 41 (Foot Above Tears) and both can be used to balance and steady the emotions, particularly those yoyo-ing between elation and despair, action and inaction. Consider for those who are unable to cry. This powerful point can bring a great release to the patient through the shedding of tears.

⊥	Δ		Location
3	7	Directly superior to the lateral canthus of the eye 2/3 of the distance from Du 24 to St 8 **3 cun** lateral to Du 24 (anterior median line) **0.5 cun** posterior to the natural anterior hairline	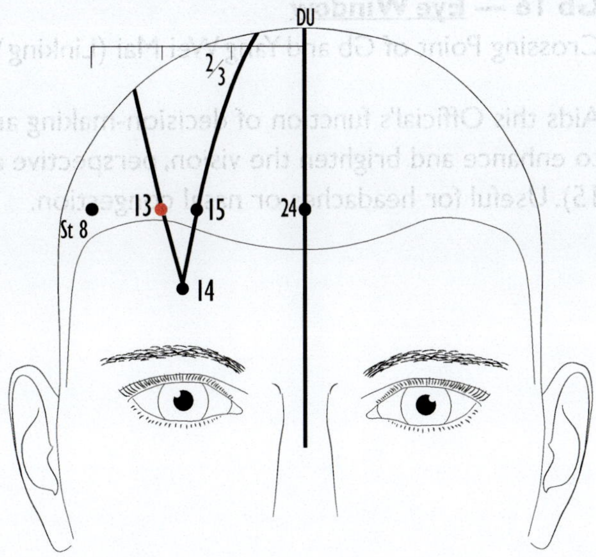
2	3	Directly superior to the centre of the pupil of the eye when the person is looking straight ahead Approx **1 cun** superior to the middle of the eyebrow/ supraorbital notch	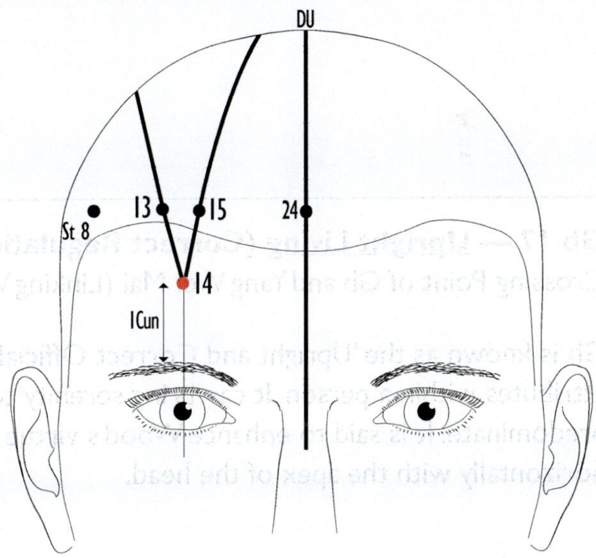
3	X	Midway between Du 24 and St 8 Directly superior to Gb 14 **0.5 cun** posterior to the natural anterior hairline **2.25 cun** lateral to Du 24	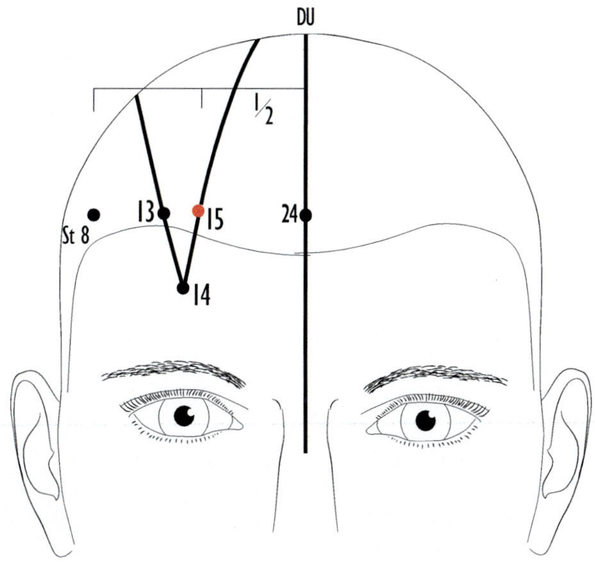

Gallbladder

Gb 16 — Eye Window

Crossing Point of Gb and Yang Wei Mai (Linking Vessel)

Aids this Official's function of decision-making and judgement. Consider for all eye disorders. Used to enhance and brighten the vision, perspective and Spirit of the patient (together with Gb 13 and 15). Useful for headaches or nasal congestion.

Gb 17 — Upright Living (Correct Regulation)

Crossing Point of Gb and Yang Wei Mai (Linking Vessel)

Gb is known as the 'Upright and Correct Official', and this point can help strengthen these attributes within a person. It can bring serenity to the Spirit particularly if fear and loneliness predominate. It is said to enhance Wood's virtue of benevolence and human kindness. Located horizontally with the apex of the head.

⊥	Δ		Location
3	5	Gb 16–19 lie on the line between Gb 15 and Gb 20. **2.25 cun** lateral to the median line. **2 cun** posterior to the natural anterior hairline **1.5 cun** posterior to Gb 15 1/3 of the distance measured from Gb 15 to Gb 18	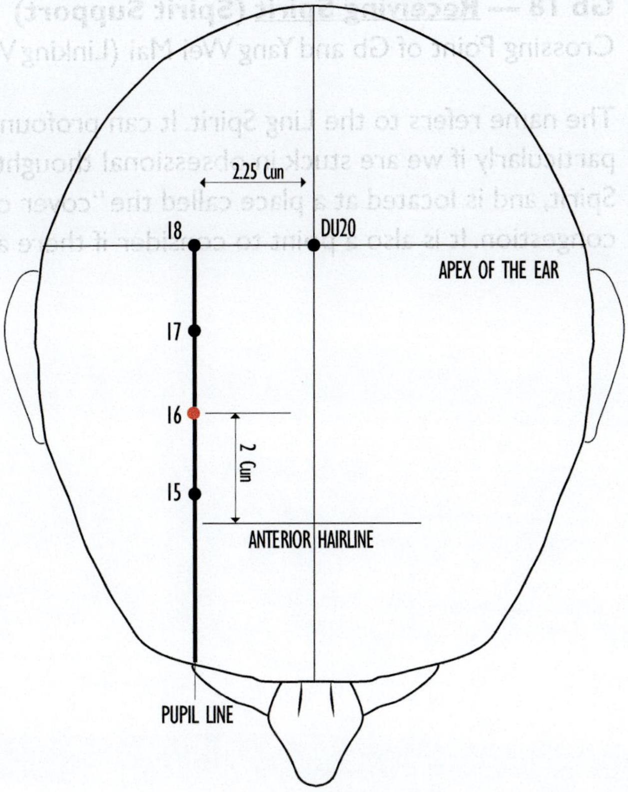
3	5	**3.5 cun** posterior to the natural anterior hairline **1.5 cun** posterior to Gb 16 **3 cun** posterior to Gb 15 (anterior median line) 2/3 of the distance measured from Gb 15 to Gb 18	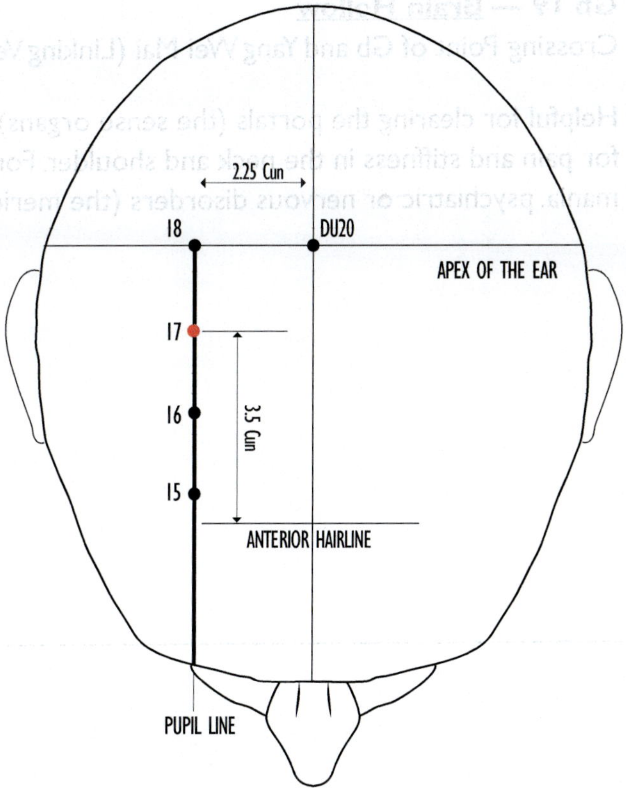

Gb 18 — Receiving Spirit (Spirit Support)
Crossing Point of Gb and Yang Wei Mai (Linking Vessel)

The name refers to the Ling Spirit. It can profoundly enhance our sensitivity and awareness, particularly if we are stuck in obsessional thought patterns. It is said to connect to the Universal Spirit, and is located at a place called the "cover of the celestial spirit". Consider for nasal congestion. It is also a point to consider if there are signs of dementia.

Gb 19 — Brain Hollow
Crossing Point of Gb and Yang Wei Mai (Linking Vessel)

Helpful for clearing the portals (the sense organs), and for local or one-sided headaches. Consider for pain and stiffness in the neck and shoulder. For disturbances of the Mind and Spirit such as mania, psychiatric or nervous disorders (the meridian traverses the brain area here).

⊥	Δ		Location
X	5	**5 cun** posterior to the natural anterior hairline Transversely level with Du 20 **4.5 cun** posterior to Gb 15 (anterior median line) **3 cun** posterior to Gb 16 / coronal suture **1.5 cun** posterior to Gb 17 Needling is permitted by some schools.	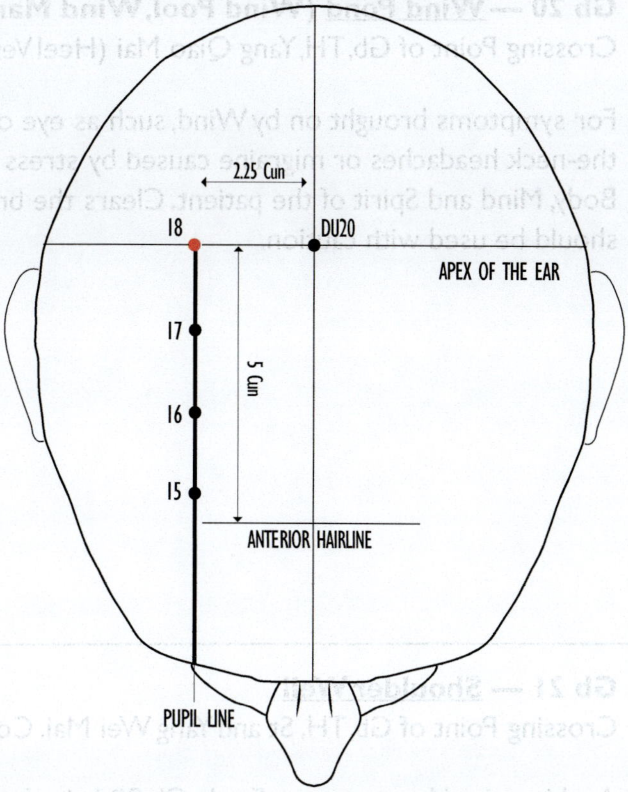
3	5	On the level of the upper border of the external occipital protuberance of the occipital bone Level with Du 17 and Bl 9 **1.5 cun** superior to Gb 20 **9.5 cun** posterior to the natural anterior hairline **2.5 cun** superior to the natural posterior hairline **2.25 cun** lateral to median line	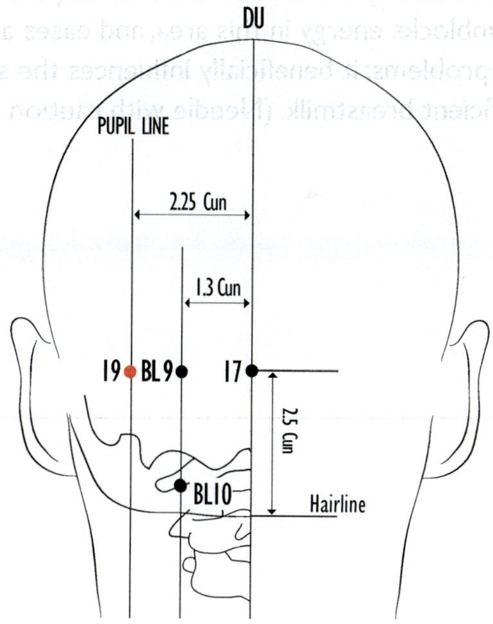

Gallbladder

Gb 20 — <u>Wind Pond</u> (Wind Pool, Wind Mansion)
Crossing Point of Gb, TH, Yang Qiao Mai (Heel Vessel) and Yang Wei Mai (Linking Vessel)

For symptoms brought on by Wind, such as eye or ear problems. Consider for localised back-of-the-neck headaches or migraine caused by stress and tension. This point can bring clarity to the Body, Mind and Spirit of the patient. Clears the brain and sense orifices. This is a powerful point and should be used with caution.

Gb 21 — <u>Shoulder Well</u>
Crossing Point of Gb, TH, St and Yang Wei Mai. Connects to Du 14, Bl 11, SI 12 and St 12

At this point Heaven meets Earth. Gb 20 is in the heavenly axis above the neck, whereas Gb 21 is in the earthly axis below it. Gb 21 helps connect and integrate the patient with their higher self, unblocks energy in this area, and eases anger and frustration. Good for arm, shoulder and neck problems; it beneficially influences the sinews and relieves muscular tension. Consider for insufficient breastmilk. (Needle with caution — located adjacent to the lungs).

⊥	Δ		Location
6	7-10	Posterior aspect of the upper neck, inferior to the occipital bone Between the lateral border of the trapezius and posterior border of the sternocleidomastoid muscles Level with Du 16 **1 cun** superior to the natural posterior hairline **2.25 cun** lateral to median line	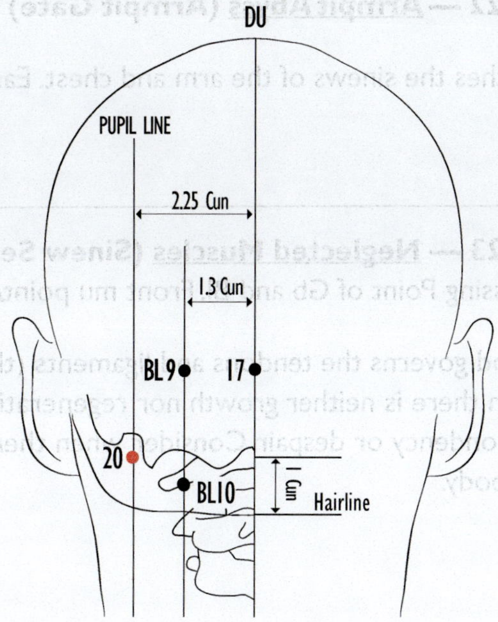
4-6	7-15	Forbidden to needle or moxa during pregnancy Do not use before the 2nd stage of labour At the highest point of the shoulder On the anterior border of the trapezius muscle Midway between Du 14 and the lateral extremity of the Acromion process of the scapula	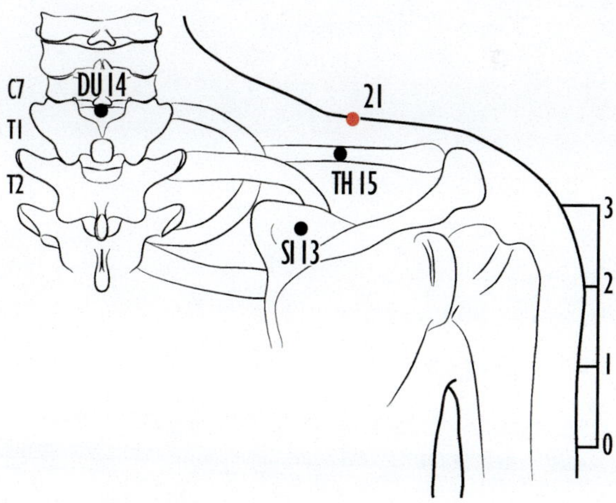

Gallbladder

Gb 22 — Armpit Abyss (Armpit Gate)

Soothes the sinews of the arm and chest. Eases restriction of movement of the arm and shoulder.

Gb 23 — Neglected Muscles (Sinew Seat)
Crossing Point of Gb and Bl. Front mu point/Alarm Point of Gb (in some texts).

Wood governs the tendons and ligaments (the sinews) which hold the muscles in place. Use when there is neither growth nor regeneration, which may lead to frustration, repressed anger, despondency or despair. Consider when there is stagnation or restricted movement in this area of the body.

⊥	Δ		Location
4-6	X	In the 4th **Intercostal Space** (occasionally in the 5th space) On the mid-axillary line Approx **3 cun** inferior to the axillary fold (apex of axilla)	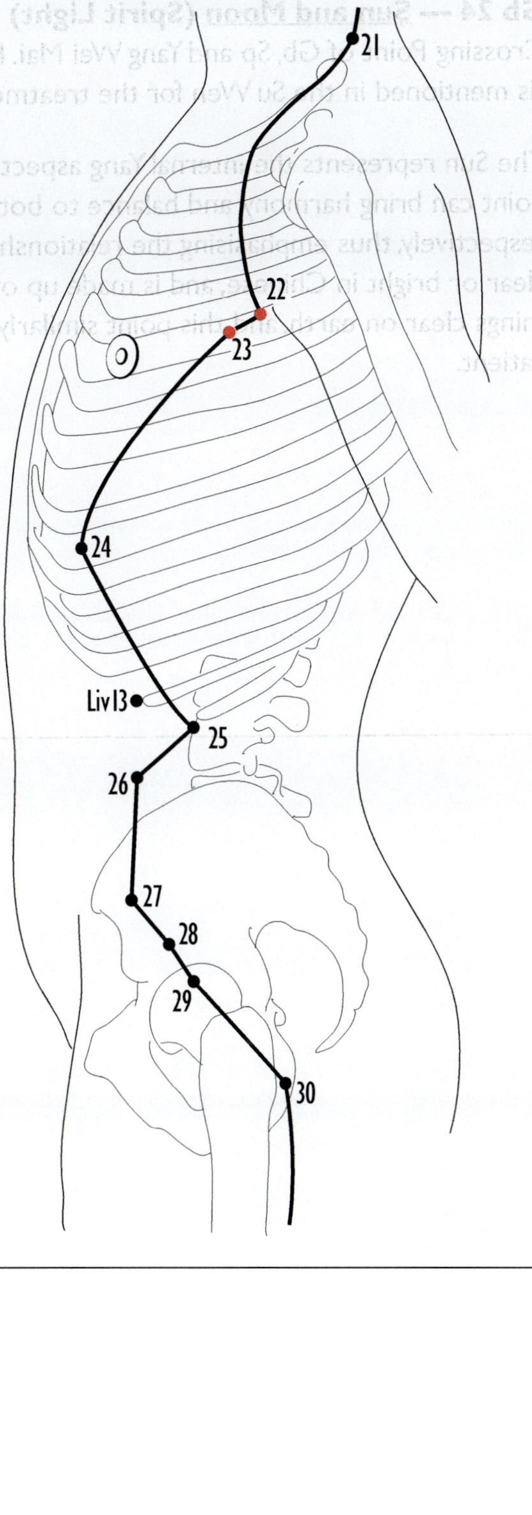
5	5	In the 4th **Intercostal Space** (occasionally in the 5th space) **1 cun** anterior to Gb 22 and **1 cun** anterior to the mid-axillary line **3 cun** inferior to the axillary fold (apex of axilla)	

Gallbladder

Gb 24 — Sun and Moon (Spirit Light)
Crossing Point of Gb, Sp and Yang Wei Mai. Front mu Point/Alarm Point of Gb. "Decisiveness point" (is mentioned in the Su Wen for the treatment of indecisiveness).

The Sun represents the internal Yang aspect within a person, and the Moon, the Yin; this wonderful point can bring harmony and balance to both. Sun and Moon correspond to the left and right eye respectively, thus emphasising the relationship of the Wood Element to the eyes. "Ming" means clear or bright in Chinese, and is made up of the characters of the Sun and Moon. Their light makes things clear on earth, and this point similarly brings clarity and decisiveness to the Mind of the patient.

⊥	Δ		Location
5	5-7	Directly inferior to the nipple In the **7th Intercostal Space** **4 cun** lateral to the anterior median line Directly inferior to Liv 14 (alt) (which is in the 6th intercostal space)	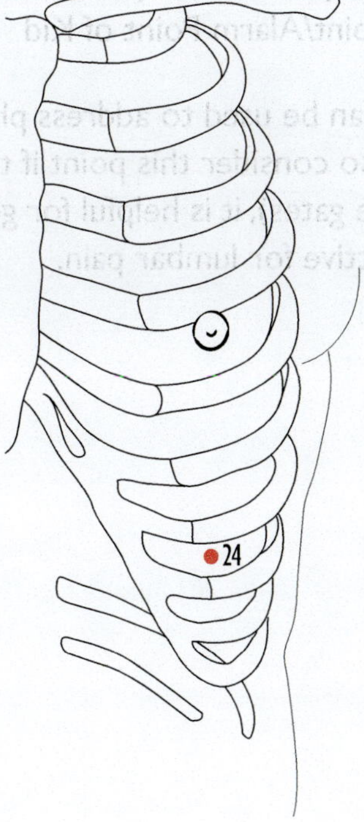

Gallbladder

Gb 25 — <u>Capital Gate</u> (Palace Door)
Front mu point/Alarm Point of Kid

This point can be used to address physical problems of the kidney, such as kidney pain or stones. It is a gate, so consider this point if there are signs of blockages in this area, Often used with Liv 13 (both are gates), it is helpful for getting things moving in a person's life if their Qi is stuck. It can also be effective for lumbar pain.

⊥	Δ		Location
7	7-12	Just inferior to the anterior tip of the 12th rib (second floating rib)	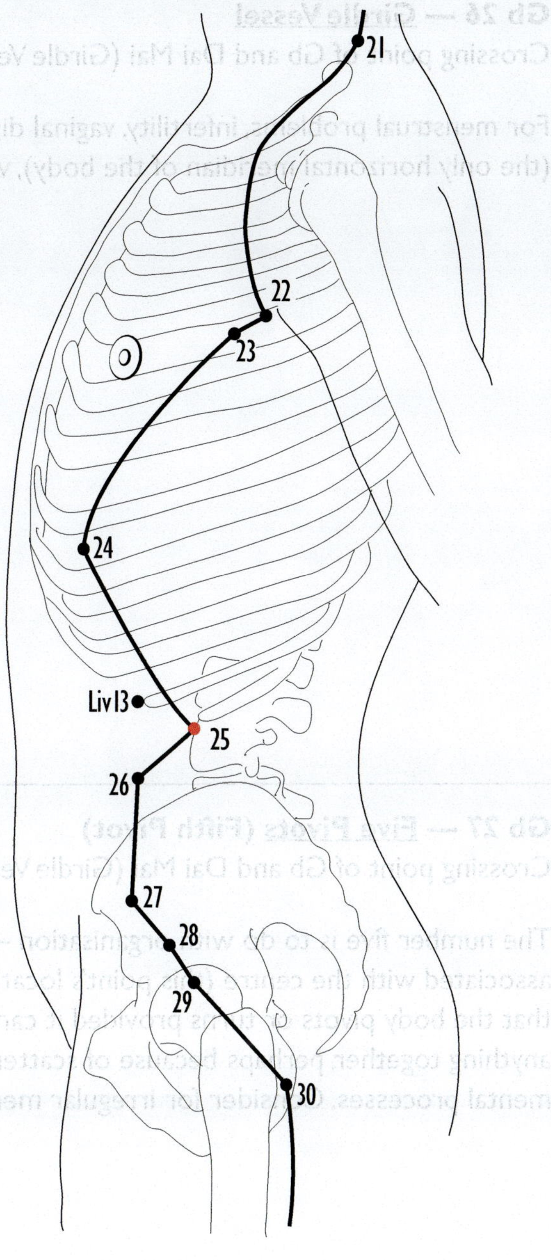

Gallbladder

Gb 26 — Girdle Vessel
Crossing point of Gb and Dai Mai (Girdle Vessel)

For menstrual problems, infertility, vaginal discharge or cystitis. This point influences the Dai Mai (the only horizontal meridian of the body), which itself regulates the uterus and menstruation.

Gb 27 — Five Pivots (Fifth Pivot)
Crossing point of Gb and Dai Mai (Girdle Vessel)

The number five is to do with organisation — something that is well regulated. Five is also associated with the centre (this point's location is on a central level), and it is around this area that the body pivots or turns provided it can retain its flexibility. Helpful where a person can't get anything together, perhaps because of scattered thinking or, conversely, if they are too rigid in their mental processes. Consider for irregular menstruation, vaginal discharge or lower abdominal pain.

⊥	△		**Location**
8	5-15	At the level of the umbilicus **Just** inferior to the anterior tip of the 11th rib (where Liv 13 is located) On a line from Gb 25 to Gb 27	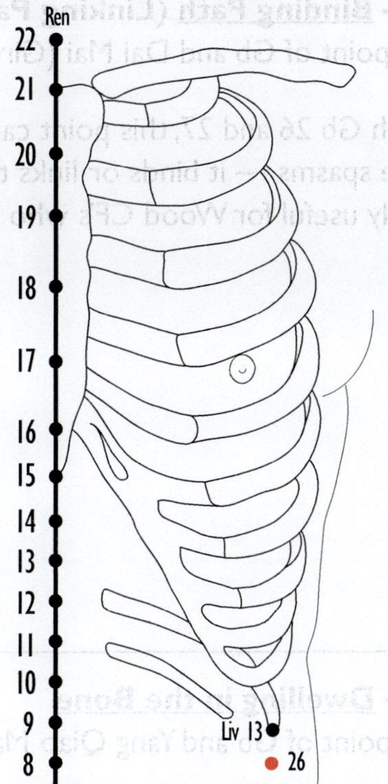
7	3-10	Just anterior to the border of the anterior superior iliac spine of the ilium **3 cun** inferior to the level of the umbilicus Transversely level with Ren 4	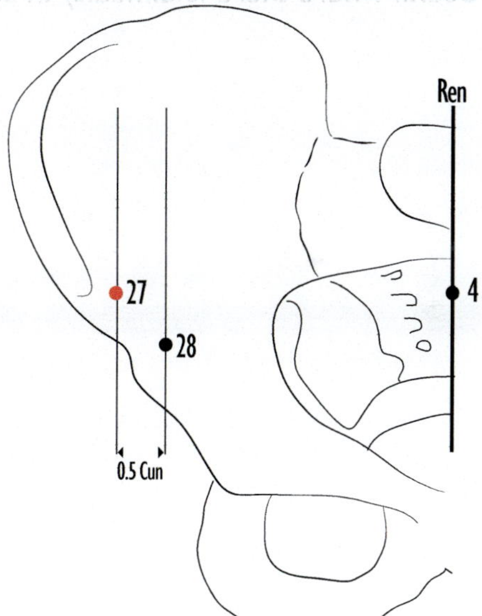

Gallbladder

Gb 28 — Binding Path (Linking Path)
Crossing point of Gb and Dai Mai (Girdle Vessel)

Along with Gb 26 and 27, this point can help in cases of irregular menstruation and vaginal or uterine spasms — it binds or links things together and keeps the meridians in their place. Particularly useful for Wood CF's who suffer with difficult periods, vaginal discharge or uterine prolapse.

Gb 29 — Dwelling in the Bone
Crossing point of Gb and Yang Qiao Mai (Heel Vessel)

A very useful point for pain in the hip or from the hip to the groin. Consider for sciatica, along with Gb 30. Useful where there is difficulty in straightening the leg. Moxa and needle effective here.

<table>
<tr><th>⊥</th><th>△</th><th></th><th>Location</th></tr>
<tr><td>8</td><td>5-7</td><td>Anterior to the border of the anterior superior iliac spine of the ilium
Inferior to Gb 27
Approx 0.5 cun medial to the level of Gb 27</td><td>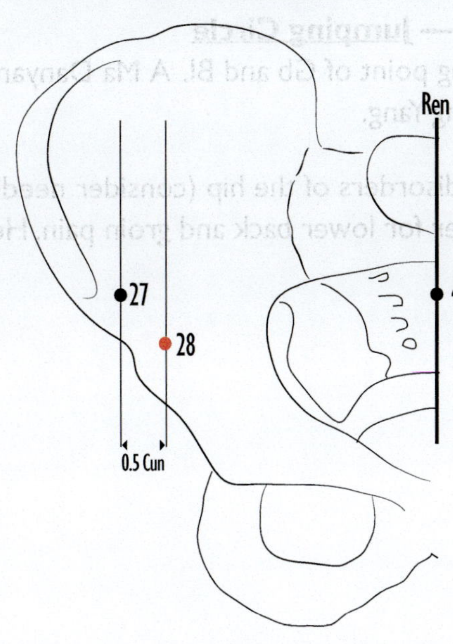</td></tr>
<tr><td>8</td><td>5-7</td><td>Midway between anterior superior iliac spine of the ilium and the prominence of the greater trochanter of the femur
Approx 3 cun posterior to Gb 28
Traditionally described as in the anterior fossa of the greater trochanter of the femur</td><td>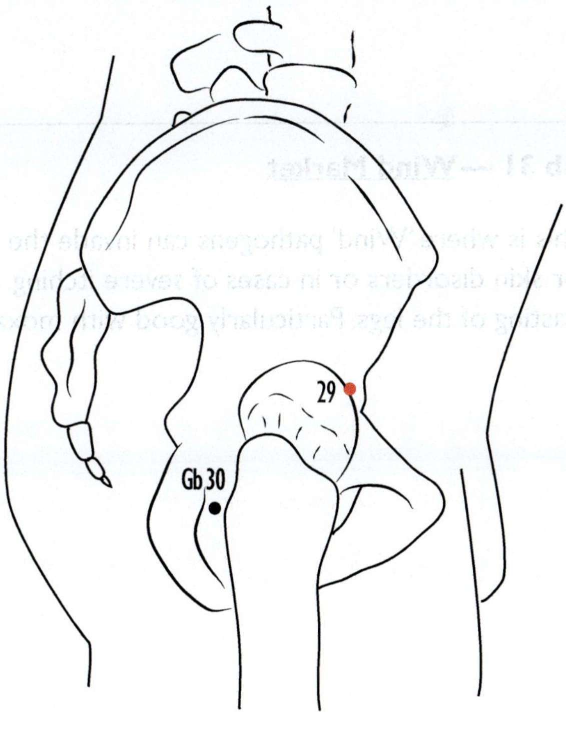</td></tr>
</table>

Gb 30 — Jumping Circle

Crossing point of Gb and Bl. A Ma Danyang Heavenly Star Point. One of the nine needles for returning Yang.

For all disorders of the hip (consider needle/moxa). For sciatic pain down Gb or Bl meridians. Consider for lower back and groin pain. Helps a person's mobility — they can jump once again.

Gb 31 — Wind Market

This is where 'Wind' pathogens can invade the system (gathering like people at a market). Consider for skin disorders or in cases of severe itching. For hip and leg problems, weakness, numbness or wasting of the legs. Particularly good with moxa.

⊥	Δ		Location
10-15	7-20	Patient is lying on side (recumbent) with lower leg extended and the thigh flexed with knee near abdomen Lateral aspect of upper thigh Posterior to prominence of the greater trochanter of the femur 1/3 of the distance between the prominence of the greater trochanter of the femur and the sacral hiatus of the sacrum (Du 2) In the middle of a triangle formed by the greater trochanter of the femur, the posterior superior iliac spine of the ilium and the ischial tuberosity of the ischium	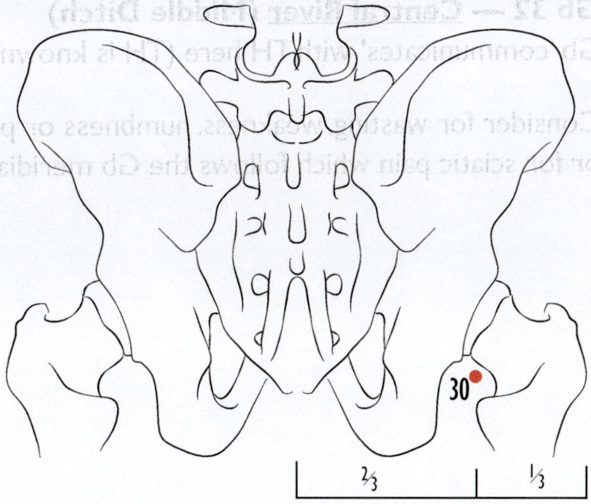
5	5	Midline of the lateral aspect of upper thigh Distal to greater trochanter of the femur In a seam between the vastus lateralis and biceps femoris muscles **7 cun** proximal to the popliteal crease	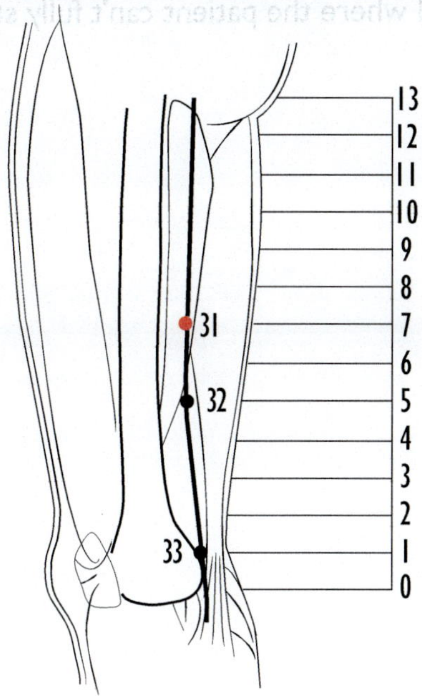

Gallbladder

Gb 32 — Central River (Middle Ditch)
Gb 'communicates' with TH here (TH is known as 'the central river').

Consider for wasting, weakness, numbness or pain in the legs. For cold in the sinews and muscles, or for sciatic pain which follows the Gb meridian.

Gb 33 — Knee Yang Border (Cold Mansion)

Can be used with good effect for knee problems — arthritis, swelling, pain or cold in the joint. Beneficial where the patient can't fully straighten their leg (Wood controls the sinews).

⊥	Δ		Location
5	5-7	Lateral aspect of thigh Distal to greater trochanter of the femur In a seam between the vastus lateralis and biceps femoris muscles **5 cun** proximal to the popliteal crease	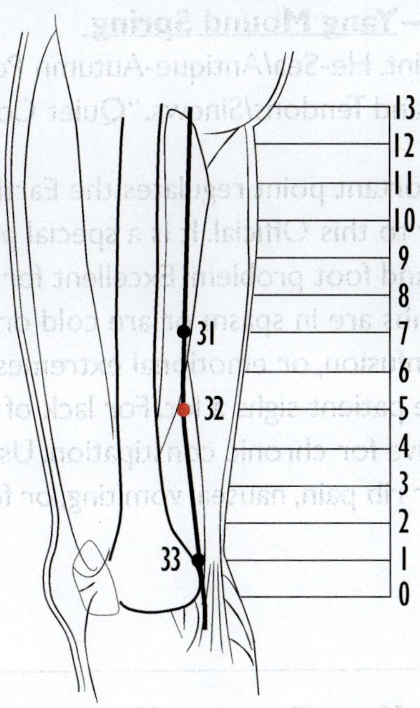
5	X	In a fossa between the tendon of the biceps femoris muscle and the femur Just proximal to the flare of the lateral epicondyle of the femur Approx **3 cun** proximal to Gb 34	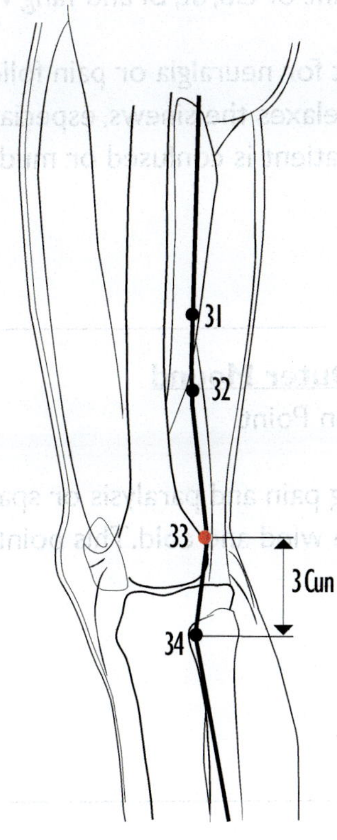

Gallbladder

Gb 34 — Yang Mound Spring

Earth Point. He-Sea/Antique-Autumn Point. Lower He-Sea Point of Gb. Influential Point for the Muscles and Tendons/Sinews. "Quiet Courage Point". A Ma Danyang Heavenly Star Point.

This important point regulates the Earth within the Wood, and as such brings strength and flexibility to this Official. It is a special point for the muscles and tendons. Consider for every type of knee and foot problem. Excellent for improving the articulation of the knee. Consider if the lower limbs are in spasm or are cold or numb. For mental disorders such as depression, irritability, anger, confusion, or emotional extremes. It is helpful for timidity and poor decision-making, or when the patient sighs a lot. For lack of coordination between Body/Mind, left/right, up/down. It can be effective for chronic constipation. Useful when the patient becomes frightened easily. Consider for lower rib pain, nausea, vomiting, or for a bitter taste in the mouth. Commonly used with Liv 3.

Gb 35 — Yang Crossing (Yang Intersection)

Crossing Point of Gb, St, Bl and Yang Wei Mai (Linking Vessel). Accumulation Point of Yang Wei Mai.

Special point for neuralgia or pain following the Gb meridian, especially neuralgia or paralysis of the tibial area. Relaxes the sinews, especially around the knee and lower leg. Helps with clarity of vision where the patient is confused or muddled in their mind.

Gb 36 — Outer Mound

Accumulation Point

For acute leg pain and paralysis or spasms of the ankle or calf. Consider where there is a strong dislike of the wind and cold. This point can help to bring clarity and perspective in a person's life.

⊥	Δ		Location
6	7-10	Forbidden from 2nd month of pregnancy Inferior and anterior to the head of the fibular **14 cun** proximal to the prominence of lateral maleolus Anatomy takes precedence Approximately level with Sp 9	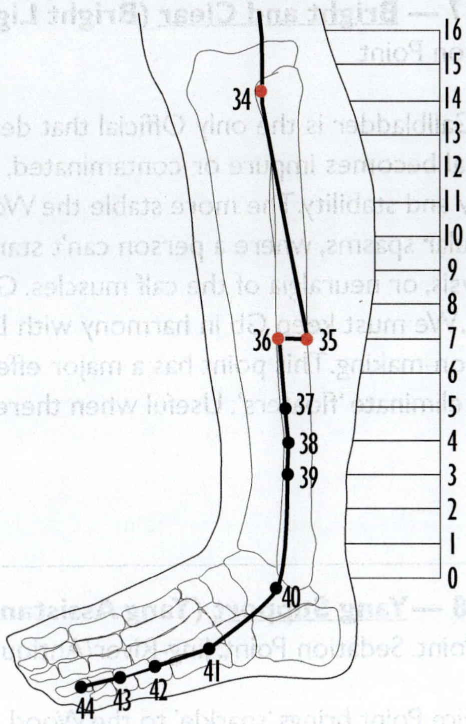
6	3-7	Posterior to posterior border of fibular **7 cun** proximal to prominence of lateral maleolus Posterior to and on a level with Gb 36	
4	3	Anterior to anterior border of fibular **7 cun** proximal to prominence of lateral maleolus Between peroneus longus and extensor digitorum longus muscles	

Gallbladder

Gb 37 — <u>Bright and Clear</u> (Bright Light)
Junction Point

The Gallbladder is the only Official that deals with pure energy and pure substance. If the Gb Official becomes impure or contaminated, we must consider treating here first. This point brings clarity and stability. The more stable the Wood, the better the coordination of the muscles, e.g. muscular spasms, where a person can't stand for long periods or where there is muscle rigidity, paralysis, or neuralgia of the calf muscles. Good for people who have had an excessive intake of drugs. We must keep Gb in harmony with Liv because of the Wood's influence on planning and decision-making. This point has a major effect on the eyes: clear-sightedness, improves eyesight, helps eliminate 'floaters'. Useful when there is a lack of spiritual or mental vision.

Gb 38 — <u>Yang Support</u> (Yang Assistance)
Fire Point. Sedation Point. Jing-River/Antique-Late Summer Point.

This Fire Point brings 'sparkle' to the Wood. Consider where there are no plans for the future — where the patient can't see clearly the way forward in their life. Useful when a person sighs a lot. This point supports our Yang aspect. For timidity, irritability or where there is no sense of growth or development. For a bitter taste in the mouth. Consider for chronic migraine. Often used with Liv 2.

Gb 39 — <u>Hanging Cup</u> (Marrow Convergence)
Crossing Point of the 3 Yang Meridians of Leg — Gb, Bl, St. Influential Point of Marrow.

For emotional 'stuckness', lack of growth or vision. Helpful for muscle weakness, pain under the ribs, joint and neck problems, or lower leg pain (it nourishes the bones and marrow and draws energy from above down to the lower limbs). Consider for loss of hearing or tinnitus.

Gb 40 — <u>Wilderness Mound</u>
Source Point. 'Unshakeable Calm Point'.

Helps bring perspective in a person's life, particularly on the Mental and Spiritual levels. If we are lost and climb a hill (in this case a burial mound), we can see where we are. Helpful for decision-making, and brings clarity. It can be effective for joint pains — hips, wrist, knees, and for sciatica and rib pain. Consider for one-sided headaches or migraines. This is a classic point to use after surgery to encourage faster healing. For those who sigh a lot. This point strengthens the Wood Official and thus a person's resolve and, as such, can be helpful for timidity.

⊥	△		Location
6	7	Anterior to anterior border of fibular **5 cun** proximal to prominence of lateral maleolus Between peroneus brevis and extensor digitorum longus muscles	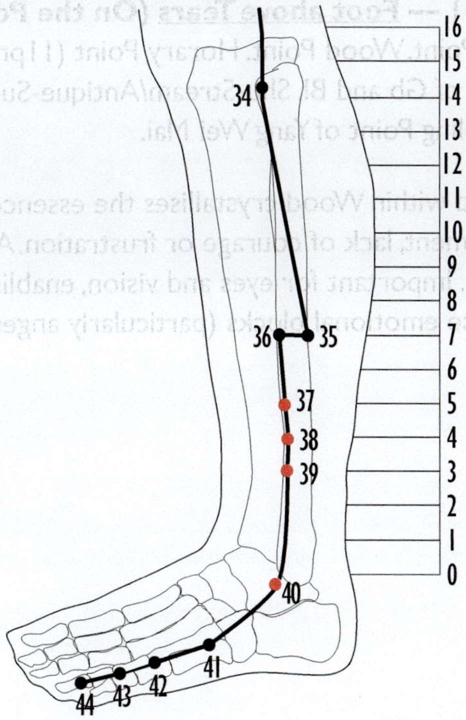
6	5-15	Anterior to anterior border of fibular **4 cun** proximal to prominence of lateral maleolus Between peroneus brevis and extensor digitorum longus muscles	
3	5-15	Between posterior border of fibular and anterior border of tendons of peroneus brevis (fibularis brevis) and peroneus longus **3 cun** proximal to prominence of lateral maleolus	
5	3-7	Lateral aspect of flexure of ankle Anterior and inferior to prominence of lateral maleolus (form a box around the maleolus — the point will be on the most lateral and most inferior part of the box) In a hollow between lateral malleolus and the tendon of the extensor digitorum longus muscle (on the opposite side would be Sp 5)	

Gallbladder

Gb 41 — <u>Foot above Tears</u> (On the Point of Weeping, Foot Overlooking Tears)
Exit Point. Wood Point. Horary Point (11pm–1am). Seasonal Horary Point — Spring. Crossing Point of Gb and Bl. Shu-Stream/Antique-Summer Point. Opening Point of Dai Mai (Girdle Vessel). Coupling Point of Yang Wei Mai.

Wood within Wood crystallises the essence of Wood and helps with decision-making, clarity, judgement, lack of courage or frustration. Aids the smooth flow of Liver energy (it connects to Liv 1). Important for eyes and vision, enabling a person to grow and move forward in their life. Can release emotional blocks (particularly anger), and as a result may also release tears.

Gb 42 — <u>Earth Five Meetings</u> (Five Terrestrial Reunions)

Five is the number for organisation, order and unity. This point restores order, balance and control to the Gb, and thus can have a unifying effect upon all the other Officials. Similar in effect to Du 20. Consider for arthritis, swelling or neuralgia of the foot, or for red and painful eyes.

⊥	△		Location
3	5	Dorsum of foot Distal to the junction of the 4th and 5th metatarsal bones Just distal and lateral to the flare of the base of the 4th metatarsal Lateral to the (fourth slip of the) tendon of extensor digitorum longus muscle	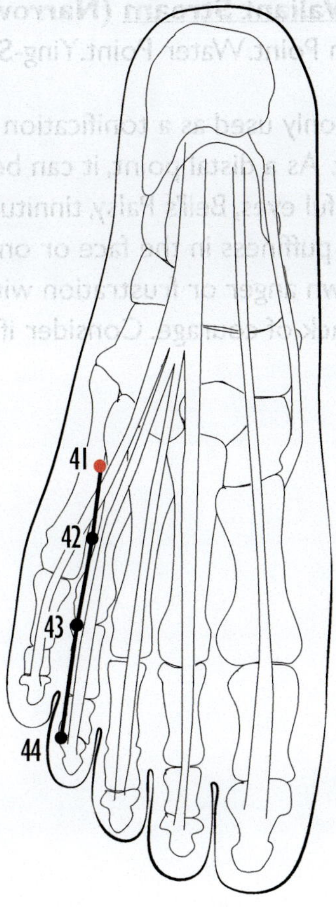
2	X	Dorsum of foot Between 4th and 5th metatarsal bones Proximal to 4th metatarso-phalangeal joint Just proximal to flare of head of 4th metatarsal bone Medial to the (fourth slip of the) tendon of extensor digitorum longus muscle	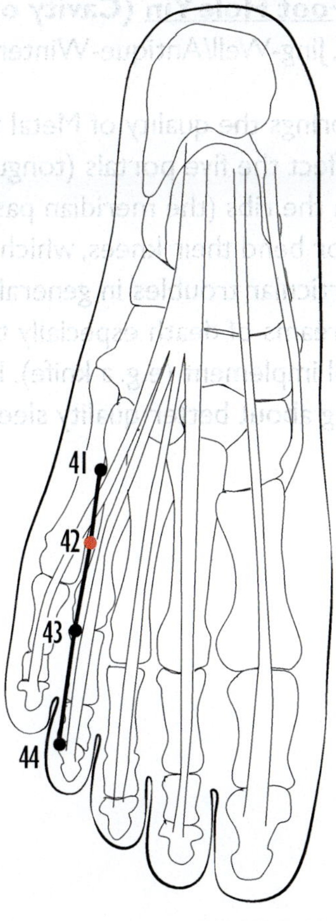

Gb 43 — Valiant Stream (Narrow Ravine)
Tonification Point. Water Point. Ying-Spring/Antique-Spring Point.

Not commonly used as a tonification point because Wood is usually more energetically abundant than Water. As a distal point, it can be beneficial for problems in the head and face, e.g. headaches, red or painful eyes, Bell's Palsy, tinnitus or dizziness. If Water is in excess, this can give rise to swelling or puffiness in the face or on the meridian pathway itself. This Water point can be sedated to cool down anger or frustration within a person or, conversely, can strengthen their resolve if there is a lack of courage. Consider if a Wood CF is too 'brittle' or rigid.

Gb 44 — Foot Hole Yin (Cavity of Yin, Foot Portal Yin, Foot Opening Yin)
Metal Point. Jing-Well/Antique-Winter Point.

This point brings the quality of Metal to the Wood. It is similar to Gb 11 (Head Hole Yin) in that both affect the five portals (tongue, nose, eyes, ears and mouth). Consider for sharp pains, especially in the ribs (the meridian passes through this area). Helpful when the patient can't raise their arms or bend their knees, which may indicate that the Metal within is too cold, stiff or rigid. Good for articular troubles in general. Metal over-controlling Wood can give rise to fright, dreams of ghosts, dreams of death especially those dreams where a person is being chased or threatened with a metal implement (e.g. a knife). This point can help to calm this type of dream disturbance, thus bringing about better quality sleep. Eases migraines that affect the eyes.

⊥	△		Location
3	3-5	Dorsum of foot Between 4th and 5th digits Distal to 4th metatarso-phalangeal joint Distal to flare of the base of the proximal phalanx of 4th digit Proximal to web margin between 4th and 5th digits	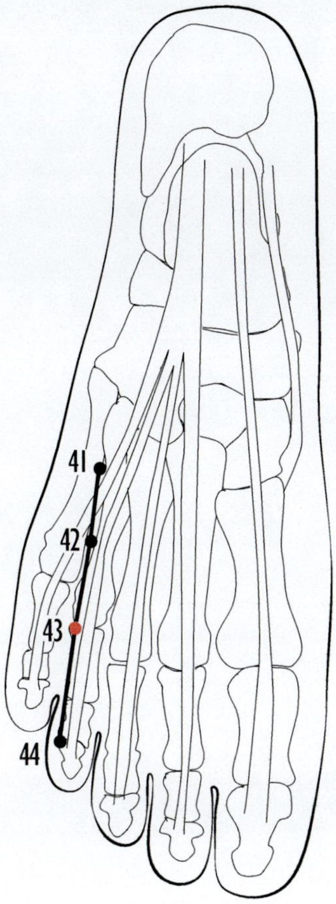
1	3-5	Lateral nail point of the 4th digit Approx **0.1 cun** proximal to corner of nail Distal to the flare of the distal phalanx	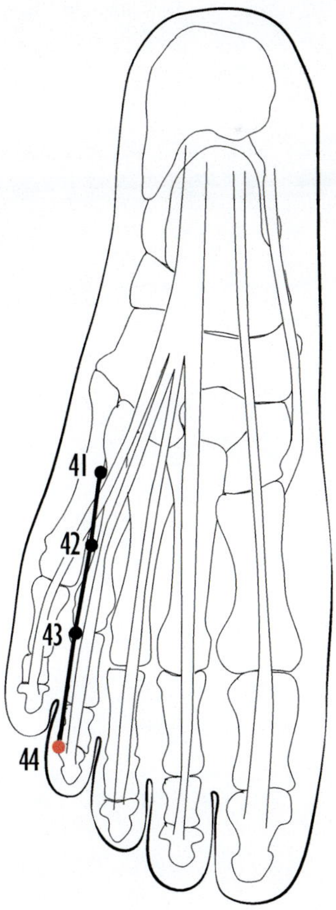

Liver

- **The Official in Charge of Strategic Planning and the Assessment of Circumstances**
- **The meridian loops through the genital area, and via its deep pathway connects to the eyes and brain. Houses the 'Hun'. Stores the Blood**
- **The emotion of Wood is anger and its taste is sour**

Liver

Liv 1 — <u>Great Esteem</u> (Great Mound, Great Clarity)
Entry Point. Wood Point. Horary Point (1–3am). Seasonal Horary Point — Spring. Jing-Well/ Antique-Winter Point. First Aid Point: unconsciousness.

Wood within Wood revitalises this Official and shakes off the dead wood. This point can produce a great surge of energy at the start of the meridian, or can strongly calm it (particularly effective between 1–3 pm). Often used with moxa. Good point for hernias, vaginal discharges, enlarged scrotum, vaginal prolapse, pain in the penis, testicles or vagina. Consider for severe, painful headaches. Beneficial for a patient lacking in self-esteem. Also helpful for those who cannot see the way forward in their mind's eye, who cannot plan or put a plan into action. They may have become stagnated, perhaps through a build-up of anger or frustration, and this point can lift them out of this situation and encourage them towards fulfilling their true potential.

Liv 2 — <u>Walk Between</u> (Moving Between, Walking Space)
Sedation Point. Fire Point. Ying-Spring/Antique-Spring Point. 'Happy Calm' Point.

Repressed emotion, particularly anger, can cause stagnation within a person, which can then lead to depression or oscillations in their mood. Excessive anger can also produce heat and hot-headedness within a person, giving rise to agitation. Certain drugs, foods or excess alcohol can also produce heat in the Liver. Liv 2 addresses these symptoms as it calms and cools the system. Furthermore, it is very useful in cases of painful or irregular menstruation, genital itching or insomnia caused by excessive dreaming. Consider for headaches and migraines.

⊥	Δ		Location
1	5-7	Lateral nail point of the 1st digit Approx **0.1 cun** proximal to the lateral corner of the nail Distal to the flare of the distal phalanx	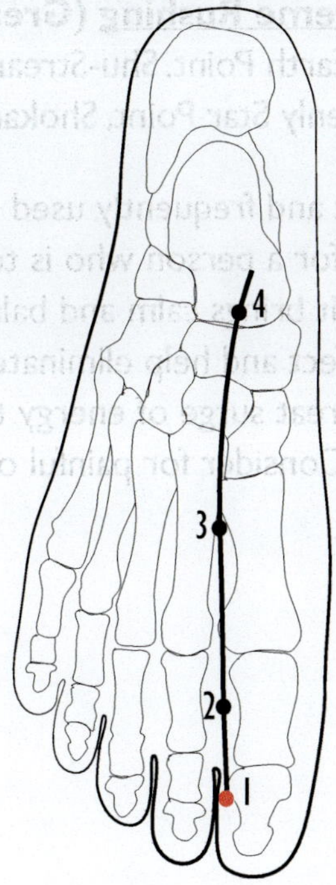
3	5-7	Between 1st and 2nd digits Distal to metatarsophalangeal joint of first digit Just distal to the flare of the base of the proximal phalanx	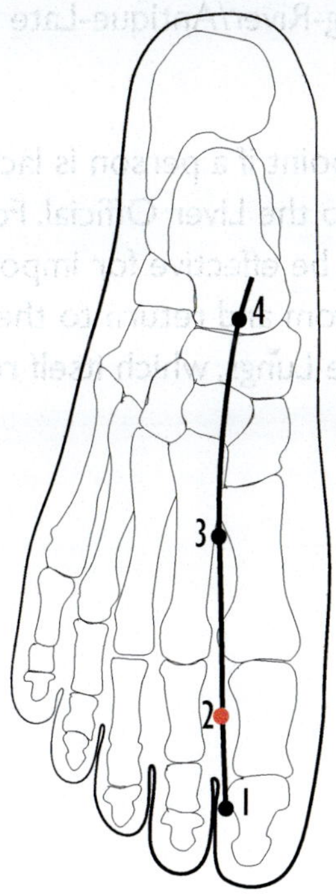

Liver

Liv 3 — <u>Supreme Rushing</u> (Great Surge, Happy Calm)
Source Point. Earth Point. Shu-Stream/Antique-Summer Point. 'Total Relaxation Point'. A Ma Danyang Heavenly Star Point, Shokanten Point. Independent point for spasms.

This important and frequently used point is indicated for many conditions. It is particularly effective when sedated for a person who is tense, over-excited, easily angered or annoyed, agitated or 'tightly-wired'. It brings calm and balance to the system. It can be combined with LI 4 to accentuate this calming effect and help eliminate toxins on both the mental and physical levels. When tonified, it can bring a great surge of energy to the meridian. Its alternative name of 'Happy Calm' describes its effect well. Consider for painful or irregular menstruation.

Liv 4 — <u>Middle Seal</u> (Central Mound, Middle Border)
Metal Point. Jing-River/Antique-Late Summer Point. Point used in the Husband/Wife treatment protocol.

Consider this point if a person is lacking in self-confidence or a sense of their own identity. It brings quality to the Liver Official. For pain and swelling in the ankles and feet, muscular wastage or paralysis. It can be effective for impotence or pain in the genital area. In Spiritual terms, the Hun is said to come from and return to the ancestral realms, and is kept in place and earthed by the P'o, the Spirit of the Lungs, which itself returns to the Earth upon death.

⊥	Δ		Location
3	3-7	<u>Forbidden in pregnancy</u>. Dorsal aspect of foot Distal to the junction of the flare of the bases of the 1st and 2nd metatarsal bones Lateral to the tendon of the extensor Hallucis longus	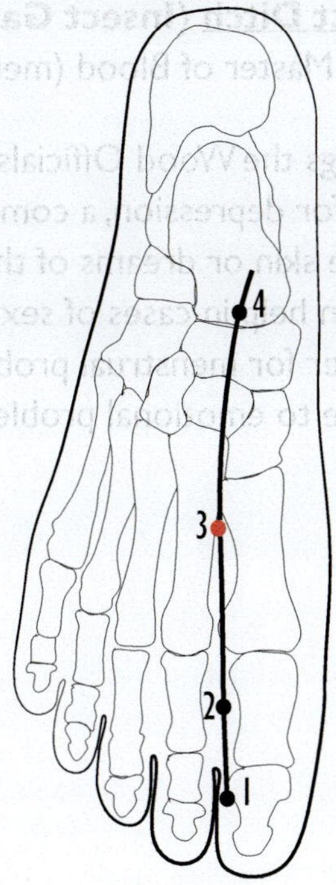
4	3-5	Anterior aspect of flexure of ankle Between medial maleolus and the tendon of the tibialis anterior muscle Level with the prominence of the Medial Maleolus	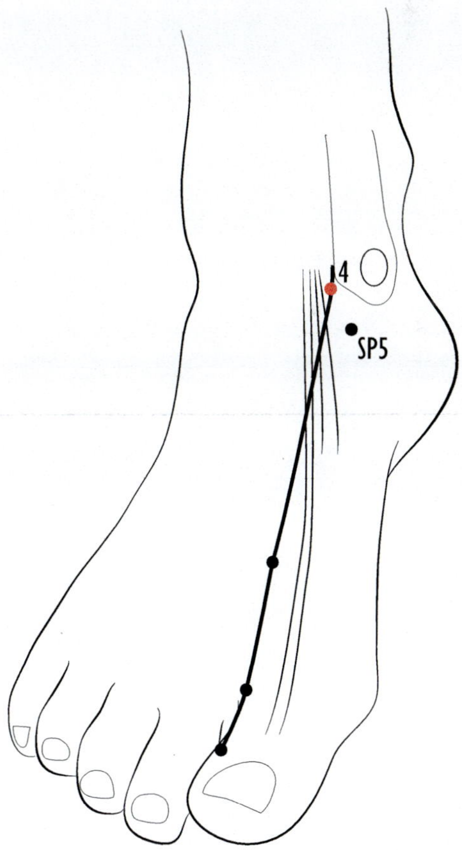

Liver

Liv 5 — <u>Insect Ditch</u> (Insect Gate, Wormwood Canal)
Junction point. Master of Blood (menstrual) point.

This point brings the Wood Officials together, restoring their stability, unity and harmony, and can be helpful for depression, a common Liver-related condition. Consider for a feeling of insects crawling on the skin or dreams of things crawling — this point clears the ditch. Connects to the genitals, and can help in cases of sexual problems such as premature ejaculation, sterility or genital itching. Consider for menstrual problems. Helpful if there is difficulty flexing the knee or for throat restrictions due to emotional problems (the deep pathway flows through here).

⊥	△		Location
3	3-7	Medial surface of tibia, near to medial border of tibia On medial border of soleus/ gastrocnemius muscle **5 cun** proximal to prominence of medial maleolus	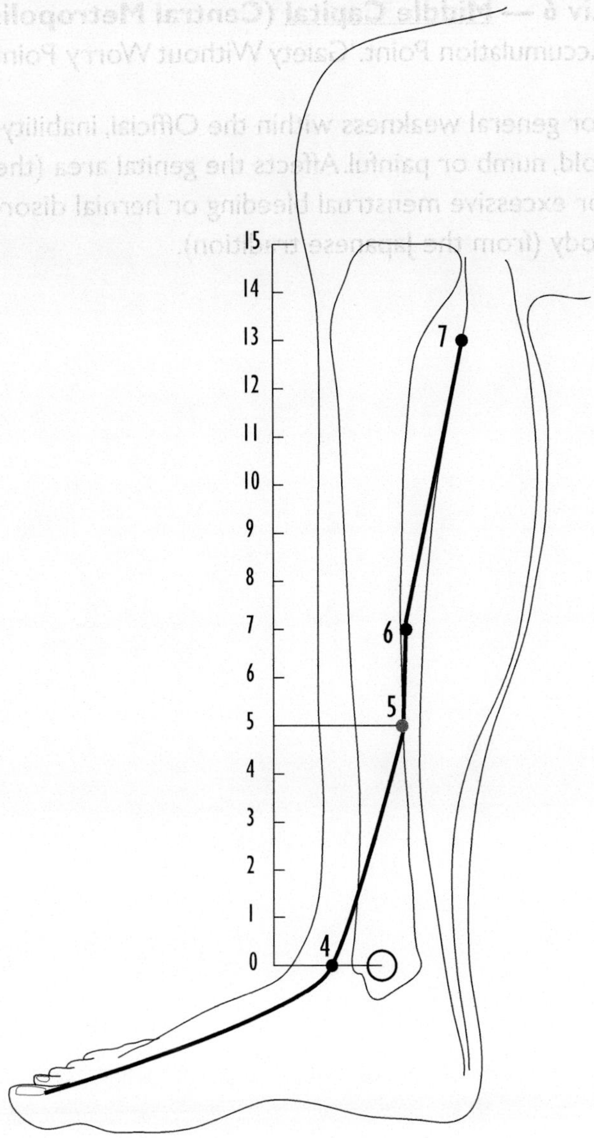

Liver

Liv 6 — <u>Middle Capital</u> (Central Metropolis)
Accumulation Point. 'Gaiety Without Worry Point'. First Aid: spasm, cramp, urinary pain.

For general weakness within the Official, inability to stand, inability to walk, or where the legs are cold, numb or painful. Affects the genital area (the meridian passes through this sector), so consider for excessive menstrual bleeding or hernial disorders. Said to be a revitalisation point for the whole body (from the Japanese tradition).

⊥	△		**Location**
3	3	Medial surface of tibia near to medial border of tibia On medial border of soleus/ gastrocnemius muscle **7 cun** proximal to prominence of medial maleolus	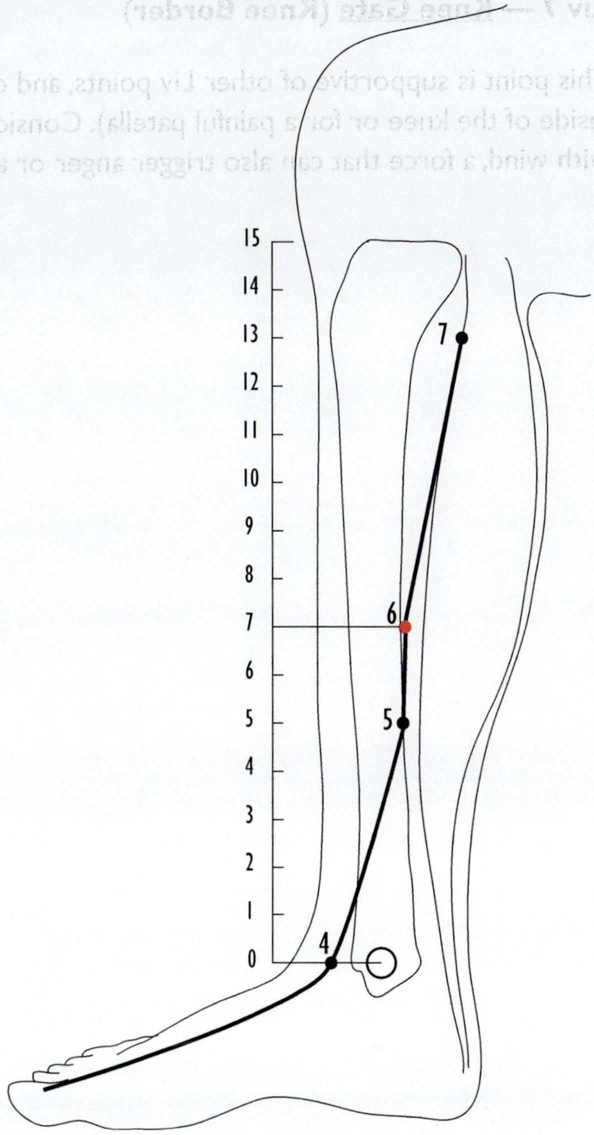

Liv 7 — Knee Gate (Knee Border)

This point is supportive of other Liv points, and can be used for knee troubles (particularly for the inside of the knee or for a painful patella). Consider for arthritis or rheumatism that gets worse with wind, a force that can also trigger anger or agitation within some people.

⊥	Δ		Location
4	5	In the medial head of the gastrocnemius muscle Approx **13 cun** proximal to the prominence of the medial maleolus **1 cun** posterior to Sp 9	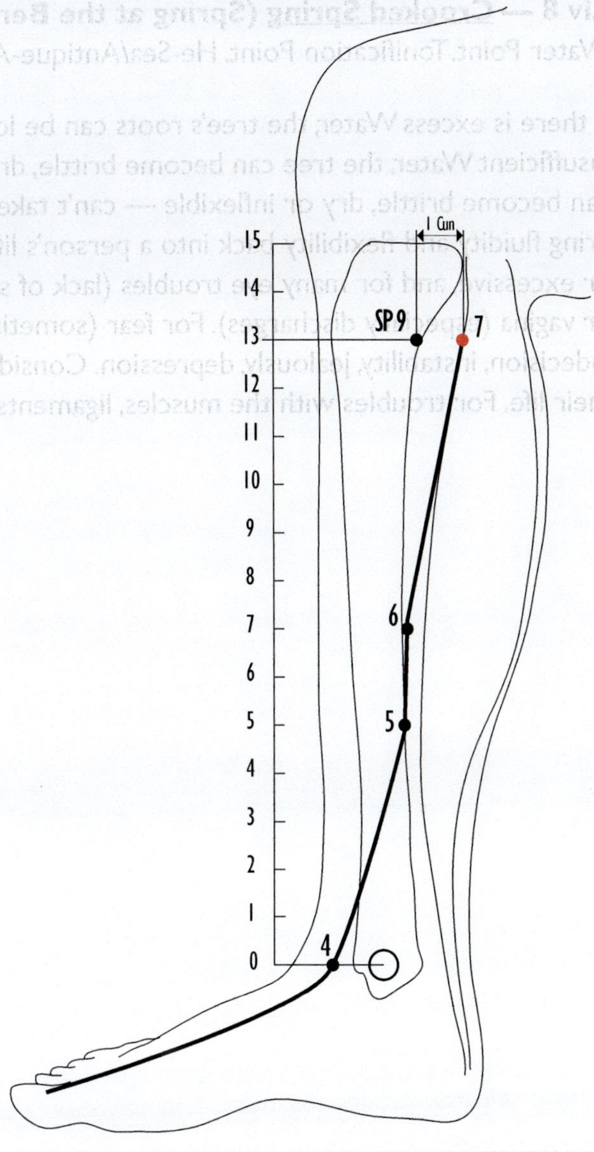

Liv 8 — Crooked Spring (Spring at the Bend)
Water Point. Tonification Point. He-Sea/Antique-Autumn Point. "Flexibility Point".

If there is excess Water, the tree's roots can be loosened and thus becomes unstable. If there is insufficient Water, the tree can become brittle, dried out, unable to yield. Similarly, the Body/Mind can become brittle, dry or inflexible — can't take one more trial or tribulation. This point can bring fluidity and flexibility back into a person's life. Consider for urinary troubles — retention or excessive, and for many eye troubles (lack of secretions). Excellent for problems in the penis or vagina (especially discharges). For fear (sometimes worse than Kidney fear), anger, irritation, indecision, instability, jealously, depression. Consider for a person who cannot tolerate change in their life. For troubles with the muscles, ligaments and tendons, particularly around the knees.

⊥	Δ		Location
6	3-5	Medial border of joint of knee Superior to medial end of popliteal crease when foot is flexed Posterior to medial condyle of the tibia Medial and anterior to the tendon of the semimembranosus muscles	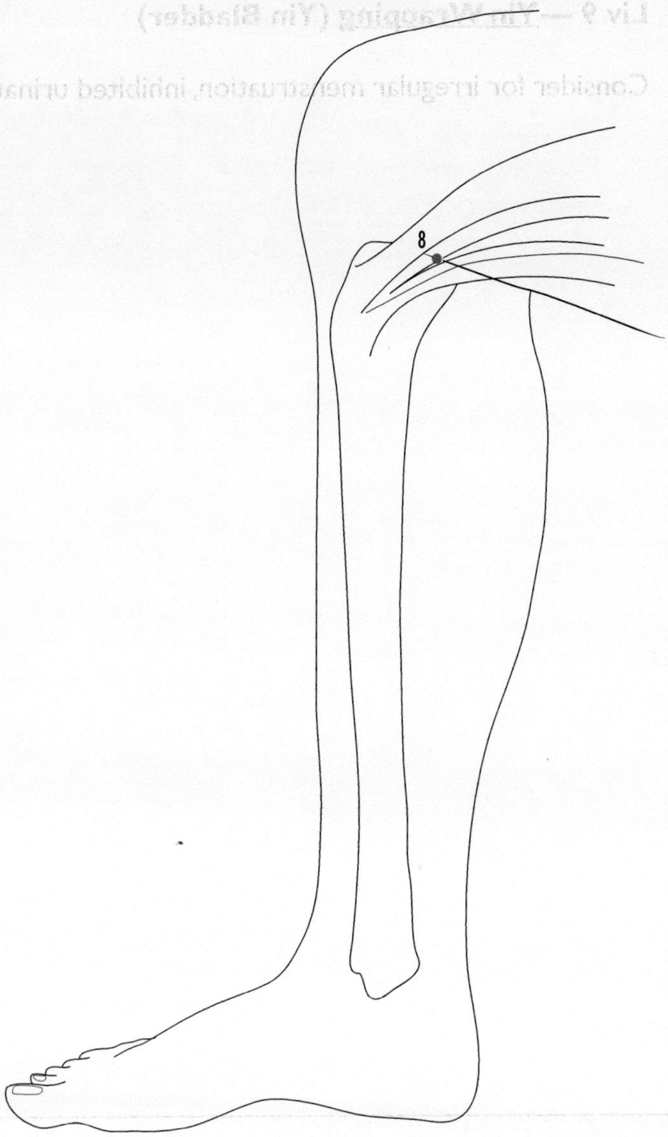

Liver

Liv 9 —Yin Wrapping (Yin Bladder)

Consider for irregular menstruation, inhibited urination or spasms in the buttocks, loins or legs.

⊥	Δ		Location
5	3	In a seam between vastus medialis and sartorius muscles **6 cun** proximal to medial popliteal crease **4 cun** proximal to medial epicondyle of the femur	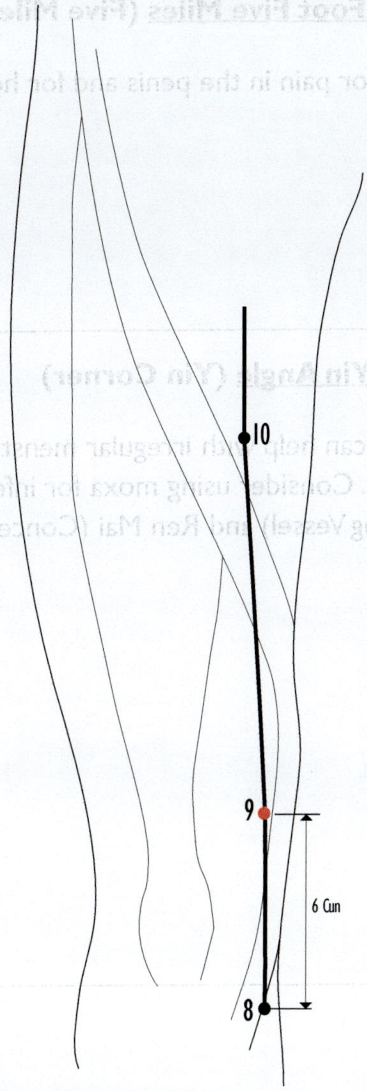

Liv 10 — <u>Foot Five Miles</u> (Five Miles)

Consider for pain in the penis and for hernias. Said to be helpful in cases of urine retention.

Liv 11 —<u>Yin Angle</u> (Yin Corner)

This point can help with irregular menstruation. Eases childbirth, because of its ability to relax the patient. Consider using moxa for infertility, if appropriate, as Liv 11 regulates the Chong Mai (Penetrating Vessel) and Ren Mai (Conception Vessel).

⊥	Δ		Location
5	3-5	Medial and superior to the sartorius muscle At the medial margin of femoral artery Inferior to the pubic tubercule Directly inferior to St 30 **2 cun** below Liv 12 (inguinal groove) **1 cun** below Liv 11	
3	3	Medial to femoral artery Inferior to the pubic tubercule **2 cun** lateral to the anterior median line of lower abdomen **1 cun** below Liv 12	

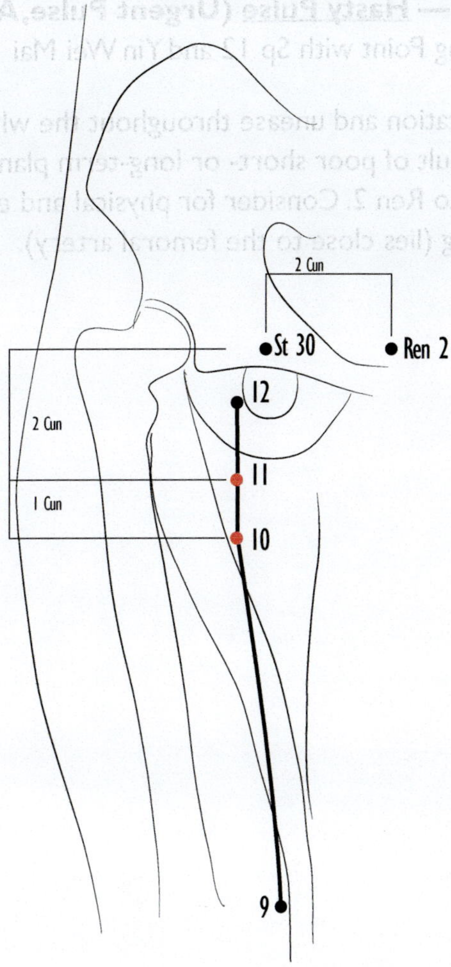

Liver

Liv 12 — <u>Hasty Pulse</u> (Urgent Pulse, Anxious Pulse)
Crossing Point with Sp 12 and Yin Wei Mai

For agitation and unease throughout the whole person where everything is done too quickly, often as a result of poor short- or long-term planning. The deep pathway passes through the testicles/vagina to Ren 2. Consider for physical and emotional problems around sexuality. Take care when needling (lies close to the femoral artery).

Liv 13 — <u>Chapter Gate</u> (Gate of Perfection. Camphorwood Gate)
Front mu point/Alarm Point for Sp. Crossing Point of Liv and Gb. Shokanten Point. Influential Point of the Yin Officials.

Liver 13 and 14 are one of only five sets of Points where one gate follows another. They are often used together, and both are Shokanten Points. Helps initiate change and transition in the patient's life so that a new chapter can begin to unfold for them. Promotes the smooth flowing of Liver Qi, thus easing frustration, stuckness and depression. Consider for digestive disorders arising from the Liver. Strongly affects the middle jiao. Strengthens and harmonises the relationship between Sp and Liv. The name Camphorwood Gate refers to a highly prized wood used in the construction of the Hall of Supreme Harmony in the Forbidden City, indicating a Point of great value. Furthermore it is here where the two Wood meridians intersect.

⊥	Δ		Location
X	3	In inguinal groove of the groin, on the femoral artery (feel pulse) On the inferolateral corner of the pubic crest **2.5 cun** lateral to the anterior median line (of the lower abdomen) Lateral and inferior to St 30	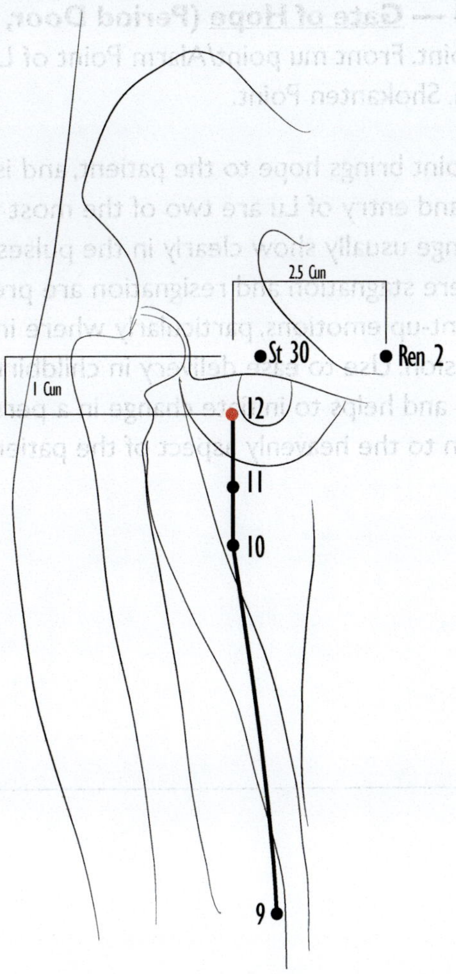
6-8	7-20	Just inferior and anterior to the tip of the 11th rib Just anterior to or on the mid-axillary line	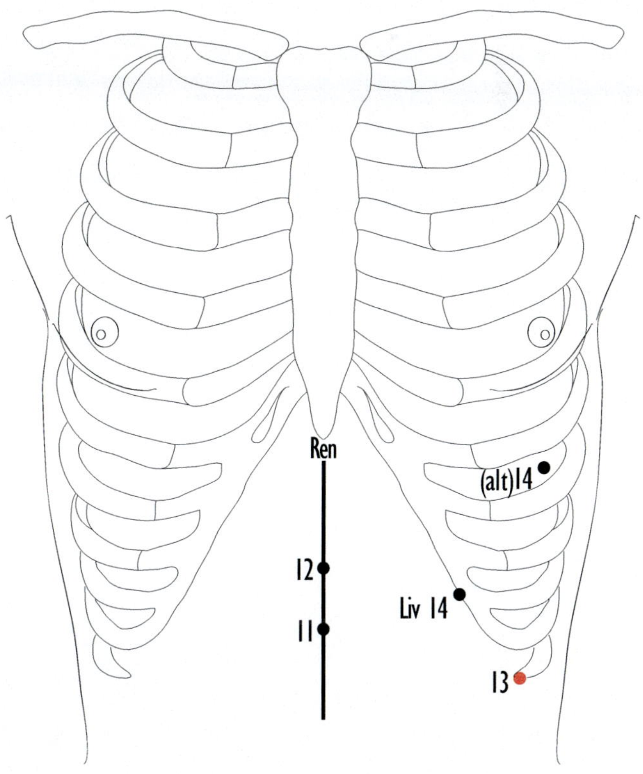

Liver

Liv 14 — Gate of Hope (Period Door, Cycle Gate)
Exit Point. Front mu point/Alarm Point of Liv. Crossing point Liv, Sp and Yin Wei Mai (Linking Vessel). Shokanten Point.

This point brings hope to the patient, and is similar in its effect to a Window of the Sky. The exit of Liv and entry of Lu are two of the most frequently used Entry-Exit points — the block and its change usually show clearly in the pulses. Consider when there is lack of creativity and vision, or where stagnation and resignation are present in a person's life. Wonderful for hypertension and pent-up emotions, particularly where internalised anger, gloom or hopelessness have led to depression. Use to ease delivery in childbirth. As with Liv 13, this point aids the free flow of Liver energy and helps to initiate change in a person's life. Connects, via a deep pathway, to the eye, and then on to the heavenly aspect of the patient at Du 20.

⊥	Δ		Location
4	5-7	Inferior to the nipple On the inferior edge of the thoracic cage Just medial to the inferior border of the 9th rib where the costal cartilage meets the 10th rib If above does not work, then use this alternative location favoured by TCM Practitioners: Directly inferior to nipple In **6th IC Space** **4 cun** lateral to midline Directly superior to Gb 24 which is in **7th IC Space**	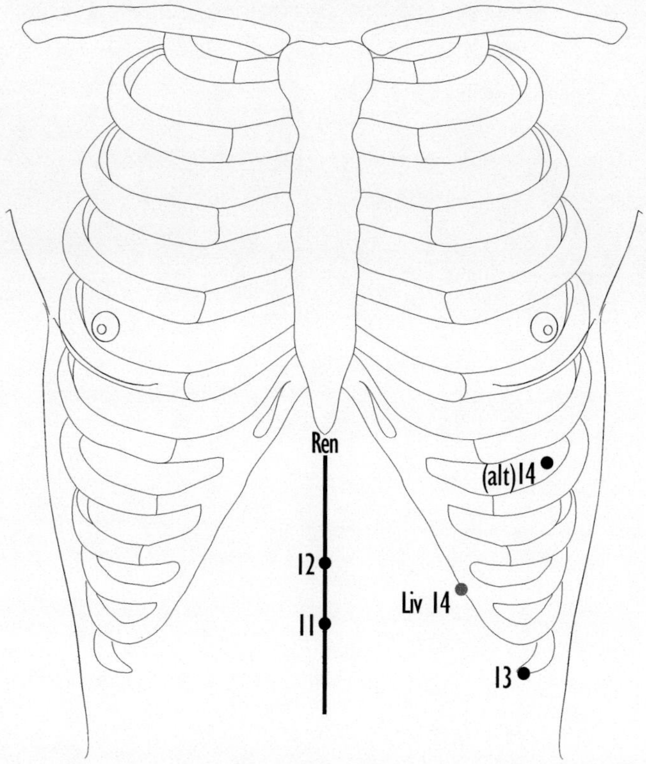

Lung

- **Receiver of Qi from the Heavens. Maintains 'rhythmic order' in the Kingdom**
- **Governs Defensive Energy (Wei Qi). Dwelling place of the P'o**
- **Holds the office of Minister and Chancellor within the Kingdom**
- **'The coming and going of this breath is the greatest miracle of all'**

Lung

Lu 1 — Central Treasury (Central Storehouse, Middle Palace)
Entry point, Front mu/Alarm point of Lu, Meeting of Tai Yin (Lu, Sp)

This entry point is the start of the energetic cycle and is where the Heavenly breaths bestow their priceless gift to the Kingdom via this Treasury. However, all Lung points help, to some degree, to receive the Heavenly Qi and to connect a person to that consciousness within. Sp and Lu connect here (Sp is the mother of Lu). This point can strengthen Lu weakness which can manifest as grief, sadness or melancholia and help bring meaning and purpose back into a patient's life. Commonly used when there is a block between Liv and Lu. Lung's 'canopy' protects the other Officials.

Lu 2 — Cloud Gate (Cloud door)

Use when a person feels like they are living 'under a cloud', and have lost connection to their heavenly aspect. This is particularly relevant following extended periods of grief, depression or sadness. Consider if the patient feels disconnected, cut off, or living a meaningless existence; this point reconnects them to the rhythms and cycles of life. Can be used with Lu 8, particularly in the Autumn. Helpful for general chest problems such as coughing or asthma.

Lu 3 — Heavenly Palace (Celestial Storehouse, Heavenly Treasury, Heaven's Residence)
Window of the Sky point. First aid: carbon monoxide poisoning.

Consider for mental confusion, severe depression, claustrophobia, agoraphobia or forgetfulness. As a Window it can lift and revitalise the spirit of a person cut off or imprisoned within themselves, often as a result of their reaction to chronic grief or sadness. Commonly used with LI 17 or LI 18.

⊥	Δ		Location
3-5	5-10	On a level with **1st IC Space** **6 cun** lateral to the anterior median line **1–1.6 cun** inferior to Lu 2 In the Pectoralis Major Muscle	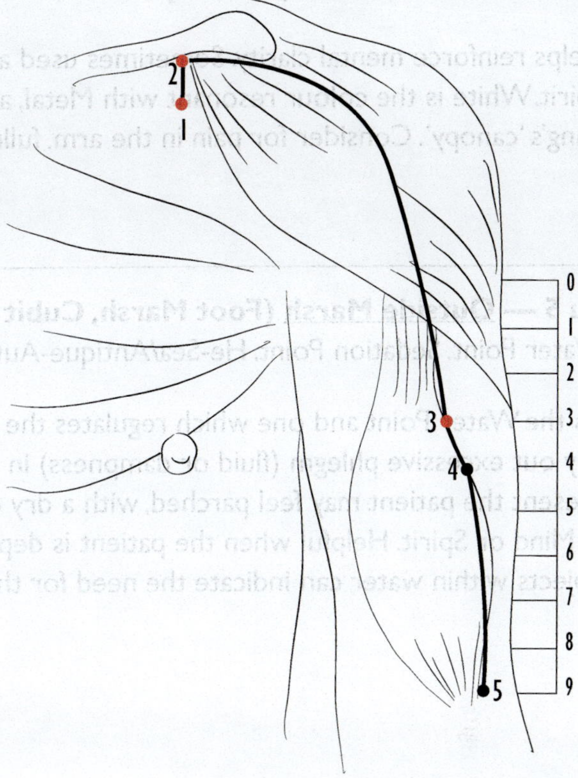
3-5	5-10	Inferior to Acromial extremity of the clavicle in the infraclavicular fossa Between upper border of the Pectoralis Major muscle and the anterior border of the deltoid muscle **6 cun** lateral to the anterior median line	
4-6	X	Anterolateral aspect of upper arm **3 cun** distal to axial crease **6 cun** proximal to the TCC and Lu 5 In the groove formed by the lateral border of the biceps brachii muscle and the humerus	

Lung

Lu 4 — <u>Valiant White</u> (Chivalry White, Pure White, Guarding White)

Helps reinforce mental clarity. Sometimes used as an adjunct to Lu 1, 2 or 3 when treating the Spirit. White is the colour resonant with Metal, and Valiant may refer to the protective nature of Lung's 'canopy'. Consider for pain in the arm, fullness in the chest or shortness of breath.

Lu 5 — <u>Outside Marsh</u> (Foot Marsh, Cubit Marsh)
Water Point. Sedation Point. He-Sea/Antique-Autumn point.

As the Water Point and one which regulates the 'Water Passages', Lu 5 can be used to expel or dry out excessive phlegm (fluid or dampness) in the lungs. Conversely, if there is too little Water present the patient may feel parched, with a dry cough, bronchitis (with much mucous), or rigid in Mind or Spirit. Helpful when the patient is depressed, weeping or sorrowful. Dreams of metal objects within water can indicate the need for this point.

Lu 6 — <u>Greatest Hole</u>
Accumulation point

For acute feelings of sorrow, loss or emptiness in a patient's life, or where grief seems to predominate. For profound feelings of grief or pain upon losing someone or something. Consider for acute chest problems or infections, e.g. bronchitis, asthma or persistent cough. Also for articular troubles of the shoulder or elbow.

⊥	Δ		Location
3-5	5	Anterolateral aspect of upper arm **4 cun** distal to axial crease **5 cun** proximal to the TCC and Lu 5 In the groove formed by the lateral border of the biceps brachii muscle and the humerus	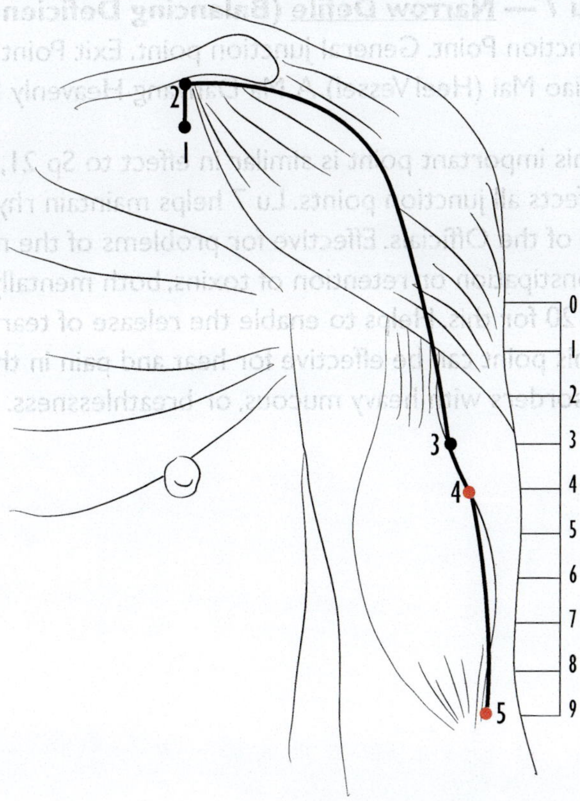
3-5	3-5	On flexure of the elbow Lateral to the tendon of the biceps brachii Arm slightly flexed	
5	5	Ulna side of the radius **7 cun** proximal to Lu 9 Between brachioradialis — medial and Flexor carpi radialis — lateral	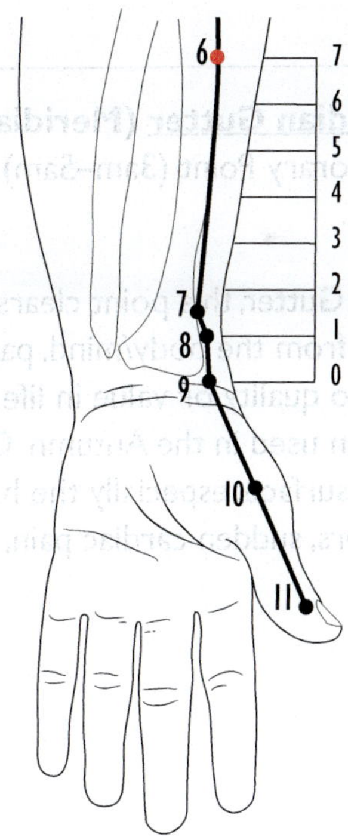

Lu 7 — Narrow Defile (Balancing Deficiencies, Broken Sequence)
Junction Point. General Junction point. Exit Point. Opening Point of Ren Mai. Coupled Point of Yin Qiao Mai (Heel Vessel). A Ma Danyang Heavenly Star Point.

This important point is similar in effect to Sp 21, as it is said to be a special junction point which affects all junction points. Lu 7 helps maintain rhythm (one role of the P'o) and balance amongst all of the Officials. Effective for problems of the mouth, throat, head and nose. Consider for constipation or retention of toxins, both mentally and physically, often combined with LI 4 and LI 20 for this. Helps to enable the release of tears if suppressed by chronic grief and sadness. This point can be effective for heat and pain in the palm of the hand, tension in the chest, chest disorders with heavy mucous, or breathlessness.

Lu 8 — Meridian Gutter (Meridian Ditch, Regulating Drain, Flowing Gutter)
Metal Point. Horary Point (3am–5am). Seasonal Horary Point — Autumn. Jing-River/Antique-Late Summer Point.

As a Meridian Gutter, this point clears and carries away garbage and poisons. It can clear stagnation and negativity from the body/mind, particularly where there is cynicism present or a feeling that there is no quality or value in life. As the Metal Point, it shakes up and cleanses the Official, especially when used in the Autumn. Consider when heat or extreme cold are out of proportion on the body's surface, especially the hands (palms hot, dry or wet). Beneficial for many lung and throat disorders, sudden cardiac pain, intermittent fever, excessive mucous or wrist pain.

⊥	△		Location
2-3	3-5	Forbidden from 6th month of pregnancy **1.5 cun** proximal to Lu 9 Proximal to root of the styloid process Between tendons of brachioradialis and abductor pollicis longus muscles	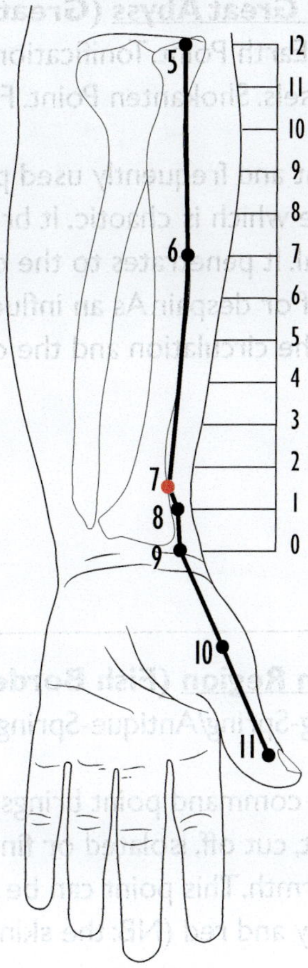
2-3	X	**1 cun** proximal to Lu 9 Level with and medial to the prominence of the styloid process of the radius Lateral aspect of the radial artery Lateral to the tendon of the flexor carpi radiali	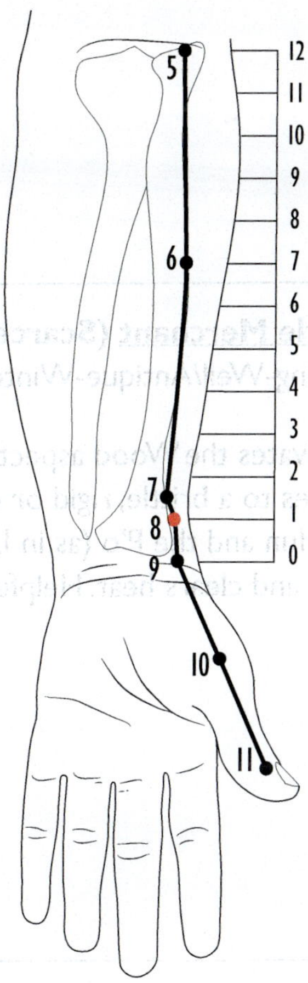

Lu 9 — Very Great Abyss (Great Abyss, Supreme Whirlpool, Corpse Reviver)
Source Point. Earth Point. Tonification Point. Shu-Stream/Antique-Summer Point. Influential Point of the Blood Vessels. Shokanten Point. First Aid: asphyxia, collapse, radiation poisoning.

This important and frequently used point can help 'revive' a person and bring clarity and order to a pulse picture which is chaotic. It brings the qualities of mother Earth, in this case the Spleen, to the child Metal. It penetrates to the deepest levels, and is indicated for someone who is in the very depths of grief or despair. As an influential reunion point of the blood vessels it has a tremendous influence on the circulation and the quality of the Blood.

Lu 10 — Fish Region (Fish Border)
Fire Point. Ying-Spring/Antique-Spring Point.

This powerful command point brings warmth to the Metal. It is particularly helpful when the patient is inert, cut off, isolated or finds difficulty making contact with others, or who is lacking in emotional warmth. This point can be tonified if the skin is cold, silvery or flaky, or sedated if the skin is hot, ugly and red (NB: the skin is our third lung, and is the largest organ of the body).

Lu 11 — Little Merchant (Scarce Trade, Young Musician)
Wood Point. Jing-Well/Antique-Winter Point. Ghost Point.

This point activates the Wood aspect within the Metal. It brings decisiveness, growth and enhanced planning abilities to a brittle, rigid or cut off Metal CF. It helps maintain the correct balance between the Hun and the P'o (as in Liv 4). Consider if the skin exhibits a silk-like sheen. Restores consciousness and clears heat. Helpful for acute sore throat or pain in the fingers.

⊥	Δ		Location
2	3	Proximal edge of the scaphoid bone Between the tendons of the flexor carpi radialis and the abductor pollicis longus muscles. Flex the wrist to find the point	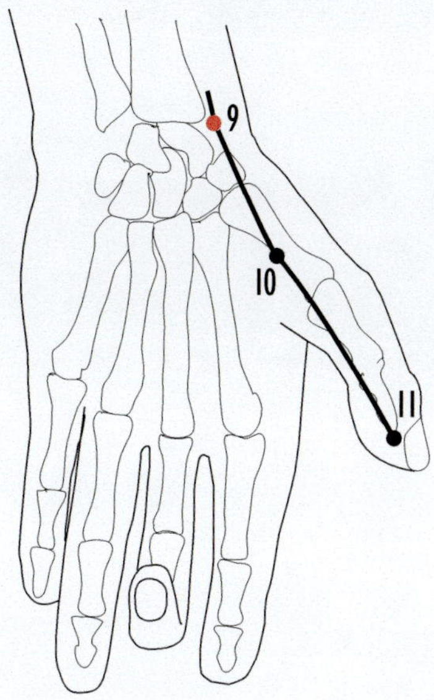
3-5	X	Radial extremity of the palmar surface of the hand Point midway between the base and head of the first metacarpal bone Lateral edge of the opponens pollicis muscle	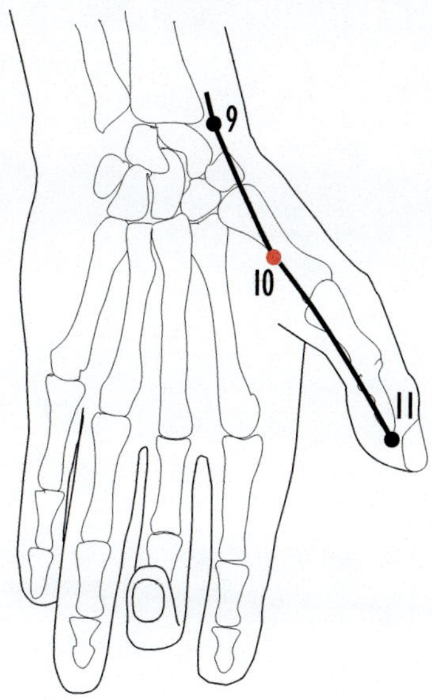
1	X	Forbidden from 7th month of pregnancy Radial nail point of the thumb Distal to the flare of the distal phalanx	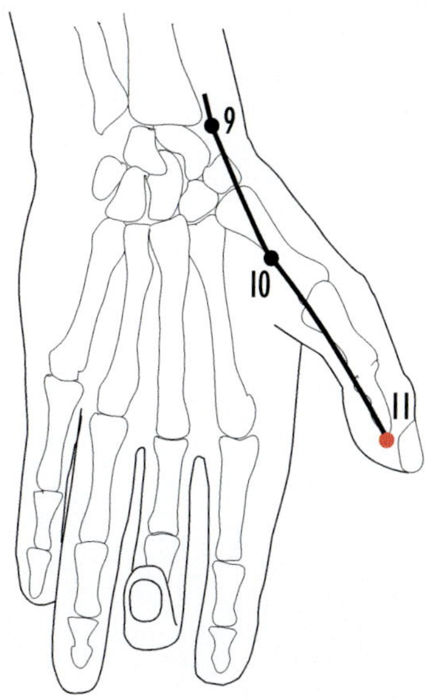

Large Intestine

- **The Official in Charge of the Drainage of the Dregs**
- **Propagates the 'correct way of living'**
- **Metal governs the nose, sense of smell, the emotion grief, the skin and body hair**

Large Intestine

LI 1 — Merchant Yang (Metal Yang)
Metal Point. Horary (5–7am). Seasonal Horary Point — Autumn. Jing-Well / Antique-Winter Point. Dental Point.

As the Metal and Horary point, Merchant Yang can revitalise the LI Official. Consider if the patient is physically cold, emotionally inert, stubborn or cynical. Helpful when they can't communicate, can't see the quality of their existence clearly, or are clogged up with rubbish. Often used with Lu 8 (Metal and Horary point) to clear out or detoxify the system, physically and mentally. Particularly effective when used in the Autumn. Useful for problems in the shoulders, fingers, arm or neck such as frozen joints. When used with LI 20, it can clear nasal congestion. Both Lu and LI are concerned with life's rhythms (an attribute of the P'o). Shang in its name is the musical note resonant with Metal (as in Lu 11 and Sp 5). Consider for dental pain along the LI meridian.

LI 2 — Second Interval (Second Section)
Water Point. Main Sedation Point. Ying-Spring/Antique-Spring Point. 'Abdominal Calm Point'.

Brings the flexibility and fluidity of Water to the Metal. Calms and cools intestinal spasm or colic. Consider for blurred vision or troubles with the inner canthus of the eye. One of the best points on the body for constipation. Helpful for lack of movement or arthritis in the fingers.

LI 3 — Third Interval (Third Section)
Wood Point. Shu-Stream/Antique-Summer point.

Although not a frequently used point, it can be helpful in cases of constipation. It is similar in its effect to LI 2. Can have a marked effect on children, especially for throat disorders, constipation or diarrhoea. For a person who has a negative view of life, this point can help bring the hope and forward-looking influence of Wood to the Metal. Local point for arthritis of the hand.

⊥	Δ		Location
I	3	The radial nail point of the second digit	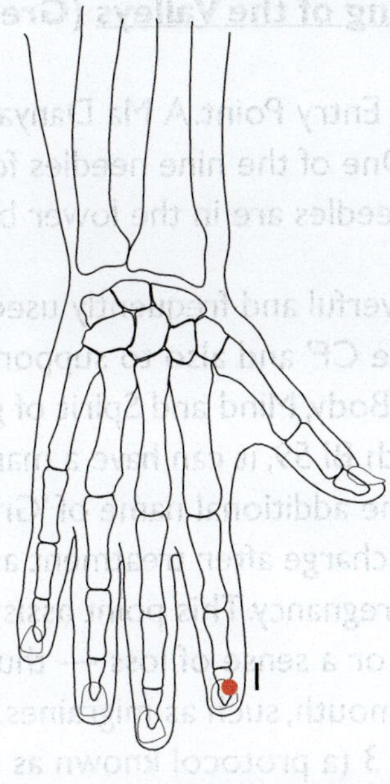
3	3	Forbidden from 9th month of pregnancy Midline of the radial surface of second digit Distal to the metacarpo-phalangeal joint Distal to the flare of the base of the proximal phalanx	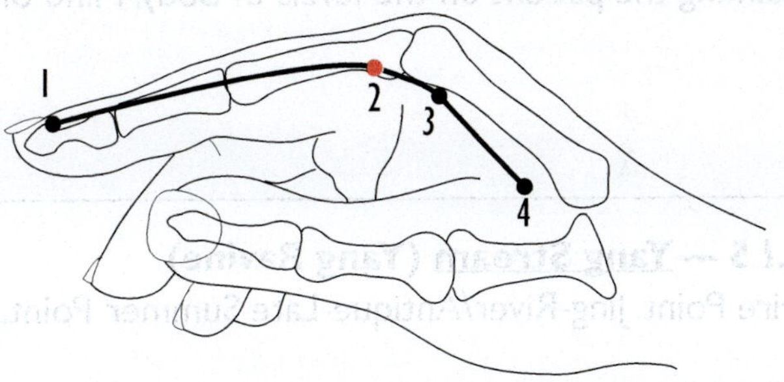
3	3	Radial side of the second digit Proximal to the metacarpo-phalangeal joint At the flare of the second metacarpal bone Between the head of the second metacarpal and the first dorsal interosseous muscle	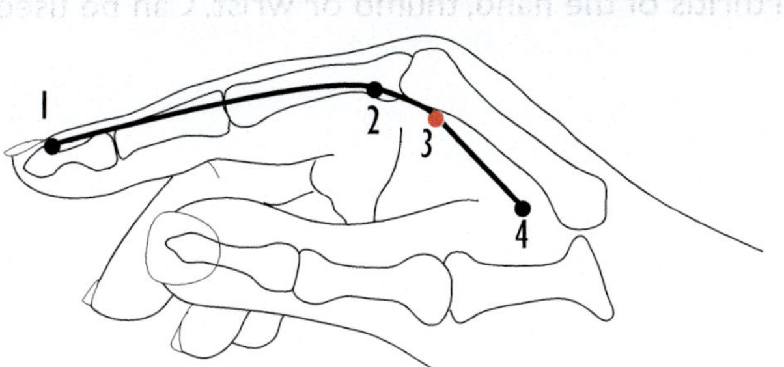

Large Intestine

LI 4 — <u>Joining of the Valleys</u> (Great Eliminator, Harmonious Valleys, Meeting of the Valleys)
Source Point. Entry Point. A Ma Danyang Heavenly Star Point. Greater Influential Point of the Face and Mouth. One of the nine needles for returning Yang. Shokanten Point. First aid: acupuncture blackout (if needles are in the lower body).

A classic, powerful and frequently used acupuncture point. As with any Source Point, it can be used to 'test for the CF' and also to support or augment the effect of other points on the meridian. It helps rid the Body, Mind and Spirit of garbage which may have accumulated over many years. When combined with Bl 59, it can have a marked effect of further removing toxins from the system. Both points have the additional name of 'Great Eliminator'. The patient may experience a physical or emotional discharge after treatment as it (eventually) brings calmness to the system. Forbidden throughout pregnancy. This point assists the patient in 'letting go' on all levels — but especially with sadness, grief or a sense of loss — thus allowing in those things of value. Consider for problems in the face and mouth, such as migraines, headaches, toothache, earache, or nasal congestion. When used with Liv 3 (a protocol known as the Four Gates), this point can have a wonderful effect of calming the patient on the levels of Body, Mind or Spirit. Strengthens the defensive Qi.

LI 5 —<u>Yang Stream</u> (Yang Ravine)
Fire Point. Jing-River/Antique-Late Summer Point.

This often neglected point can have a remarkable effect on certain mental disorders. It is said to be helpful for people who see ghosts and spirits — when it is commonly sedated. Also for 'mad' people who want to throw off their clothes. Often used together with LI 4 for their purifying and enlivening effects. Consider for tinnitus, deafness, skin disorders, incoherent speech, stuttering, pain/ arthritis of the hand, thumb or wrist. Can be used to warm a cold or inert Metal CF.

⊥	△		Location
5	5-7	Forbidden in pregnancy Between the proximal ends of the first and second metacarpal bones Distal to the flare of the radial surface on the radial side of the base of the second metacarpal bone	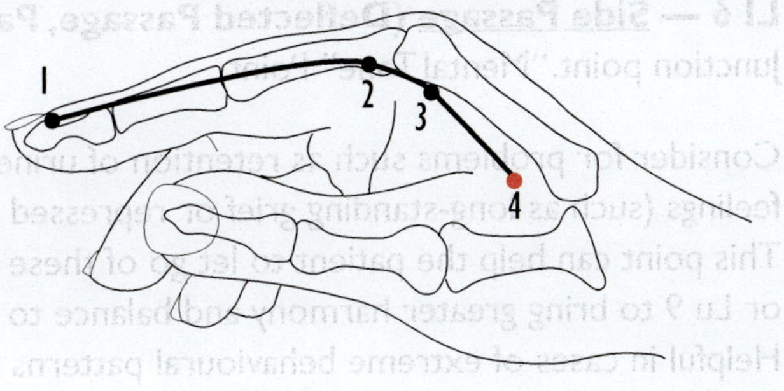
3	5	Between the tip of the Styloid process of the radius and scaphoid bone On the flexure of the wrist Between the tendons of the extensor pollicis longus and brevis muscles	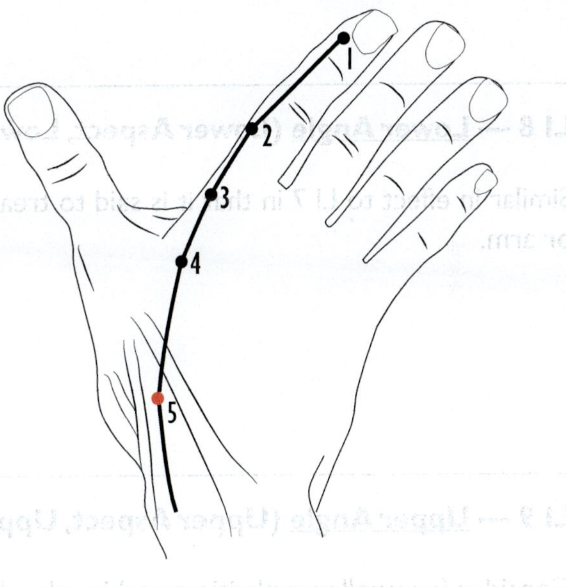

Large Intestine

LI 6 — <u>Side Passage</u> (Deflected Passage, Page of History, Slanting Passage)
Junction point. "Mental Tone" Point.

Consider for problems such as retention of urine or faeces, or where a person is holding on to feelings (such as long-standing grief or repressed emotions) no longer relevant to the present time. This point can help the patient to let go of these and move on in their life. Can be used with Lu 7 or Lu 9 to bring greater harmony and balance to the Metal Element, both mentally and spiritually. Helpful in cases of extreme behavioural patterns or mental confusion. Patients can be dirty or unkempt or, conversely, overly obsessive about cleanliness. Consider for wrist and forearm pain.

LI 7 — <u>Warm Current</u> (Warm Flow)
Accumulation point

This point can be used to warm a Metal CF who is physically or emotionally cold, inert, withdrawn or despairing, and it can take a lot of moxa — up to 30. It is said to treat madness, the seeing of ghosts, mania and hysteria. It nourishes, strengthens and invigorates the meridian. Consider for acute conditions associated with this Official.

LI 8 — <u>Lower Angle</u> (Lower Aspect, Lower Ridge)

Similar in effect to LI 7 in that it is said to treat mania and hysteria. Consider for pain in the elbow or arm.

LI 9 — <u>Upper Angle</u> (Upper Aspect, Upper Ridge)

Consider for swollen, arthritic or aching shoulder or arm. For loss of sensation in the limbs or cold and numb feelings in the bones. If this point is spontaneously tender it means you've probably got 'Brain Fatigue', i.e. the body's way of telling you to slow down!

⊥	△		Location
3	5-7	Ulna aspect of the radius **3 cun** proximal to LI 5 On the intersection formed by the ulna side of the radius and the seam of the extensor pollicis brevis and abductor pollicis longus muscles. Waggle thumb and feel between muscle and bone	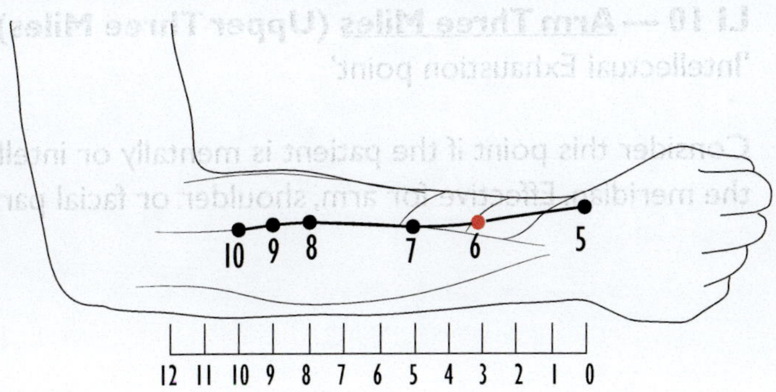
3	5-30	**5 cun** proximal to LI 5 Between the extensor digitorum and extensor carpi radialis muscles To expose this seam flex and extend the digits. Keep wrist stiffand move fingers	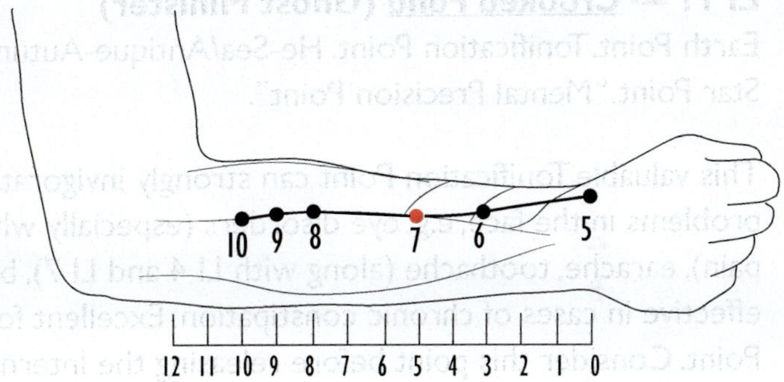
4	6	**8 cun** from LI 5 In the seam between extensor digitorum and extensor carpi radialis Mark the point with the arm at 90° across body	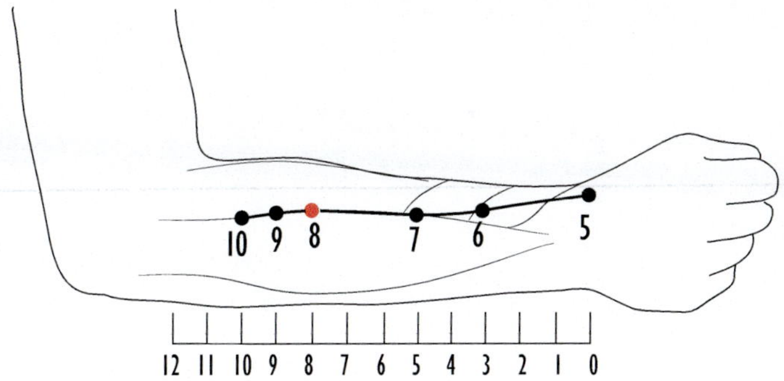
4	5-10	**9 cun** from LI5 In the seam between extensor digitorum and extensor carpi radialis Mark the point with the arm at 90° across body	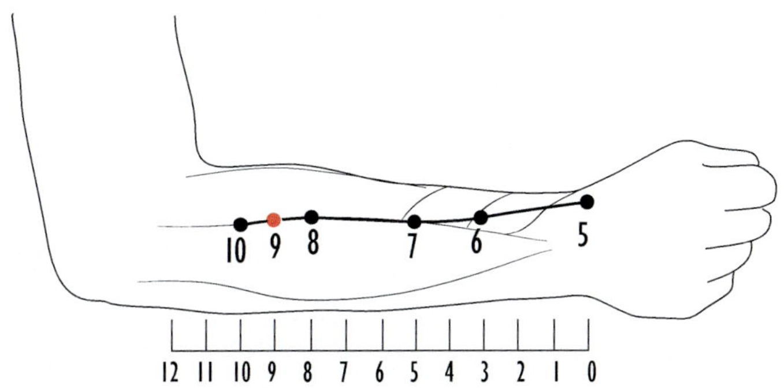

Large Intestine

LI 10 — <u>Arm Three Miles</u> (Upper Three Miles)
'Intellectual Exhaustion point'

Consider this point if the patient is mentally or intellectually exhausted. It stimulates sluggish Qi in the meridian. Effective for arm, shoulder or facial paralysis as a result of a stroke.

LI 11 — <u>Crooked Pond</u> (Ghost Minister)
Earth Point. Tonification Point. He-Sea/Antique-Autumn Point. Ghost Point. A Ma Danyang Heavenly Star Point. "Mental Precision Point".

This valuable Tonification Point can strongly invigorate the meridian. It can be considered for problems in the face, e.g. eye disorders (especially when accompanied by extreme redness and pain), earache, toothache (along with LI 4 and LI 7), bronchitis and hay fever. This point may be effective in cases of chronic constipation. Excellent for bringing stability to the LI — it's the Earth Point. Consider this point before releasing the Internal Dragons if a degree of possession is suspected (it is a Ghost Point). For problems of the shoulder, upper arm and forearm.

⊥	Δ		Location
5	5-10	Forbidden from 9th month of pregnancy **10 cun** from LI 5 In the seam between extensor digitorum and extensor carpi radialis Mark the point with the arm at 90° across body	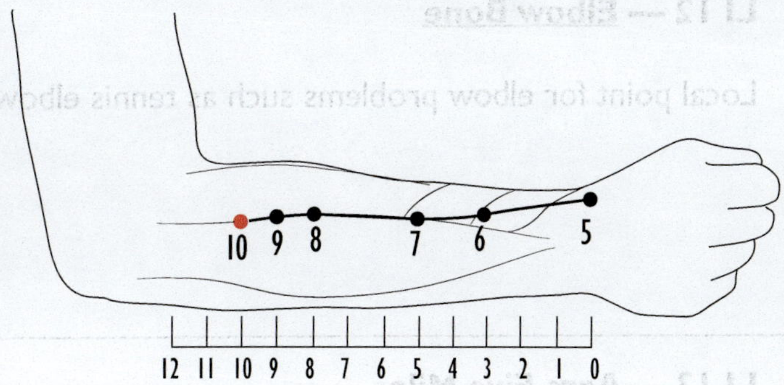
5-8	5-10	Halfway between the lateral edge of the tendon of the biceps brachii muscle and the lateral epicondyle of the humerus Towards the lateral edge of the transverse Cubital crease when flexed Mark the point with the arm at 90° across body	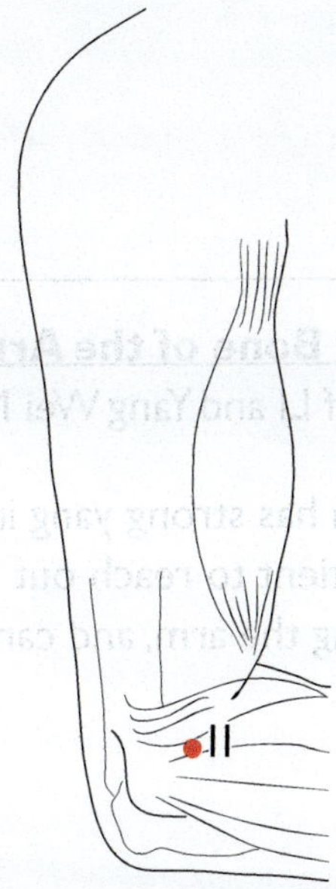

Large Intestine

LI 12 — <u>Elbow Bone</u>

Local point for elbow problems such as tennis elbow.

LI 13 — <u>Arm Five Miles</u>

Local point for elbow problems or for pain along the channel.

LI 14 — <u>Outer Bone of the Arm</u> (Thoroughfare to the Head)
Crossing Point of LI and Yang Wei Mai

This point, which has strong yang influences, can help with mental clarity and expansiveness, and can allow the patient to reach out for inspiration. Local point for arm and shoulder problems, e.g. difficulty in raising the arm, and can be used with LI 15, LI 16 and TH 14 for this.

LI 15 — <u>Shoulder Joint</u>
Crossing point of LI and Yang Qiao Mai (Heel Vessel). First Aid: Shock.

This point connects to the head, neck, brain and spine along with Du 14 and St 12, and as such is effective for mental clarity and for invigorating the system. Often used for problems of the upper arm and shoulders. Consider Moxa here for a frozen shoulder. For excessive sweating, particularly under the arm. Beneficial when the system has been shocked or concussed.

⊥	Δ		Location
3	3	Superior to lateral epicondyle of humerus **1 cun** proximal to LI 11 on the lateral border of the humerus Anterior border of the triceps brachii muscle, when arm is at 90° across body	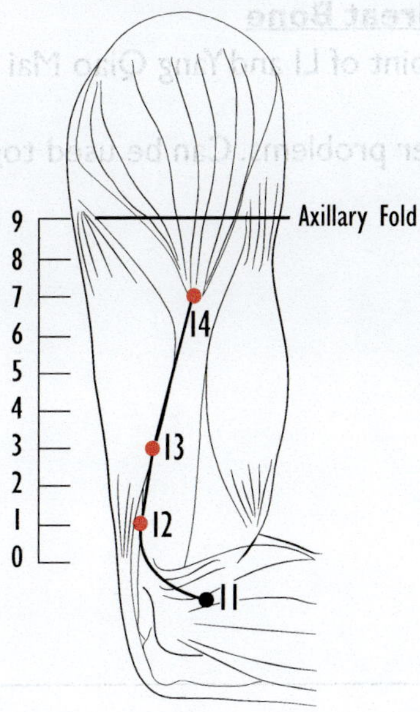
X	7	Superior to lateral epicondyle of humerus On the line joining LI 11 and LI 15 **3 cun** proximal to LI 11 on the lateral border of the humerus Between anterior border of the triceps brachii muscle and the lateral border of the humerus when arm is at 90° across body	
3	3-7	Superior to the lateral epicondyle of the humerus On a line joining LI 11 and LI 15 Approx **7 cun** proximal to flexure of elbow at LI 11 At the intersection ('V') of the deltoid into the humerus	
6	7	Lateral aspect of shoulder Inferior to the Acromion Between Acromion process of scapular bone and greater tuberosity of the humerus At the centre of the upper portion of the deltoid muscle	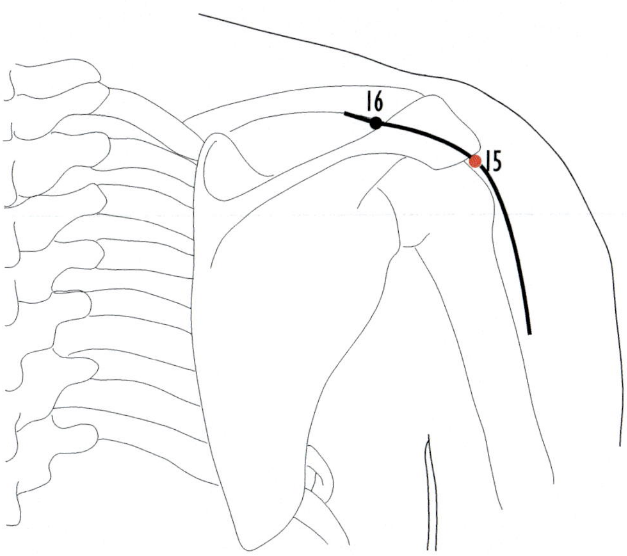

LI 16 — Great Bone

Crossing point of LI and Yang Qiao Mai (Heel Vessel)

For shoulder problems. Can be used together with LI 15. Consider using Moxa here.

LI 17 — Heavenly Vessel

This is a powerful Spirit point, similar in effect to a Window of the Sky. Brings clarity to the Mind and Spirit, especially if a patient is overwhelmed by sadness or grief. It can help a person to let go of grief, loss or sadness so that they may move on in life.

⊥	Δ		Location
6	3-7	Superior aspect of shoulder In the depression between the acromial extremity of clavicle and the scapular spine	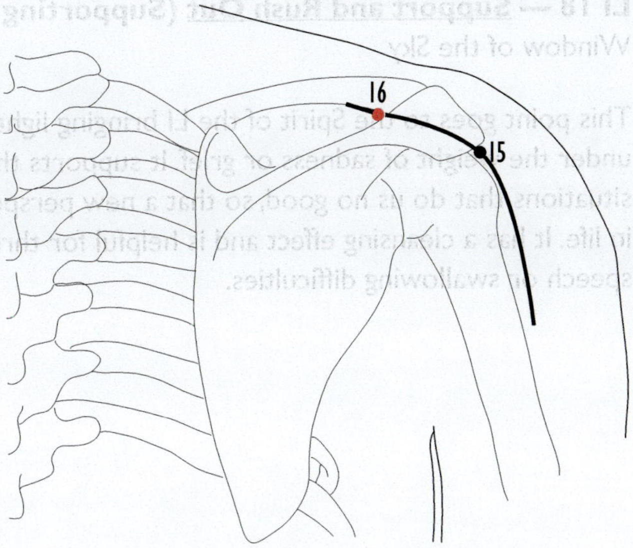
3	3-7	Just below the level of the prominence of the laryngeal cartilage On the posterior border of the clavicular head of the sternocleidomastoid muscle Approx **1 cun** inferior to LI 18	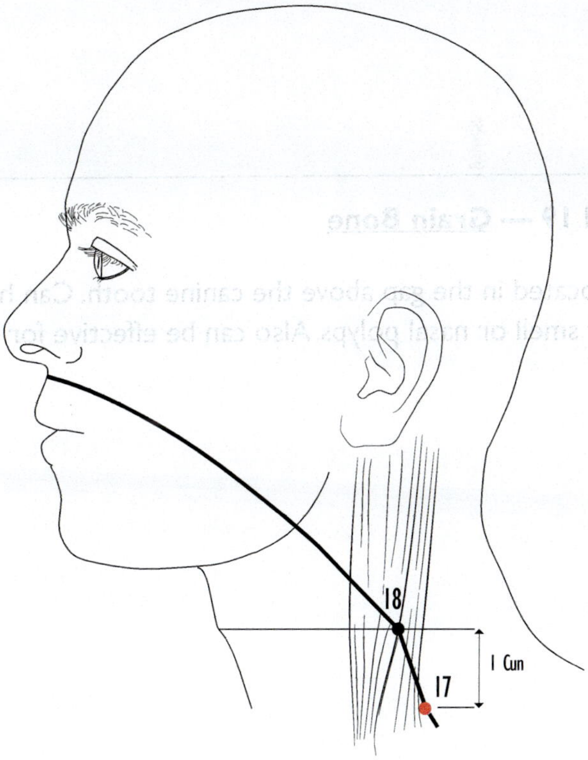

Large Intestine

LI 18 — <u>Support and Rush Out</u> (Supporting Process, Support the Prominence)
Window of the Sky

This point goes to the Spirit of the LI bringing light, clarity and perspective to a patient suffering under the weight of sadness or grief. It supports the LI's process of 'letting go' of thoughts and situations that do us no good, so that a new perspective may come in and the patient can move on in life. It has a cleansing effect and is helpful for throat problems such as excessive mucous, cough, speech or swallowing difficulties.

LI 19 — <u>Grain Bone</u>

Located in the gap above the canine tooth. Can help with nasal problems, rhinitis, loss of the sense of smell or nasal polyps. Also can be effective for local dental problems or facial paralysis.

⊥	Δ		Location
4	3	In the seam between the sternal and clavicular heads of the sternocleidomastoid muscle At the level of the prominence of the laryngeal cartilage Approx **1 cun** superior to LI 17	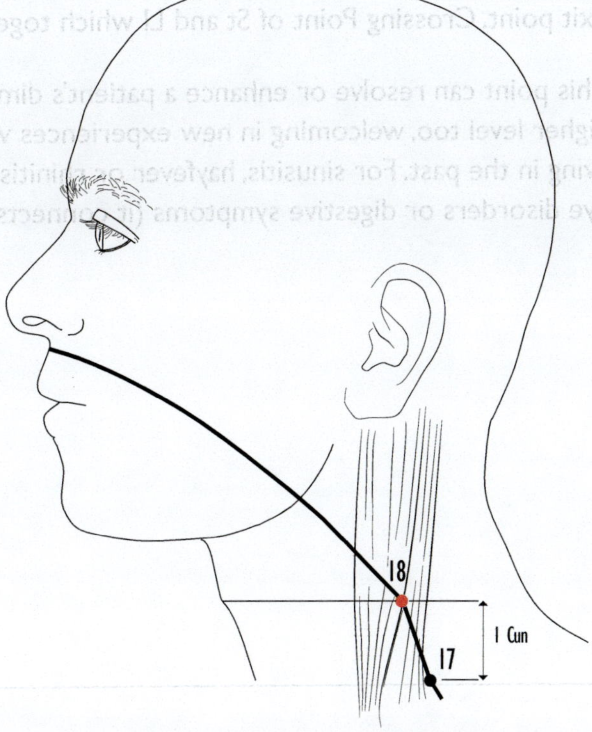
1-3	X	Directly inferior to the lateral margin of the nostril Level with and **0.5 cun** lateral to Du 26 (2/3 way up from lip at midline under nose)	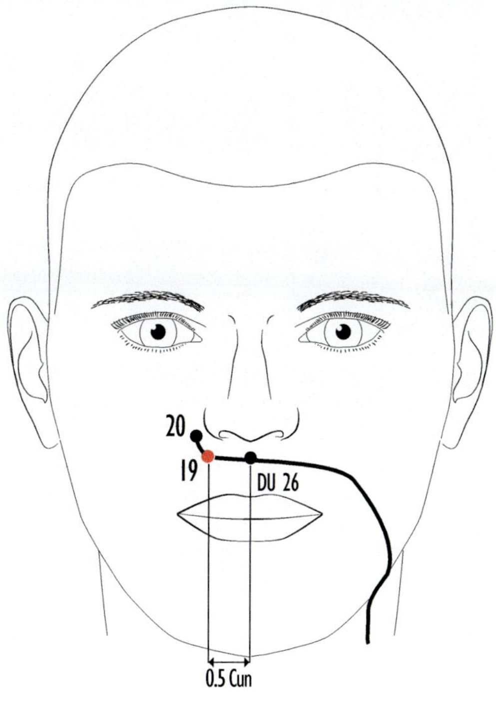

Large Intestine

LI 20 — <u>Welcome Fragrance</u> (Receiving Fragrance)
Exit point. Crossing Point of St and LI which together form the 'Yang Ming' channel.

This point can resolve or enhance a patient's diminishing sense of smell. It is said to work on a higher level too, welcoming in new experiences whilst enabling a person to recall old ones without living in the past. For sinusitis, hayfever or rhinitis. Consider for facial paralysis, trigeminal neuralgia, eye disorders or digestive symptoms (it connects to St).

⊥	△		Location
1-3	X	Level with lateral part of the nasal wing of the nostril In the nasolabial groove — laughter line Superior to the root of the canine tooth	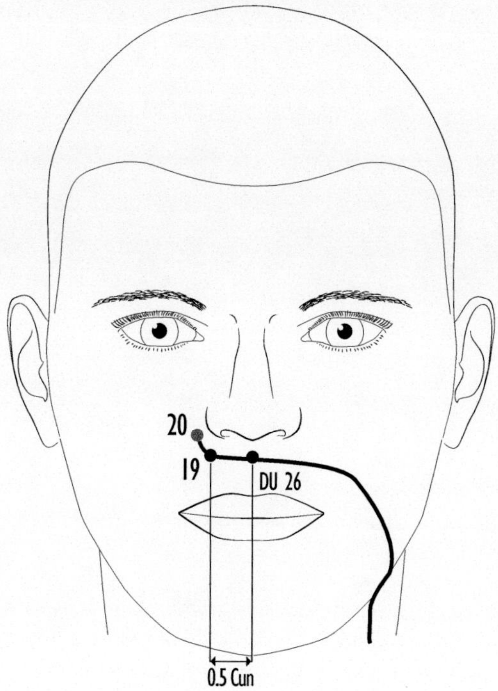

Stomach

- **The Official in Charge of Rotting and Ripening**
- **Earth governs the flesh, lips and mouth and the ability to taste things**
- **Earth confers the ability to give and receive sympathy**

Stomach

St 1 — <u>Receive Tears</u> (Containing Tears, Weeping Support)
Entry point. Crossing Point of St, Yang Qiao Mai (Heel Vessel) and Ren Mai.

This is the start of the meridian which is concerned with receiving and digesting things — food, drink, information, feelings. This point can help a person move on in their life if they are stuck mentally or emotionally, particularly with overthinking. For eye disorders such as conjunctivitis, myopia, the early stages of cataracts or glaucoma.

St 2 — <u>Four Whites</u> (Grain Gate)
Sometimes used as a secondary Entry Point to avoid bruising. Point of Yang Qiao Mai (Heel Vessel). Shokanten Point.

Consider for orbital neuralgia, feeling of smoke in the eyes, poor distant vision, trigeminal neuralgia, sinusitis, rhinitis or facial paralysis. Its alternative name of Grain Gate refers to the mouth which is the 'Gate of the Stomach' (stoma, a Greek word, also means "the mouth").

⊥	Δ		Location
1-3	X	Inferior to the centre of the pupil with the eyes looking straight ahead Between the eyeball and the infraorbital margin formed by the zygomatic bone and the maxilla bone Superior to the zygomatic notch	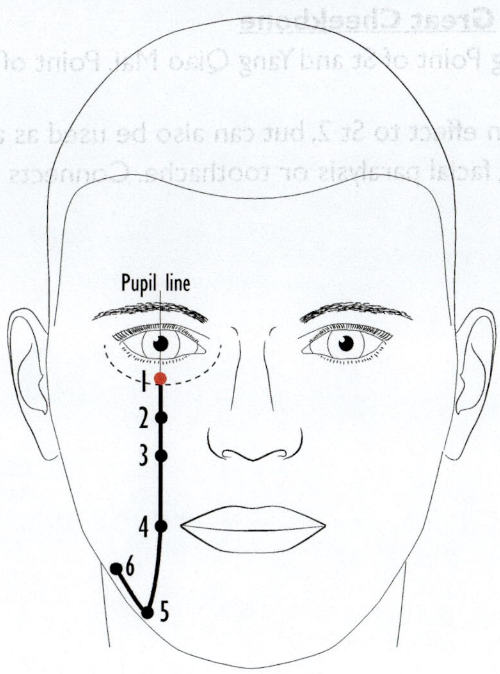
1-3	3	In the infraorbital foramen of the maxilla bone Inferior to St 1 Traditionally **1 cun** below the centre of the pupil	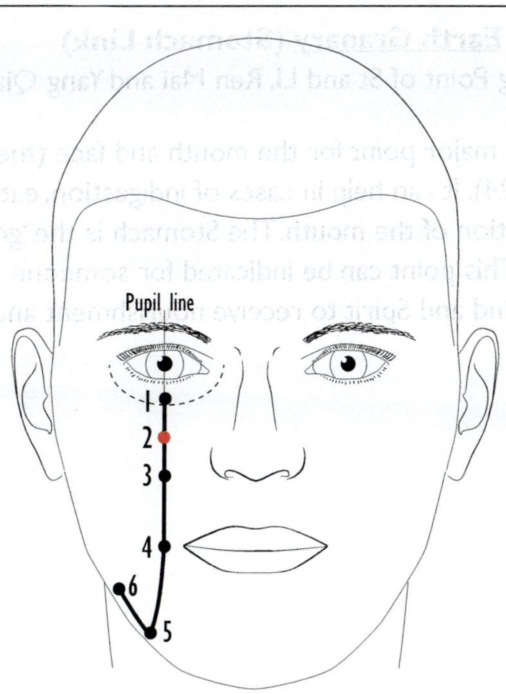

Stomach

St 3 — <u>Great Cheekbone</u>

Crossing Point of St and Yang Qiao Mai. Point of Yang Qiao Mai (Heel Vessel).

Similar in effect to St 2, but can also be used as a local point for a swollen jaw, spasm of the facial muscles, facial paralysis or toothache. Connects to Du 26 and encircles the mouth.

St 4 — <u>Earth Granary</u> (Stomach Link)

Crossing Point of St and LI, Ren Mai and Yang Qiao Mai (Heel Vessel)

This is a major point for the mouth and face (the deep pathway encircles the mouth and connects to Ren 24). It can help in cases of indigestion, eating disorders, facial paralysis, trigeminal neuralgia or deviation of the mouth. The Stomach is the 'granary organ'; it receives and stores the Five Grains. This point can be indicated for someone who has no sense of their own harvest; helps the Body, Mind and Spirit to receive nourishment and satisfaction.

⊥	Δ		Location
1-3	5	On the maxilla bone Directly inferior to the centre of the pupil Level with the inferior border of the nostrils	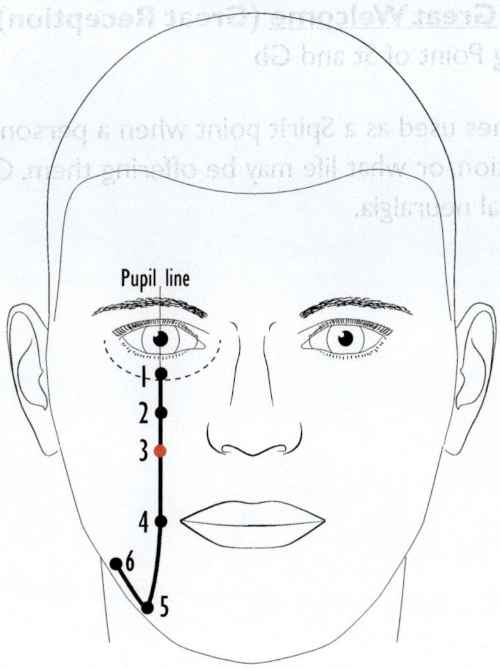
1-3	5	Forbidden from 5th month of pregnancy On the maxilla bone Directly inferior to the centre of the pupil Level with the corner of the mouth Traditionally **0.4 cun** lateral to the corner of the mouth	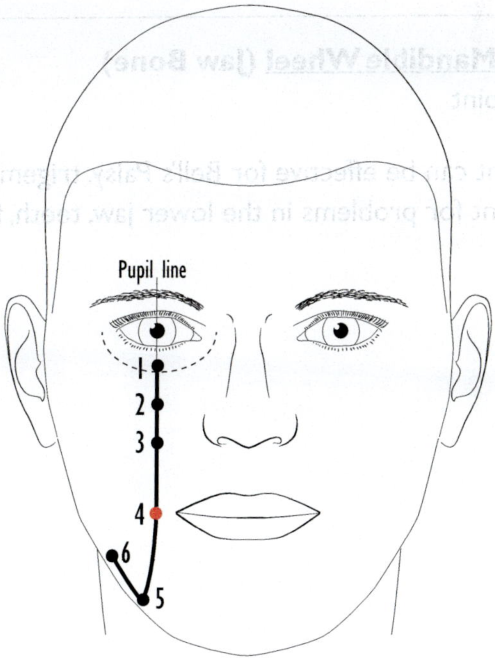

St 5 — Great Welcome (Great Reception)
Crossing Point of St and Gb

Sometimes used as a Spirit point when a person is closed off and unable to receive nourishment, information, or what life may be offering them. Consider for pain in the jaw, frequent yawning or trigeminal neuralgia.

St 6 — Mandible Wheel (Jaw Bone)
Ghost Point

This point can be effective for Bell's Palsy, trigeminal neuralgia or neuralgia of the face. Used as a local point for problems in the lower jaw, teeth, face, neck or throat.

⊥	Δ		Location
3-5	3-5	On the mandible bone In the groove on the anterior border of the masseter muscle when the teeth are clenched	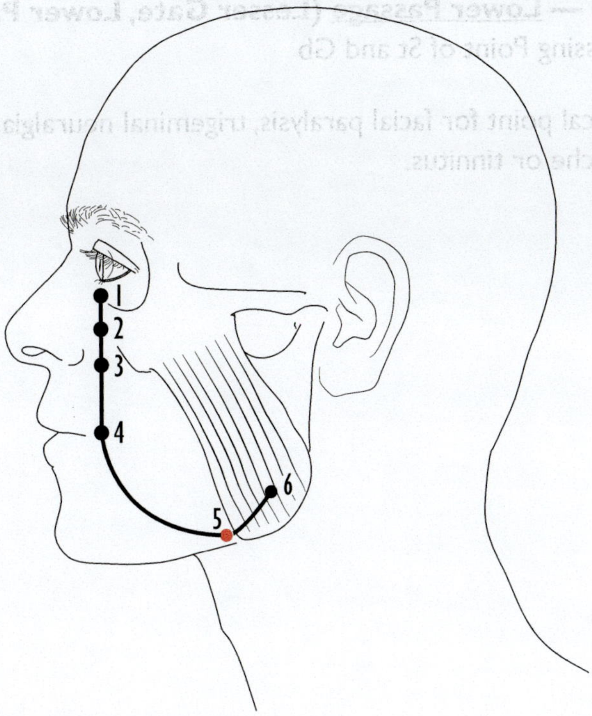
3	7	On the mandible bone On the prominence of the masseter muscle when the teeth are clenched One finger width or **0.8 cun** anterior and superior to the angle of the mandible bone	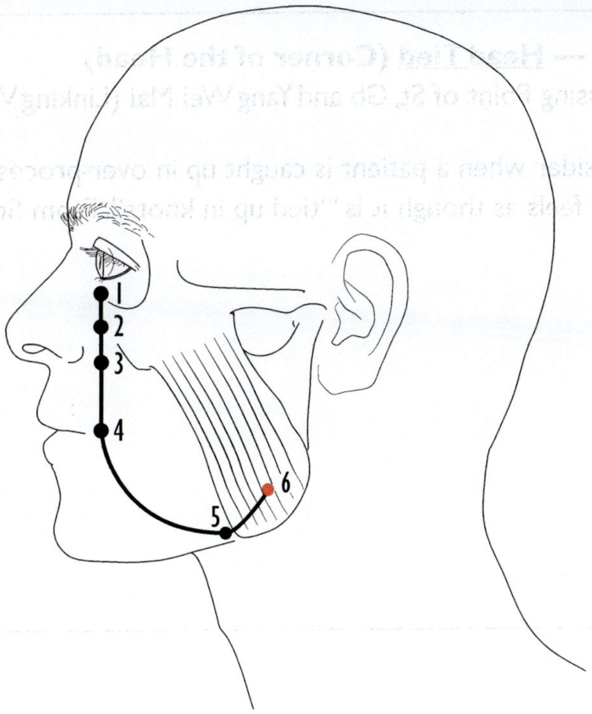

Stomach

St 7 — Lower Passage (Lesser Gate, Lower Pass)
Crossing Point of St and Gb

A local point for facial paralysis, trigeminal neuralgia, jaw or ear problems such as otitis, deafness, earache or tinnitus.

St 8 — Head Tied (Corner of the Head)
Crossing Point of St, Gb and Yang Wei Mai (Linking Vessel)

Consider when a patient is caught up in over-processing, overthinking, mental turmoil or where the head feels as though it is "'tied up in knots". From St 8 there is a deep pathway to Du 24.

⊥	Δ		Location
3	X	Inferior to the zygomatic arch of the temporal bone Anterior to the condyle of the mandible bone (when the mouth is closed) Directly superior to St 6	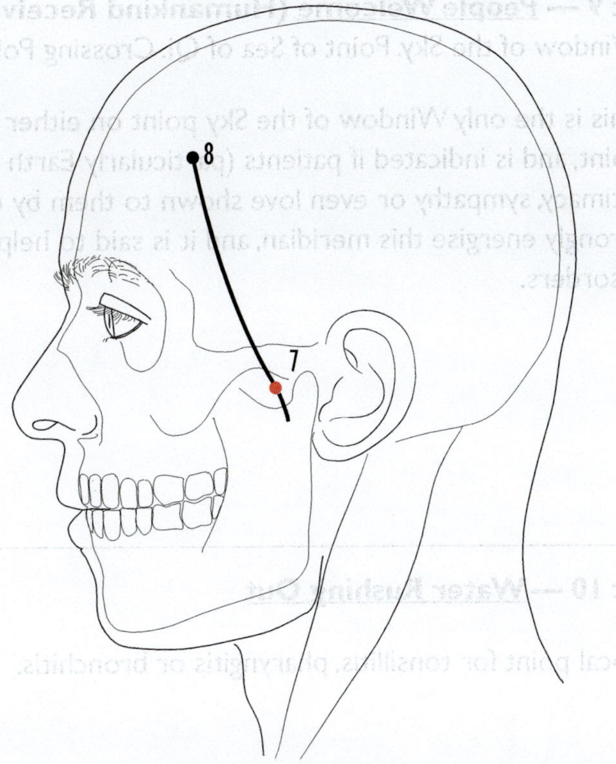
3	X	At the corner of the forehead On a vertical line directly superior to the lateral canthus of the eye **0.5 cun** posterior to the natural anterior hair line **4.5 cun** lateral to the anterior median line	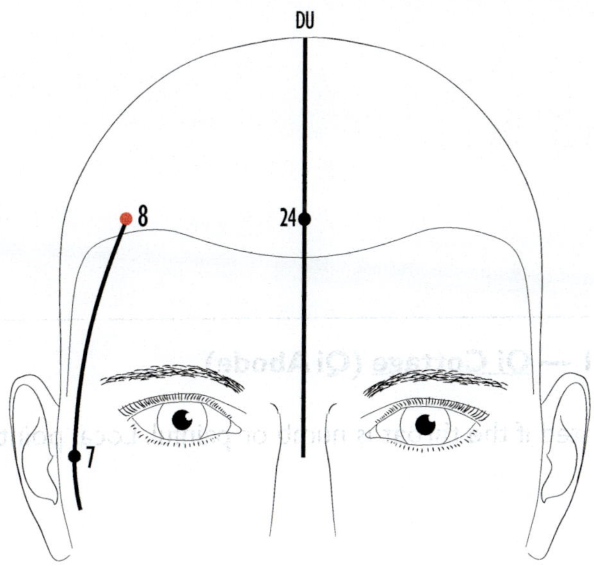

Stomach

St 9 — <u>People Welcome</u> (Humankind Receiving)
Window of the Sky. Point of Sea of Qi. Crossing Point of St and Gb.

This is the only Window of the Sky point on either of the two Earth Officials. St 9 is a powerful point, and is indicated if patients (particularly Earth CF's) have difficulty in accepting the concern, intimacy, sympathy or even love shown to them by other people. As a point of the Sea of Qi it can strongly energise this meridian, and it is said to help regulate blood pressure. Local point for throat disorders.

St 10 — <u>Water Rushing Out</u>

Local point for tonsillitis, pharyngitis or bronchitis.

St 11 — <u>Qi Cottage</u> (Qi Abode)

Indicated if the throat is numb or painful. Local point for cough.

⊥	Δ		Location
1-3	X	Anterior border of sternocleidomastoid muscle (SCM) In the seam between the sternal head of the SCM and the prominence of the laryngeal cartilage Approximately at level of prominence of the laryngeal cartilage	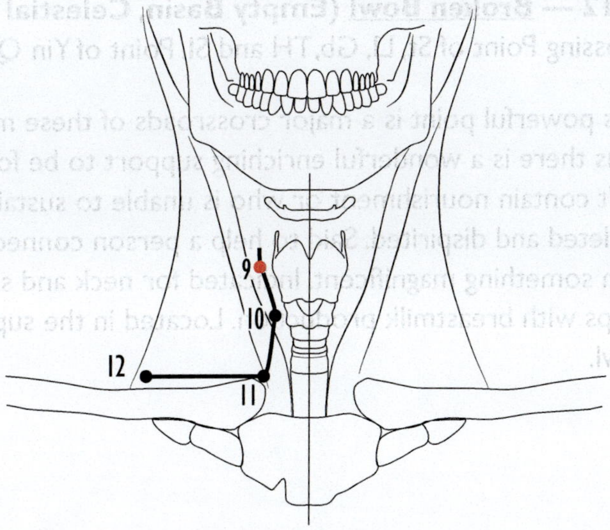
1-3	X	In the seam between the sternal head of the SCM muscle and the cricoid cartilage At the level of the cricoid cartilage Midway between St 9 and St 11	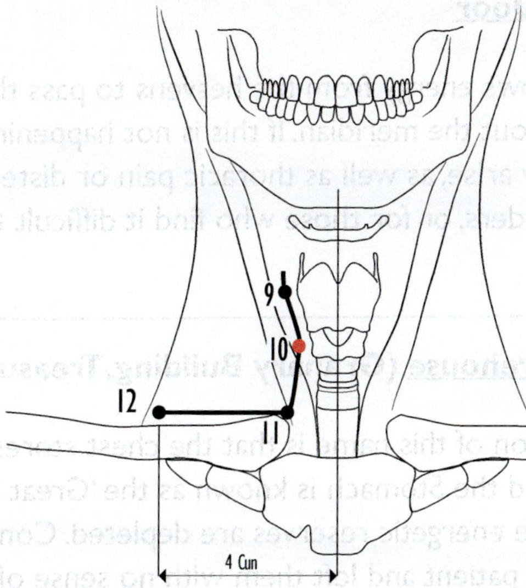
3	3	Anterior aspect of neck — at the root of the neck Superior border of sternal end of the clavicle Between the sternal and clavicular heads of the SCM	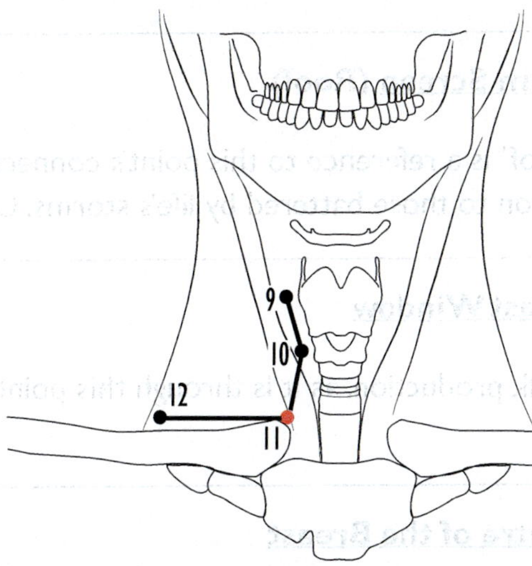

Stomach

St 12 — Broken Bowl (Empty Basin, Celestial Cover)
Crossing Point of St, LI, Gb, TH and SI. Point of Yin Qiao Mai (Heel Vessel)

This powerful point is a major crossroads of these meridians on their deep pathway journeys. Thus there is a wonderful enriching support to be found here, so consider for a patient who can't contain nourishment or who is unable to sustain themselves, and as a result becomes very depleted and dispirited. Said to help a person connect with their higher self, and thus be filled with something magnificent. Indicated for neck and shoulder pain, or for chest or throat problems. Helps with breastmilk production. Located in the supraclavicular notch, giving the impression of a bowl.

St 13 — Qi Door

This Door allows energy from the heavens to pass through to the Lungs. It allows Qi to flow freely throughout the meridian. If this is not happening, respiratory disorders such as asthma or bronchitis may arise, as well as thoracic pain or distension of the chest. Consider for chronic digestive disorders, or for those who find it difficult to receive sympathetic concern from others.

St 14 — Storehouse (Granary Building, Treasury Room)

One explanation of this name is that the chest stores or contains the Heart and Lungs. The breast stores milk, and the Stomach is known as the 'Great Storehouse'. Here is a point one can call upon when the energetic reserves are depleted. Consider when overthinking or overwork has exhausted the patient and left them with no sense of harvest in life.

St 15 — Room Screen (Roof)

The name 'Roof' is a reference to this point's connection with the Lungs (also called a canopy), giving protection to those battered by life's storms. Consider for respiratory disorders.

St 16 — Breast Window

Helpful for milk production, as it is through this point that Qi and milk pass into the breast.

St 17 — Centre of the Breast

Moxa and Needle Forbidden

⊥	Δ		Location
3	3	Anterior aspect of shoulder Superior to clavicle bone In the centre of the supraclavicular fossa In a palpable notch (inwards) **4 cun** lateral to anterior median line (Ren Mai)	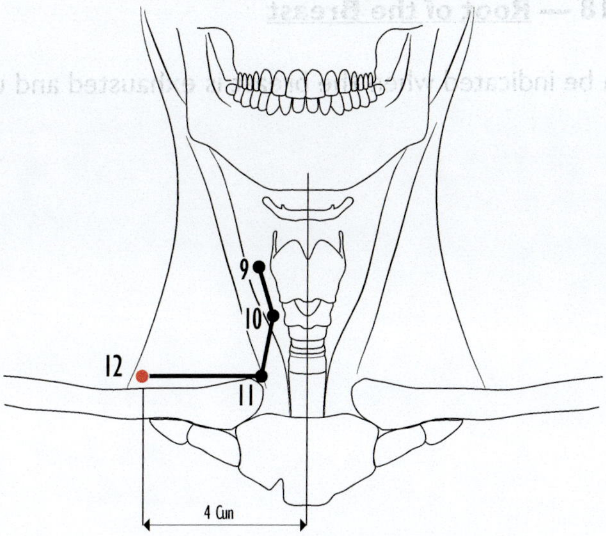
3	5	Just inferior to the clavicle in a palpable notch On the pectoralis major muscle Directly inferior to St 12 **4 cun** lateral to anterior median line (Ren Mai)	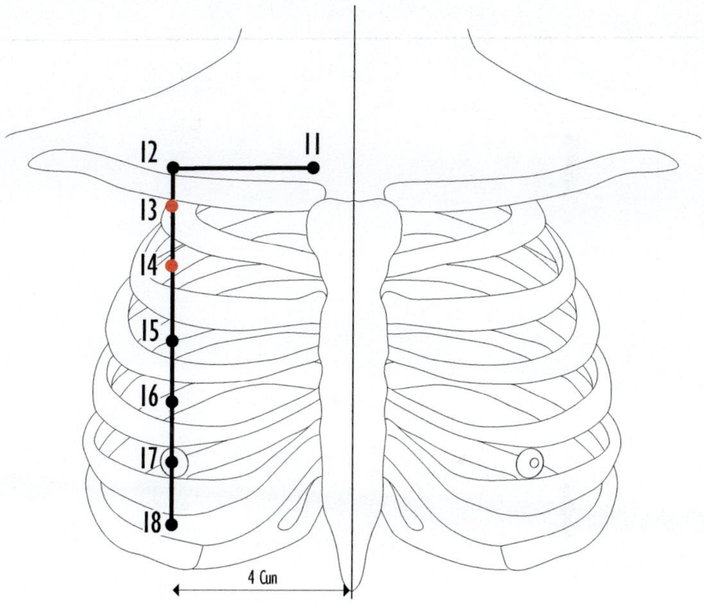
3	5	Inferior to the clavicle On the pectoralis major muscle, In the **1st IC Space** **4 cun** lateral to anterior median line (Ren Mai)	
3	5	On the pectoralis major muscle, In the **2nd IC Space** **4 cun** lateral to anterior median line (Ren Mai)	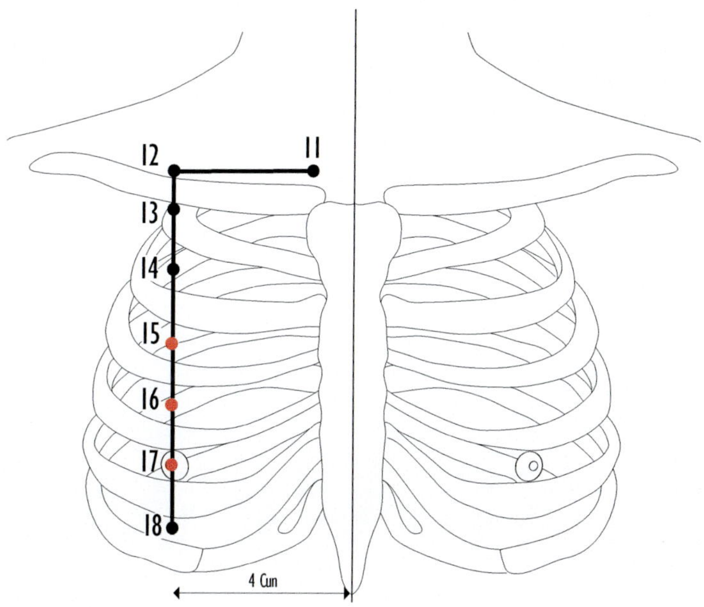
3	5	On the pectoralis major muscle, in the **3rd IC Space** **4 cun** lateral to anterior median line (Ren Mai)	
X	X	In the centre of the nipple	

Stomach

St 18 — Root of the Breast

Can be indicated when the breast is exhausted and unable to produce sufficient milk.

⊥	△		Location
3	3-5	In the 5th **IC Space** **4 cun** lateral to anterior median line (Ren Mai)	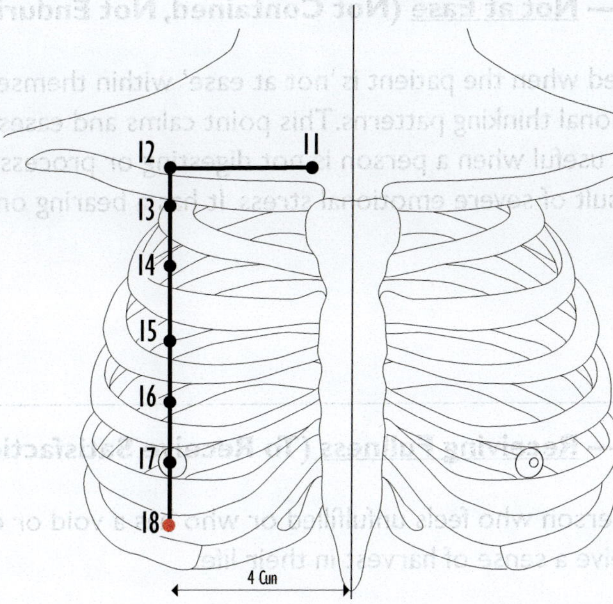

Stomach

St 19 — <u>Not at Ease</u> (Not Contained, Not Enduring)

Indicated when the patient is 'not at ease' within themselves, and is tied up with worry or with obsessional thinking patterns. This point calms and eases an anxious and insecure patient. It can also be useful when a person is not digesting or processing their food and drink properly, perhaps as a result of severe emotional stress. It has a bearing on the rhythms of life.

St 20 — <u>Receiving Fullness</u> (To Receive Satisfaction)

For a person who feels unfulfilled or who has a void or emptiness within, and as a result is unable to receive a sense of harvest in their life.

St 21 — <u>Bridge Gate</u> (Connecting Gate, Beam Gate)

If this 'Gate' is closed, a person can find it difficult to digest or assimilate things either physically or mentally. This point can help with the digestion of food and also with 'stuck in the mud' thinking processes where integration of the BMS is proving difficult. This is particularly relevant in times of transition in a person's life. Often used with St 22 and St 24. This point is on a level with Ren 12 (Alarm Point of St).

St 22 — <u>Border Gate</u>

The three gates (St 21, St 22, St 24) help regulate the St Official and are said to encourage physical, mental and spiritual digestion.

⊥	Δ		Location
5	3-7	On the lateral border of the rectus abdominis muscle **2 cun** lateral to the anterior median line **6 cun** superior to the level of the centre of the umbilicus Level with Ren 14	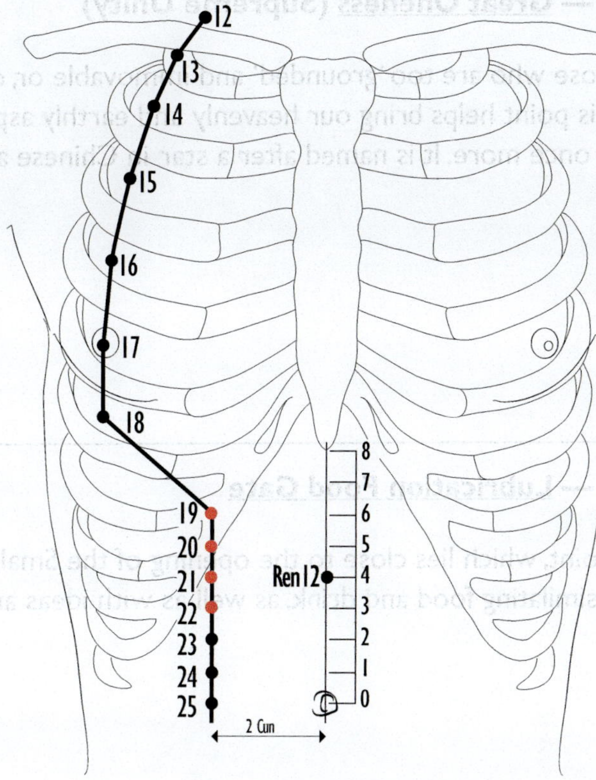
5	3-7	On the lateral border of the rectus abdominis muscle **2 cun** lateral to the anterior median line **5 cun** superior to the level of the centre of the umbilicus Level with Ren 13	
7	5-15	On the lateral border of the rectus abdominis muscle **2 cun** lateral to the anterior median line **4 cun** superior to the level of the centre of the umbilicus Level with Ren 12	
8	5-15	On the lateral border of the rectus abdominis muscle **2 cun** lateral to the anterior median line **3 cun** superior to the level of the centre of the umbilicus **5 cun** inferior to the level of the xiphisternal joint Level with Ren 11	

Stomach

St 23 — Great Oneness (Supreme Unity)

For those who are too 'grounded' and immovable or, conversely, are insecure or feel no harvest in life. This point helps bring our heavenly and earthly aspects together, so we can feel integrated and whole once more. It is named after a star in Chinese astrology that relates to the abdomen.

St 24 — Lubrication Food Gate

This point, which lies close to the opening of the Small Intestine, helps with digesting, processing and assimilating food and drink, as well as with ideas and information. Can be combined with Sp 16.

St 25 — Heavenly Pivot (Celestial Pivot. This point has at least nine other names**)**
Front mu/Alarm Point for LI. Point to Release the Internal Dragons. Shokanten Point.

This important point is at the centre of one's being — above is heaven, below is earth. It's the central pivot of our heavenly and earthly Qi. It is also the name of the central star in the northern Big Dipper (aka the Plough) — the other six stars rotate around it. Great for Earthing a person who is experiencing a lot of ups and downs, mood swings, mania, anxiety or mental instability. Said to be helpful for women who are preoccupied with gynaecological problems such as conception, infertility, or are experiencing menstrual disorders. Often paired with Sp 15 in order to enhance its stabilising action. Its name is recorded in a manuscript from the 1st century BCE.

St 26 — Outside Mound

Local point for pain around the umbilicus or for intestinal spasm

⊥	Δ		Location
8	5-10	On the lateral border of the rectus abdominis muscle **2 cun** lateral to the anterior median line **2 cun** superior to the level of the centre of the umbilicus Level with Ren 10	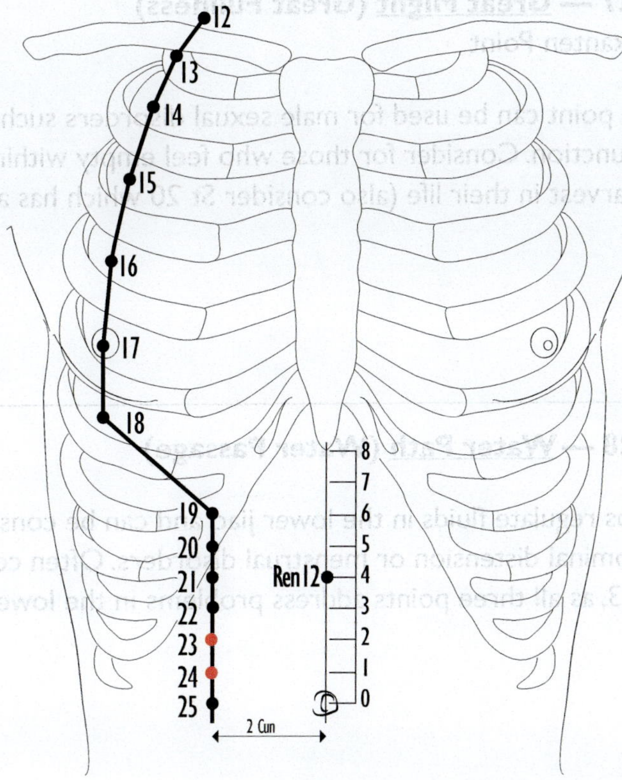
8	5-15	On the lateral border of the rectus abdominis muscle **2 cun** lateral to the anterior median line **1 cun** superior to the level of the centre of the umbilicus Level with Ren 9	
5	5-20	On the lateral border of the rectus abdominis muscle **2 cun** lateral to the anterior median line Level of the centre of the umbilicus **8 cun** inferior to the level of the xiphisternal joint Level with Ren 8	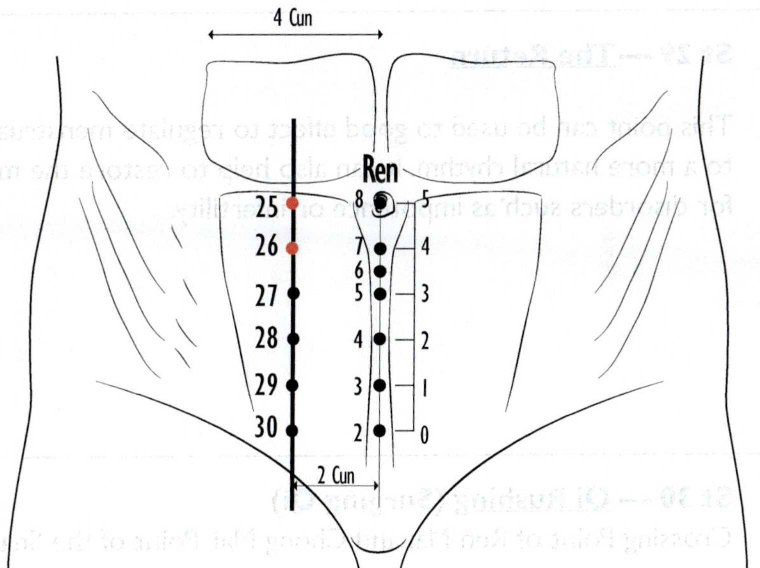
8-10	5	On the lateral border of the rectus abdominis muscle **2 cun** lateral to the anterior median line **1 cun** inferior to the level of the centre of the umbilicus Level with Ren 7	

Stomach

St 27 — <u>Great Might</u> (Great Fullness)
Shokanten Point

This point can be used for male sexual disorders such as premature ejaculation or erectile dysfunction. Consider for those who feel empty within and who are unable to experience a sense of harvest in their life (also consider St 20 which has a similar effect).

St 28 — <u>Water Path</u> (Water Passage)

Helps regulate fluids in the lower jiao and can be considered for retention of urine, lower abdominal distension or menstrual disorders. Often combined with Ren 4 and sometimes with Sp 13, as all three points address problems in the lower jiao.

St 29 — <u>The Return</u>

This point can be used to good effect to regulate menstruation so that the cycle may be returned to a more natural rhythm. It can also help to restore the male and female reproductive functions for disorders such as impotence or infertility.

St 30 — <u>Qi Rushing</u> (Surging Qi)
Crossing Point of Ren Mai and Chong Mai. Point of the Sea of Nourishment.

This powerful point can help with genital and sexual disorders such as infertility and impotence. Often combined with St 36 (which together form the Sea of Nourishment) and which can be wonderful for nourishing the Body and Mind where there has been a history of chronic malnutrition.

⊥	△		Location
8-10	5-10	On the lateral border of the rectus abdominis muscle **2 cun** lateral to the anterior median line **2 cun** inferior to the level of the centre of the umbilicus Level with Ren 5	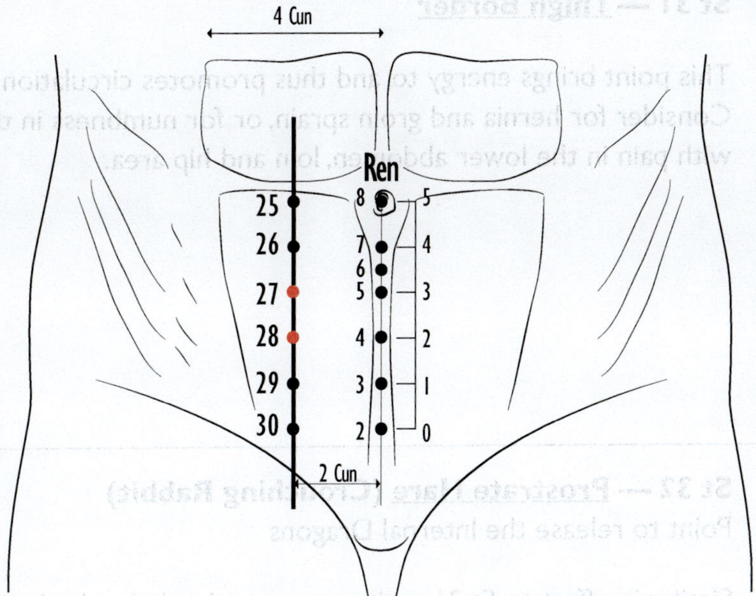
8	5-10	On the lateral border of the rectus abdominis muscle **2 cun** lateral to the anterior median line **3 cun** inferior to the level of the centre of the umbilicus Level with Ren 4	
5	5-10	On the lateral border of the rectus abdominis muscle **2 cun** lateral to the anterior median line **4 cun** inferior to the level of the centre of the umbilicus Level with Ren 3	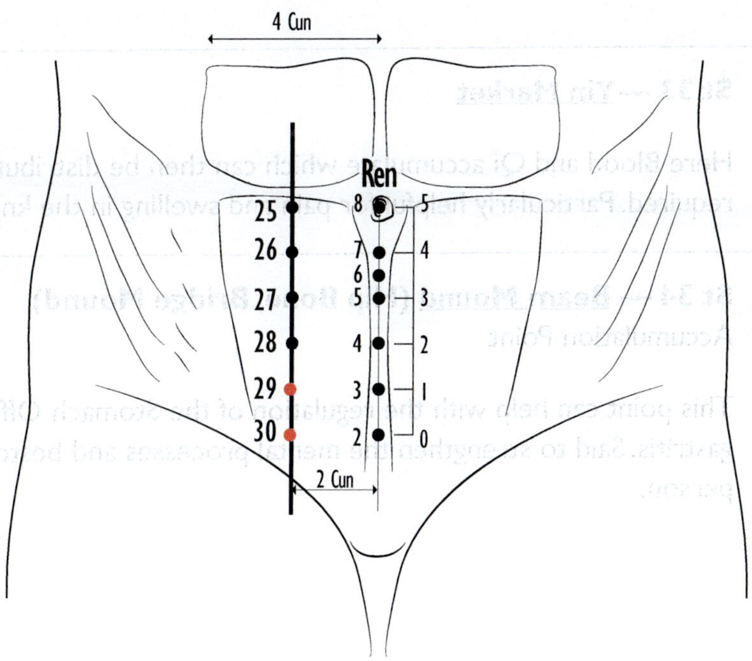
3	7	On the lateral border of the rectus abdominis muscle **2 cun** lateral to the anterior median line **5 cun** inferior to the level of the centre of the umbilicus Level with Ren 2	

Stomach

St 31 — Thigh Border

This point brings energy to, and thus promotes circulation in the hip, groin and lower limbs. Consider for hernia and groin sprain, or for numbness in the lower limbs. Furthermore, it can help with pain in the lower abdomen, loin and hip area.

St 32 — Prostrate Hare (Crouching Rabbit)
Point to release the Internal Dragons

Similar in effect to St 31 — it promotes circulation in the lower limbs. The name derives from its anatomical location in an area which resembles a crouching hare with its ears lying along its back.

St 33 — Yin Market

Here Blood and Qi accumulate which can then be distributed, as in a Market, to wherever they are required. Particularly helpful for pain and swelling in the knee or pain in the lower back.

St 34 — Beam Mound (Hip Bone, Bridge Mound)
Accumulation Point

This point can help with the regulation of the Stomach Official in cases of hiccups, nausea and gastritis. Said to strengthen the mental processes and bestow a greater sense of perspective upon a person.

St 35 — Calf Nose (Knee Eye)

This point is indicated for knee problems and lower leg paralysis. The additional use of Moxa here can also be helpful for knee problems. Calf Nose is named after its resemblance to the animal's nostrils when the knee is bent.

⊥	Δ		Location
6	3-7	Anterior aspect of upper thigh On a line connecting the anterior superior iliac spine and the superolateral corner of the patella bone In the seam between the rectus femoris and vastus lateralis muscles Approx **14 cun** proximal to the popliteal crease	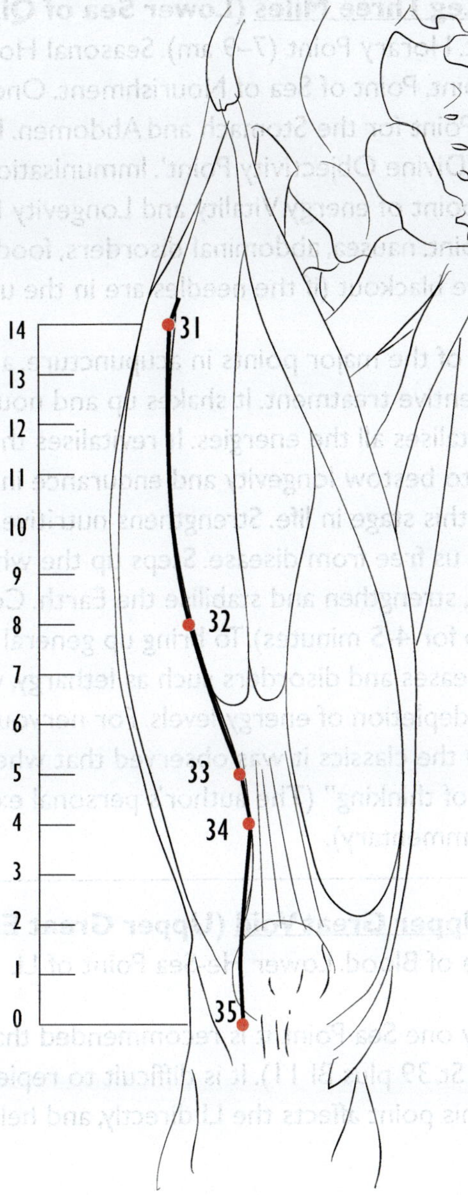
6	3-7	Anterior aspect of upper thigh On a line connecting the anterior superior iliac spine and the superolateral corner of the patella bone In the seam between the rectus femoris and vastus lateralis muscles Approx **8 cun** proximal to the popliteal crease	
4	3-5	**5 cun** proximal to the knee flexure Between the rectus femoris and the vastus lateralis muscles.	
4	3-5	Anterior aspect of upper thigh On a line connecting the anterior superior iliac spine and the superolateral corner of the patella bone In the seam between the rectus femoris and vastus lateralis Approx **4 cun** proximal to the popliteal crease	
3	3	On flexure of knee, inferolateral corner of patella Lateral border of patellar ligament	

St 36 — <u>Leg Three Miles</u> (Lower Sea of Qi, Lower Three Miles)
Earth Point. Horary Point (7–9 am). Seasonal Horary Point — Late Summer. He-Sea/Antique-Autumn Point. Point of Sea of Nourishment. One of nine needles for returning Yang. Greater Influential Point for the Stomach and Abdomen. Lower He-Sea Point of St. A Ma Danyang Heavenly Star Point. 'Divine Objectivity Point'. Immunisation Point (use Moxa daily). Centre Reunion Particular point of energy. Vitality and Longevity Point. Stimulates parathyroids.
First Aid point: nausea, abdominal disorders, food poisoning, travel sickness, morning sickness, acupuncture blackout (if the needles are in the upper body).

This is one of the major points in acupuncture, and can be considered for many illnesses as well as for preventive treatment. It shakes up and nourishes all the Officials. It is connected to all the Seas; it revitalises all the energies. It revitalises the entire Body and Mind. This point is restorative, and is said to bestow longevity and endurance in old age as well as being effective for declining eyesight at this stage in life. Strengthens nutritive and defensive Qi, and thus the immune system. Helps keep us free from disease. Steps up the white blood cell count when used with Moxa. Helps to enhance, strengthen and stabilise the Earth. Consider for nausea or abdominal disorders (press with thumb for 4-5 minutes). To bring up general energy levels, one can Moxa 7–20 times. For any 'lack of' diseases and disorders such as lethargy, weakness (especially after a long illness), coldness or chronic depletion of energy levels. For nervousness or extreme agitation. Helps to lower blood pressure. In the classics it was observed that when "Used after the age of 30, can change a person's whole way of thinking" (The author's personal experience of its effect accords with this Ming Dynasty commentary).

St 37 — <u>Upper Great Void</u> (Upper Great Emptiness)
Point of Sea of Blood. Lower He-Sea Point of LI.

If you tonify one Sea Point it is recommended that you tonify the others (i.e. all the Seas of Blood, in this case St 39 plus Bl 11). It is difficult to replenish the Sea of Nourishment if the Sea of Blood is deficient. This point affects the LI directly, and helps in cases of constipation or diarrhoea.

St 38 — <u>Branch Opening</u> (Narrow Opening)

This point can be used for stagnation or blockage in the Stomach meridian caused by this 'Branch Opening' being closed. It is also helpful for loss of sensation in the limbs (indicating the point is closed), general weakness of the legs, or for pain and stiffness in the shoulder joint.

⊥	Δ		Location
5-8	7-20	Forbidden from 8th month of pregnancy Anterolateral aspect of lower leg Lateral to anterior crest of tibia bone Inferior to inferior border of tibial tuberosity of tibia Approx **13 cun** proximal to prominence of lateral maleolus Approx **3 cun** below St 35 Approx **1 cun** inferior to the level of Gb 34	
5	3-7	Anterior aspect of lower leg Lateral to anterior crest of tibia bone Medial border of tibialis anterior muscle **10 cun** proximal to prominence of lateral maleolus	
5	3-7	Anterior aspect of lower leg Lateral to anterior crest of tibia bone Medial border of tibialis anterior muscle **8 cun** proximal to prominence of lateral maleolus	

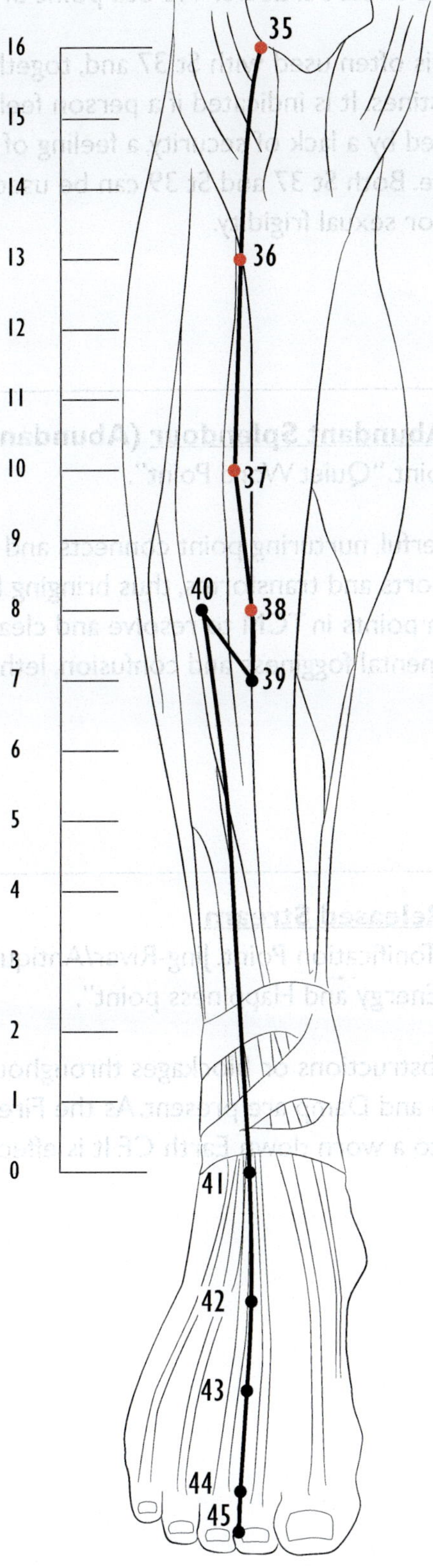

Stomach

St 39 — Lower Great Void (Lower Great Emptiness)
Point of Sea of Blood. Lower He-Sea point of SI.

This point is often used with St 37 and, together, they influence the functioning of the Small and Large Intestines. It is indicated if a person feels a void or emptiness within their being, often accompanied by a lack of security, a feeling of being unearthed or of being disconnected from their centre. Both St 37 and St 39 can be used together to promote conception and to help with emotional or sexual frigidity.

St 40 — Abundant Splendour (Abundant Prosperity, Rich and Prosperous)
Junction point. "Quiet Word Point".

This wonderful, nurturing point connects and enhances the Official who rots and ripens to the one that transports and transforms, thus bringing balance and harmony to the Earth Element. It is one of the main points in TCM to resolve and clear Damp and Phlegm from the system, and thus can help with mental fogginess and confusion, lethargy, poor memory, worry or obsessive thinking.

St 41 — Released Stream
Fire Point. Tonification Point. Jing-River/Antique-Late-Summer Point. Point to release the Internal Dragons. "Energy and Happiness point".

Releases obstructions or blockages throughout the length of the Stomach meridian, particularly when Cold and Damp are present. As the Fire point, it can help restore a sense of joy and happiness to a worn down Earth CF. It is effective for pain or arthritis in the ankle or foot.

⊥	Δ		Location
5	3-7	Anterior aspect of lower leg Lateral to anterior crest of tibia bone Medial border of tibialis anterior muscle **7 cun** proximal to prominence of lateral maleolus	
3	3-5	Anterior aspect of lower leg **8 cun** proximal to prominence of lateral maleolus Approx **1 cun** lateral to St 38, palpate for the lateral border of tibialis anterior muscle	
5	3-7	Anterior aspect of flexure of ankle Between tendons of Extensor Hallucis Longus muscle and Extensor Digitorum Longus muscle	

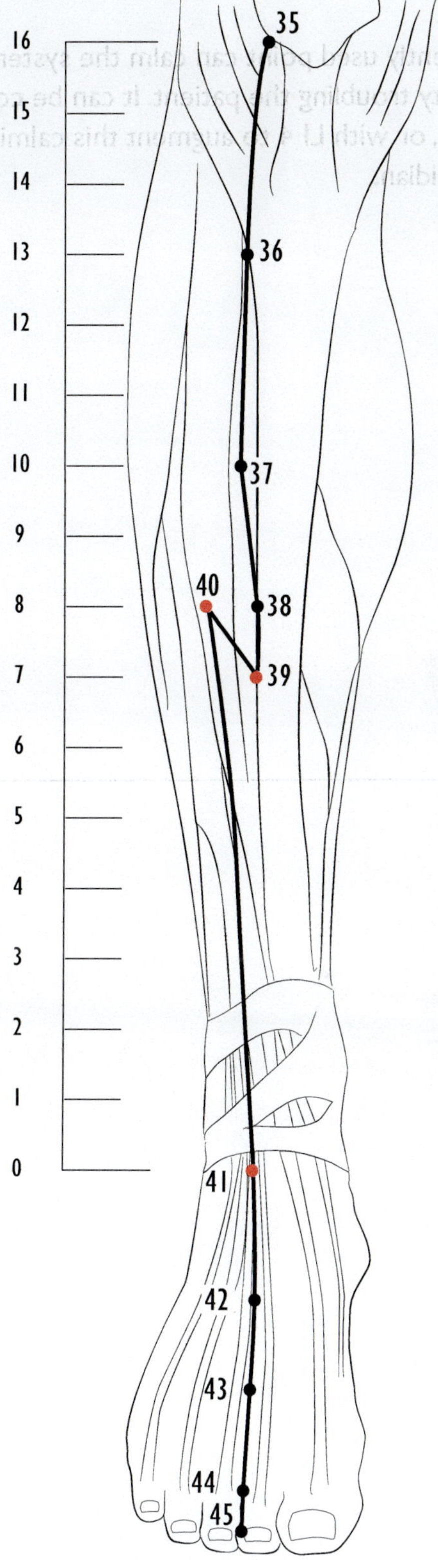

St 42 — <u>Rushing Yang</u> (Surging Yang)
Source Point. Exit Point. Shokanten Point. "Perfect Calm Point".

This frequently used point can calm the system if there is worry, anxiety, mania, overthinking or instability troubling the patient. It can be combined with TH 4 for general harmonisation of the system, or with LI 4 to augment this calming effect. Conversely, it can be used to invigorate the whole meridian.

⊥	Δ		Location
3	3-5	Dorsum of foot Between tendons of extensor digitorum longus and extensor Hallucis longus muscles In hollow between navicular bone, intermediate cuniform bone and lateral cuniform bone Halfway between St 41 and St 43 In an indentation formed when the foot and toes are dorsiflexed	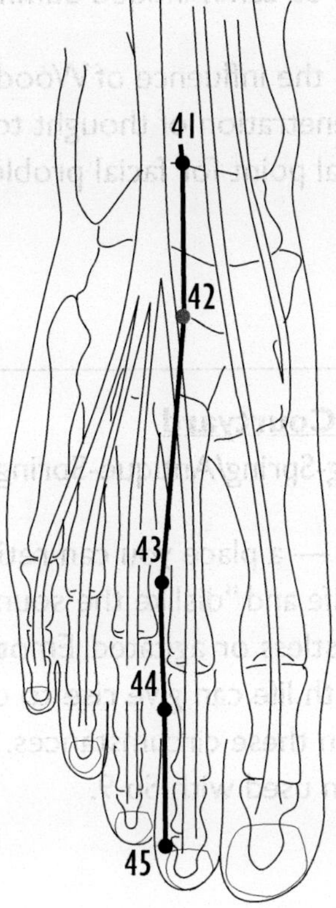

Stomach

St 43 — <u>Sinking Valley</u> (Sunken Valley)
Wood point. Shu-Stream/Antique-Summer Point.

This point brings the influence of Wood to the meridian, thus refreshing it and bestowing clarity and enhanced penetration of thought to the patient. For pain or swelling of the foot or heel. Can be used as a distal point for facial problems such as oedema.

St 44 — <u>Inner Courtyard</u>
Water point. Ying-Spring/Antique-Spring Point. A Ma Danyang Heavenly Star Point.

Inner Courtyard — a place you can retire to, to get away from everyone and everything when you are fed up with life and "dislike the sound of the human voice". Consider this point if the patient is overheated, restless or agitated. Emotional response to resentment, hurt feelings or general dissatisfaction with life can give rise to overeating but never feeling satisfied — this cooling point can be effective in these circumstances. For a swollen abdomen, trigeminal neuralgia, facial paralysis or sinusitis. Often used with Sp 9.

St 45 — <u>Hard Bargain</u> (Harsh Exchange, Hard Payment, Severe Mouth)
Metal Point. Sedation Point. Jing-Well/Antique-Winter Point. "Cruel Payment Point".
First Aid: indigestion and hangover.

Being the sedation point, this point can be used to calm the Mind and Spirit. Effective for insomnia and agitation, problems of the mouth, particularly deviation of the mouth or clenched jaws.

⊥	△		Location
3	3	Dorsum of foot At junction of 2nd and 3rd metatarsal bones Just distal to the flare of the base of the 2nd metatarsal bone	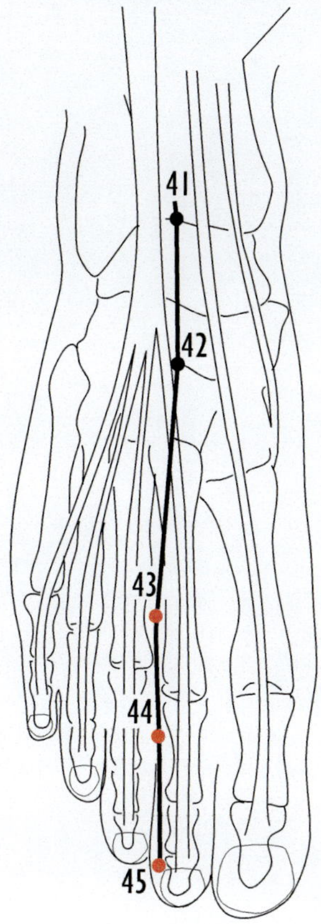
3	3	Dorsum of foot Between 2nd and 3rd digits Proximal to web margin Just distal to the flare of the base of the proximal phalanx of the 2nd digit	
1	3	Forbidden from 6th month of pregnancy Lateral nail point of the 2rd digit Approx **0.1 cun** prox to corner of nail Distal to the flare of the distal phalanx	

Spleen

- **The Official in Charge of Transformation and Transportation**
- **It is the dwelling place of the 'Yi'. Governs the thinking processes**
- **The two Earth Officials 'guard the storehouses and granaries'**

Spleen

Sp 1 — Hidden White (Mysterious White, Yin White, Retired White)
Wood Point. Entry Point. Jing-Well/Antique-Winter Point. Ghost Point.

This Wood point helps to stimulate the Spleen Qi if there are signs of stagnation or clogging up such as paralysis, obsessive or stuck thinking, overweight and overeating (especially when worry and depression dominate). For menstrual disorders, particularly if prolonged, as Sp 'holds' the Blood (one can use direct moxa here to strengthen this action). Brings clarity of thought and helps focus and concentration (Wood penetrating Earth). Calms the mind and eases mania or excessive dreaming. "White" probably indicates the Spleen's Mother connection to the son Metal (Lungs).

Sp 2 — Great Capital (Great Metropolis)
Fire Point. Tonification Point. Ying-Spring/Antique-Spring Point.

This Fire point invigorates the Spleen Official bringing warmth, light-heartedness and expansiveness to someone who is bogged down in thoughts, too serious, self-absorbed or stuck in a rut. For general fatigue, heavy cold limbs, insomnia or restless dreaming. Connects Fire and Earth. It can be compared to the central position held by the Earth element, with this Fire point playing an active role in the many exchanges and interactions that take place within a capital city. Often used in combination with St 41.

⊥	Δ		Location
1	X	Forbidden from 1st month of pregnancy Medial nail point of the 1st digit Approx **0.1 cun** proximal to the lateral corner of the nail. Distal to the flare of the distal phalanx	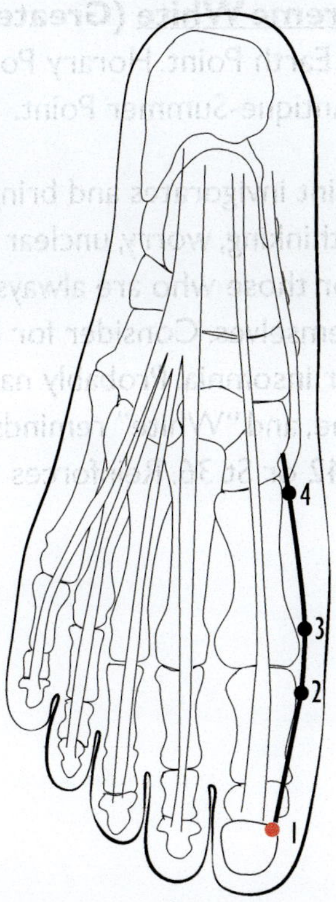
3	3-5	Forbidden from 2nd month of pregnancy Medial surface of first digit Distal to metatarsophalangeal joint of first digit Just distal to the flare of the base of the proximal phalanx Approximately at the junction of the change in skin colour	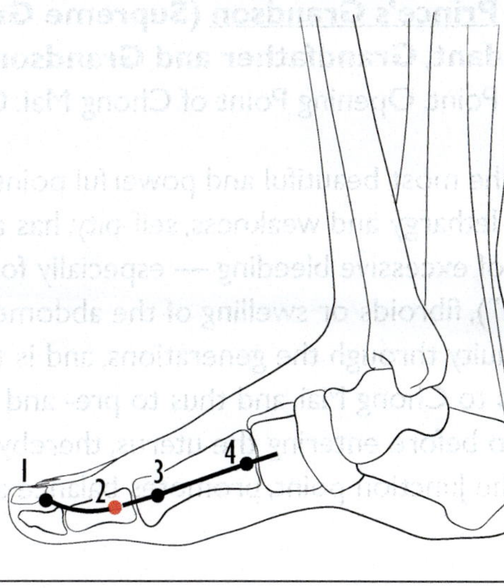

Spleen

Sp 3 — Supreme White (Greater White, Extreme Whiteness, Great Brightness)
Source Point. Earth Point. Horary Point (9–11am). Seasonal Horary Point — Late Summer. Shu-Stream/Antique-Summer Point. "Cerebral Calm Point". "Equilibrium and Joy Point".

This Earth point invigorates and brings stability to the Spleen and, as such, can be effective in cases of overthinking, worry, unclear thinking or poor memory. Helps the Spleen to self-regulate, particularly for those who are always giving out to others, over-mothering and thus becoming exhausted themselves. Consider for Damp conditions such as tiredness, coldness, lack of perspective or insomnia. Probably named after the bright and illuminating planet Venus which has the same name, and "White" reminds us that Earth connects to and nourishes Metal. Commonly used with St 42 or St 36. Reinforces the Transforming and Transporting actions of the Spleen.

Sp 4 — Prince's Grandson (Supreme Grandchild, Yellow Emperor, Ancestor and Descendant, Grandfather and Grandson)
Junction Point. Opening Point of Chong Mai. Coupled Point of Yin Wei Mai.

One of the most beautiful and powerful points in the body. Consider where a patient has long-standing lethargy and weakness, self-pity, has a weak digestion, is anxious or depressed. Helps in cases of excessive bleeding — especially for painful, irregular periods (Sp "holds the Blood together"), fibroids or swelling of the abdomen. This Point's name (Gong Sun) has the connotation of continuity through the generations, and is the family name of the Yellow (Earth) Emperor. It connects to Chong Mai, and thus to pre- and post-heavenly Qi. The meridian passes through the three Jiao before entering the uterus, thereby regulating menstruation. Helps circulation in the legs and, as the Junction point, promotes balance and equilibrium within the Earth Element.

⊥	Δ		Location
3	3-5	Medial surface of foot Proximal to the first metatarsophalangeal joint Proximal and inferior to the flare of the head of the 1st metatarsal bone	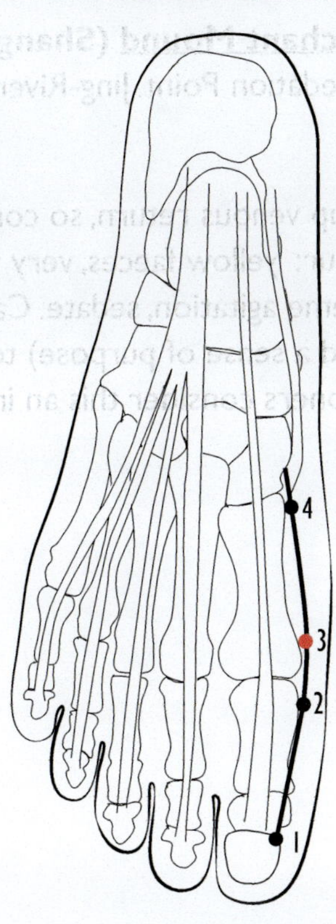
3	3	Distal and inferior to the base of the 1st metatarsal bone Just distal to the flare of the base of the 1st metatarsal bone Approx **1 cun** proximal to Sp 3.	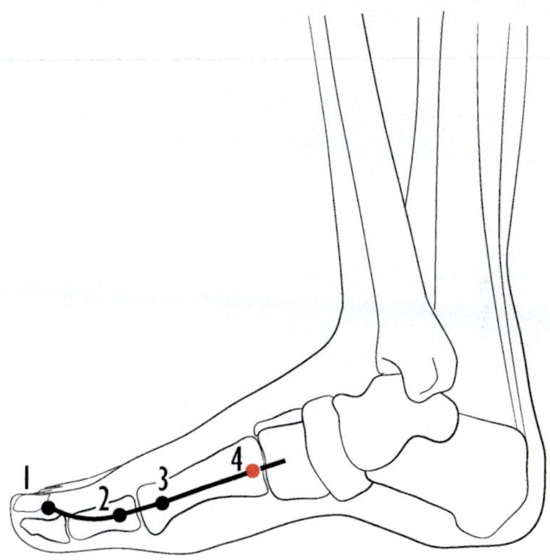

Sp 5 — Merchant Mound (Shang Hill)
Metal Point. Sedation Point. Jing-River/Antique-Late Summer Point. "Calm Sleep Point". Reunion of Veins Point.

Helps speed up venous return, so consider for varicose veins or haemorrhoids. For problems involving colour: yellow faeces, very yellow urine, very yellow vaginal discharges or jaundice. In cases of extreme agitation, sedate. Can be tonified to bring the influence of Metal (structure, inspiration and a sense of purpose) to the Spleen Official. Local point for ankle and knee problems. TCM practitioners consider this an important point for resolving Damp.

⊥	Δ		Location
3	3-7	Medial aspect of the ankle Anterior and inferior to the prominence of medial maleolus Medial to the tendon of the tibialis anterior muscle	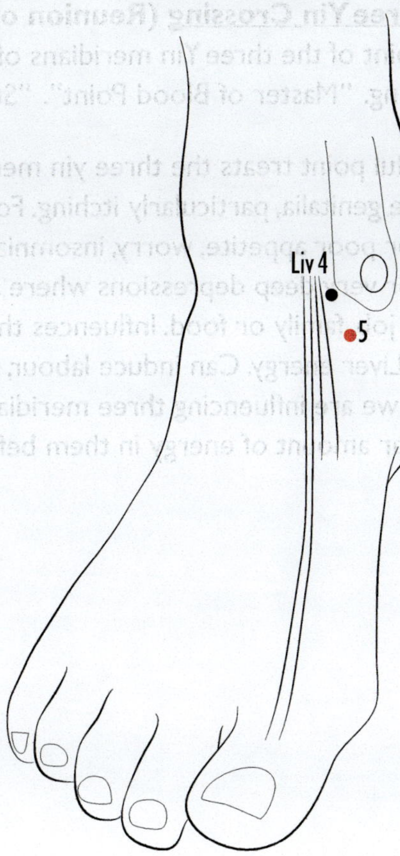

Sp 6 — Three Yin Crossing (Reunion of Three Yin)
Crossing Point of the three Yin meridians of the leg — Sp, Liv, Kid. One of the nine needles for returning Yang. "Master of Blood Point". "Strengthener and Calmer Point".

This powerful point treats the three yin meridians simultaneously. For female or male disorders involving the genitalia, particularly itching. For excessive discharges and most menstrual disorders. Consider for poor appetite, worry, insomnia or fear, as it can have a profound effect on calming the BMS. For very deep depressions where a person is desperate, wants to run away, wants to "throw up" job, family or food. Influences the Blood and urinary function. Helps with irritability as it smooths Liver energy. Can induce labour, as it affects the uterus (forbidden during pregnancy). Remember, we are influencing three meridians with this point, so we need to ensure that all three have a similar amount of energy in them before tonifying or calming.

⊥	△		Location
4	3-10	Forbidden during pregnancy Medial aspect of lower leg Posterior border of the medial aspect of the tibia bone Between the tibia bone and the soleus muscle **3 cun** proximal to prominence of medial maleolus	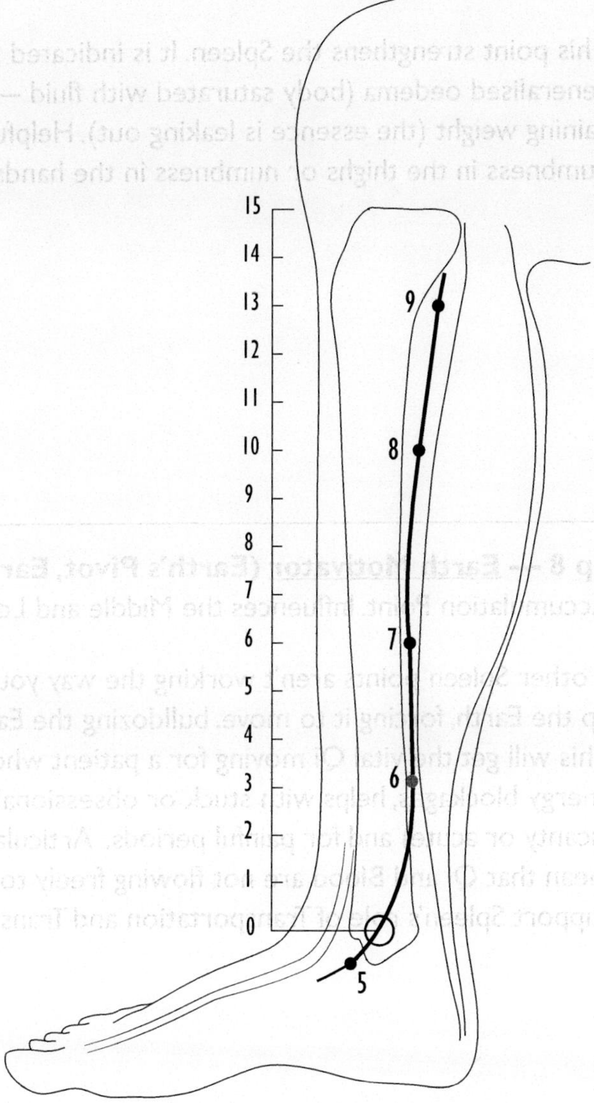

Spleen

Sp 7 — Leaky Valley

This point strengthens the Spleen. It is indicated for swollen ankles, swollen feet, swollen abdomen, generalised oedema (body saturated with fluid — a sign of damp). For people who eat without gaining weight (the essence is leaking out). Helpful for general fatigue. Consider for cold and numbness in the thighs or numbness in the hands or feet.

Sp 8 — Earth Motivator (Earth's Pivot, Earth's Crux)
Accumulation Point. Influences the Middle and Lower Jiao.

If other Spleen points aren't working the way you feel they should, consider using Sp 8 — it shakes up the Earth, forcing it to move, bulldozing the Earth and turning it over, thus allowing it to receive. This will get the vital Qi moving for a patient who is sluggish; all pulses can change. Breaks down energy blockages, helps with stuck or obsessional thinking patterns. For irregular menstruation, (scanty or acute) and for painful periods. Articular troubles and restrictions of movement can mean that Qi and Blood are not flowing freely to the parts of the body that need them. Helps support Spleen's role of Transportation and Transformation.

Sp 9 —Yin Mound Spring
Water Point. He-Sea/Antique-Autumn Point.

This Water point can be used to regulate the balance of fluids within the Earth. It can be effective if the Earth has too much water in it and has thus become waterlogged. This presence of 'excessive Damp' can not only cause oedema of the legs or abdomen, retention of urine or diarrhoea, but can also result in being mentally 'bogged down' or woolly-headed. The patient may crave sympathy or understanding, which can be indicated by their need for others to "feel sorry for me". Can be excellent for knee problems (along with St 35). Tenderness of this point on women may indicate the presence of hormonal problems.

⊥	Δ		Location
4	X	Medial aspect of lower leg Posterior border of the medial aspect of the tibia bone Between the tibia bone and the soleus muscle **6 cun** proximal to prominence of medial maleolus	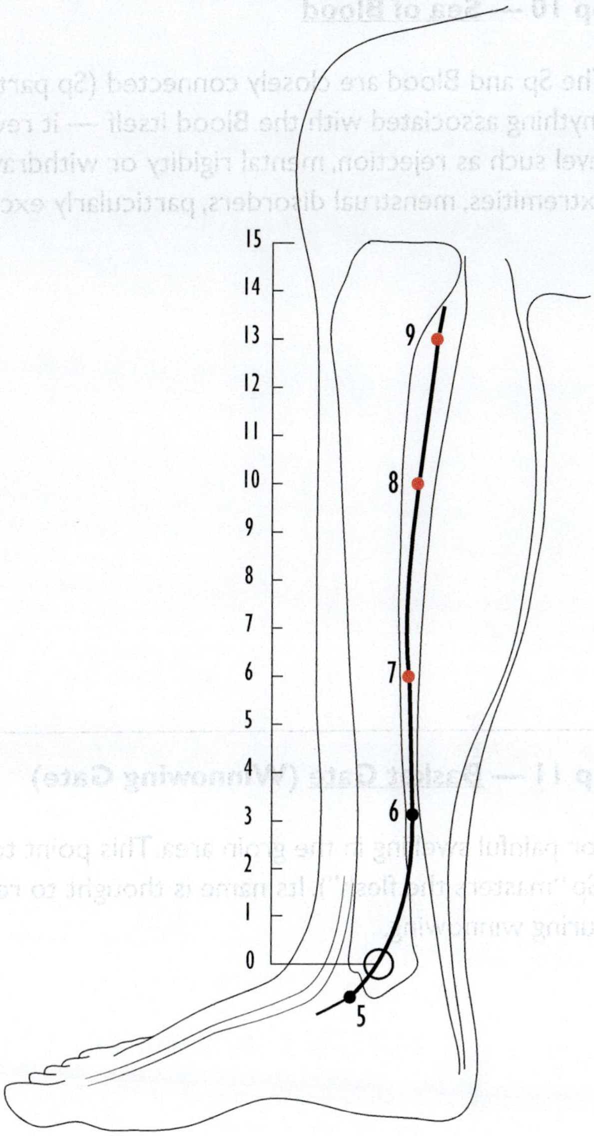
4	3-7	Medial aspect of lower leg **10 cun** proximal to prominence of medial maleolus Posterior border of the medial aspect of the tibia bone Between the tibia bone and the soleus muscle	
5-8	X	Medial aspect of lower leg **13 cun** proximal to prominence of medial maleolus Posterior border of the medial aspect of the tibia bone Inferior border of the medial condyle of the tibia Level with Gb 34	

Spleen

Sp 10 — Sea of Blood

The Sp and Blood are closely connected (Sp partly forms it and 'holds' it). Consider this point with anything associated with the Blood itself — it revitalises and nourishes it. For coldness on a mental level such as rejection, mental rigidity or withdrawal. For poor circulation, lack of energy, cold extremities, menstrual disorders, particularly excessive bleeding or painful periods.

Sp 11 — Basket Gate (Winnowing Gate)

For painful swelling in the groin area. This point tonifies the Spleen and thus the flesh of the body (Sp "masters the flesh"). Its name is thought to refer to the shape the thighs make whilst squatting during winnowing.

⊥	Δ		Location
3-5	3-10	Medial aspect of upper thigh On the prominence of the vastus medialis (one of the quadriceps muscles) when the foot is flexed **4 cun** proximal to the medial popliteal crease	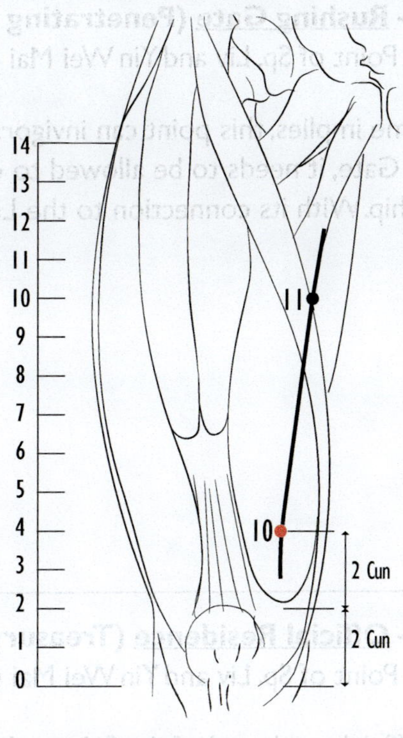
5	3	Medial aspect of upper thigh In a groove between medial border of the sartorius muscle and the gracilis muscle **10 cun** proximal to the medial popliteal crease	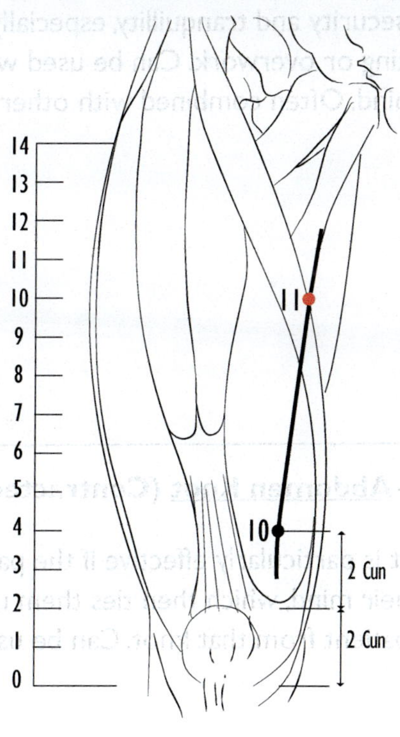

Spleen

Sp 12 — <u>Rushing Gate</u> (Penetrating Gate, Surging Gate)
Crossing Point of Sp, Liv and Yin Wei Mai (Linking) Vessel

As its name implies, this point can invigorate and clear obstructions in the Sp channel. Being a (second) Gate, it needs to be allowed to open and close effectively. Consider for hernia, pain in the groin or hip. With its connection to the Liv, this point can help smooth the flow of Blood and Qi.

Sp 13 — <u>Official Residence</u> (Treasury Dwelling, Bowel Abode)
Crossing Point of Sp, Liv and Yin Wei Mai (Linking Vessel)

As the 'official residence' of the Spleen, this point calms, enhances and stabilises the Official. It brings security and tranquillity, especially if the patient is scattered as a result of agitation, overthinking or overwork. Can be used with Sp 14 if the patient is knotted up in their abdomen or in their mind. Often combined with other abdominal points such as Ren 3–5 or Kid 12–13.

Sp 14 — <u>Abdomen Knot</u> (Contracted Belly)

This point is particularly effective if the patient is constantly worrying — churning things over and over in their mind, which then ties them up in knots. It also works at a deeper Spirit level, to help free the patient from that knot. Can be used for extreme emotional anxiety.

⊥	Δ		Location
7	5	Level with the superior border of symphysis pubis Lateral edge of femoral artery Superior to the lateral end of the inguinal groove **3.5 cun** lateral to anterior median line (Ren Mai) Level with Ren 2	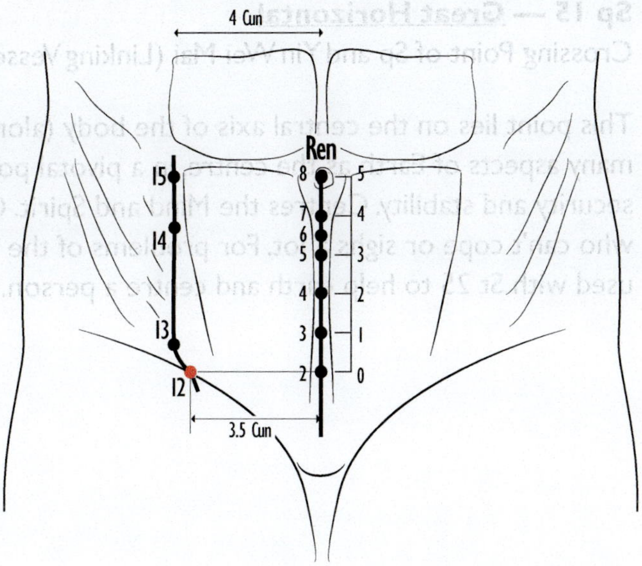
7	5-10	Lateral edge of rectus abdominis muscle Superior to inguinal ligament **4 cun** lateral to anterior median line (Ren Mai) **0.5 cun** lateral to and **0.7 cun** superior to Sp 12 **0.7 cun** superior to superior border of symphysis pubis at Ren 2 **4.3 cun** inferior to the level of the centre of the umbilicus or Sp 15	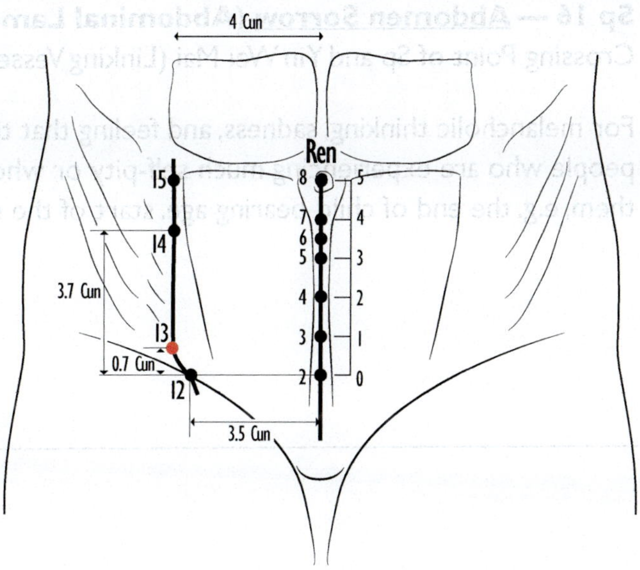
7	5-15	Lateral edge of rectus abdominis muscle **4 cun** lateral to anterior median line (Ren Mai) **3.7 cun** superior to Sp 12 **1.3 cun** inferior to the level of the centre of the umbilicus or Sp 15	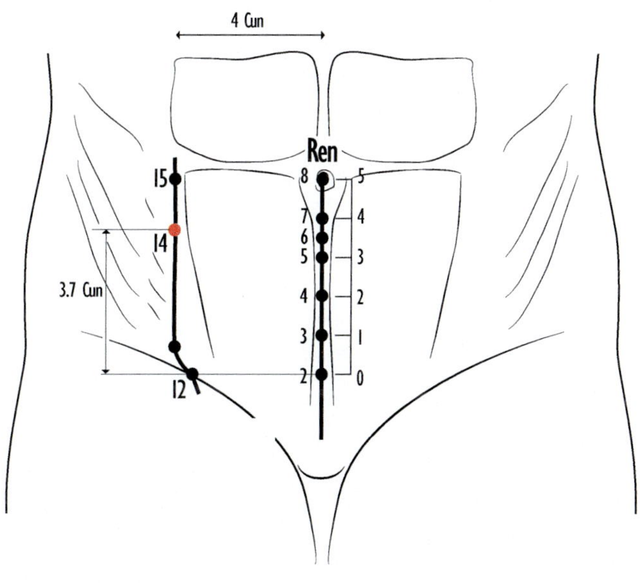

Spleen

Sp 15 — Great Horizontal
Crossing Point of Sp and Yin Wei Mai (Linking Vessel)

This point lies on the central axis of the body (along with Ren 8, Kid 16 and St 25), and epitomises many aspects of Earth as the centre, in a pivotal position. Calms anxiety and agitation; brings security and stability. Centres the Mind and Spirit. Consider for someone on the verge of tears, who can't cope or sighs a lot. For problems of the bowels such as diarrhoea or constipation. Often used with St 25 to help earth and centre a person.

Sp 16 — Abdomen Sorrow (Abdominal Lament)
Crossing Point of Sp and Yin Wei Mai (Linking Vessel)

For melancholic thinking, sadness, and feeling that there is no harvest in life. Consider for those people who are experiencing much self-pity or who feel bereft at the effect of life's changes upon them, e.g. the end of child-bearing age, start of the menopause or declining interest in sex.

⊥	△		Location
10	5-10	Lateral edge of rectus abdominis muscle **4 cun** lateral to anterior median line (Ren Mai) **4 cun** lateral to the level of the centre of the umbilicus **4 cun** lateral to Ren 8	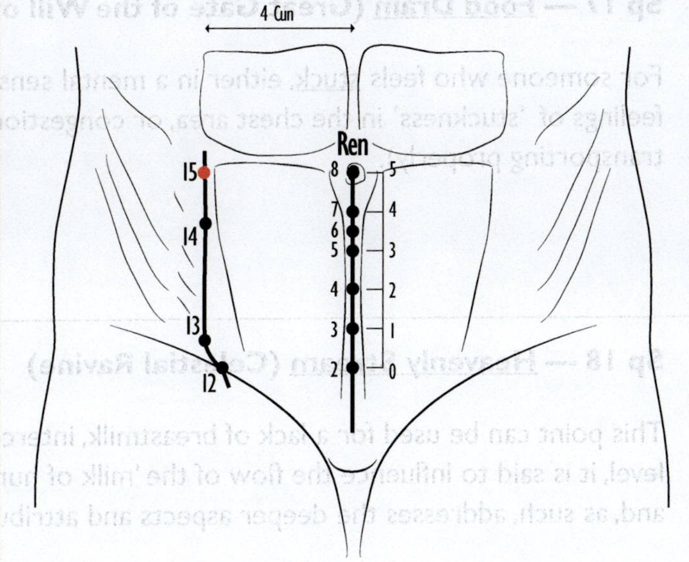
7	5-10	Lateral edge of rectus abdominis muscle **4 cun** lateral to anterior median line (Ren Mai) **3 cun** superior to Sp 15 Level with Ren 11	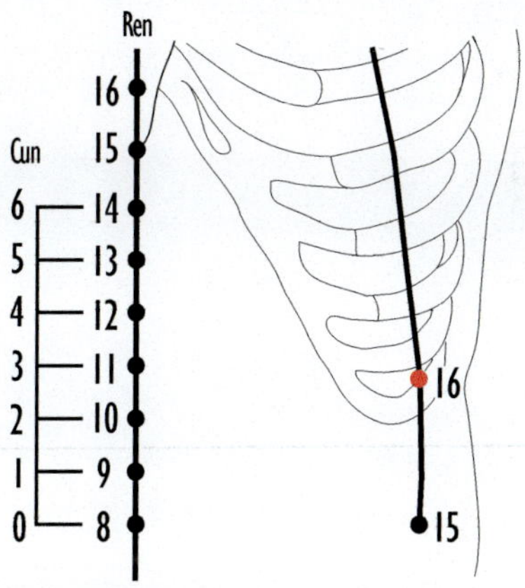

Spleen

Sp 17 — Food Drain (Great Gate of the Will of Heaven)

For someone who feels stuck, either in a mental sense (e.g. obsessions) or physically such as feelings of 'stuckness' in the chest area, or congestion of the lungs (indicating that the Sp is not transporting properly).

Sp 18 — Heavenly Stream (Celestial Ravine)

This point can be used for a lack of breastmilk, intercostal pain or mastitis. On a more spiritual level, it is said to influence the flow of the 'milk of human kindness', nourishment and understanding and, as such, addresses the deeper aspects and attributes of the Earth element.

⊥	△		Location
3	5	In the 5th **IC Space** **6 cun** lateral to anterior median line (Ren Mai)	
3	5	In the 4th **IC Space** **6 cun** lateral to anterior median line (Ren Mai) Approx **1 cun** lateral to Pc 1	

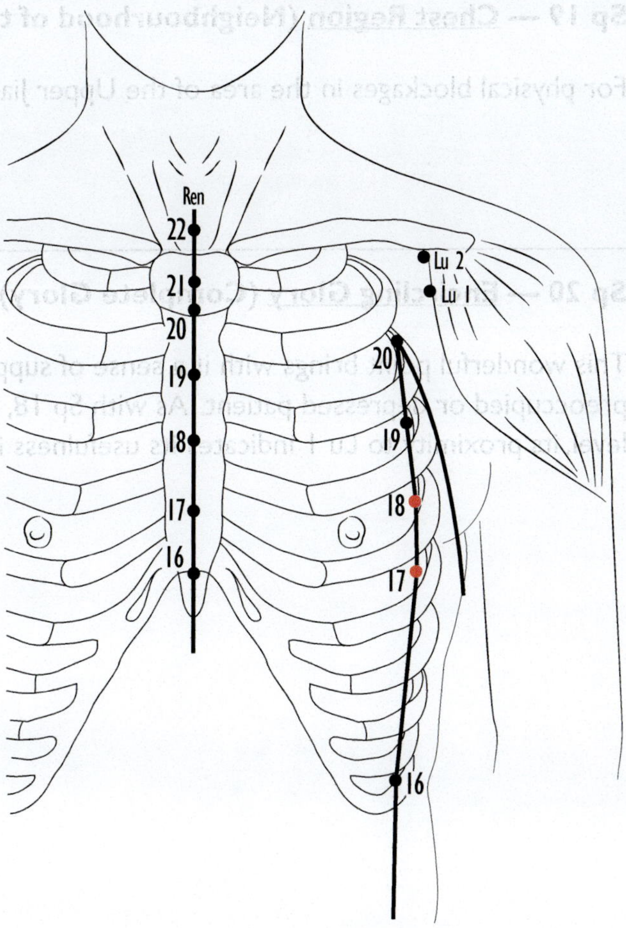

Spleen

Sp 19 — Chest Region (Neighbourhood of the Breast)

For physical blockages in the area of the Upper Jiao.

Sp 20 — Encircling Glory (Complete Glory)

This wonderful point brings with it a sense of support, security and stability to a worried, preoccupied or depressed patient. As with Sp 18, it addresses the Spirit of the Earth. On a physical level, its proximity to Lu 1 indicates its usefulness in helping with some lung problems.

⊥	Δ		Location
3	5	In the **3rd IC Space** **6 cun** lateral to anterior median line (Ren Mai)	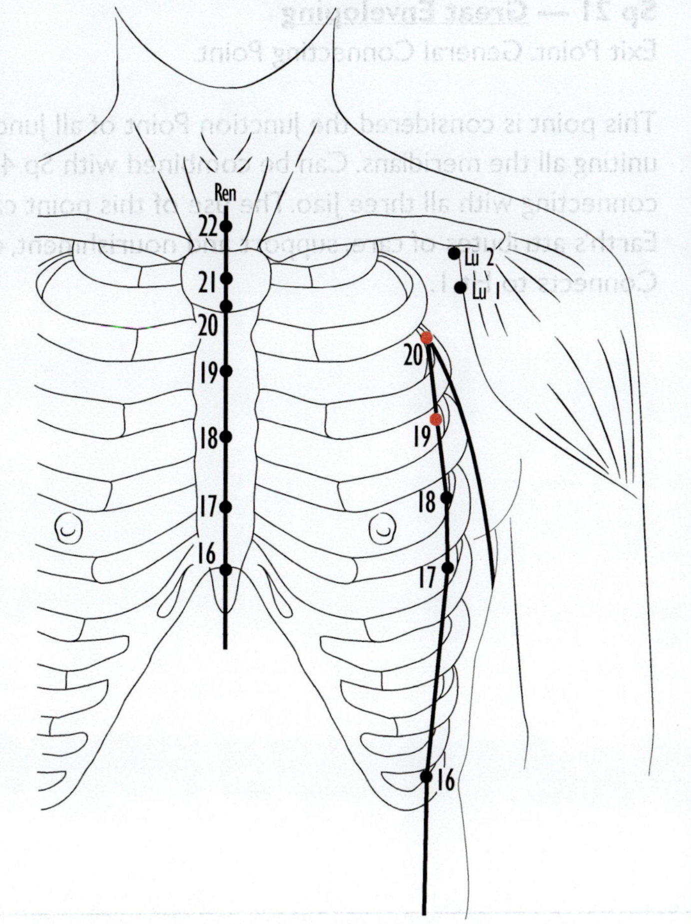
3	5	In the **2nd IC Space** **6 cun** lateral to anterior median line (Ren Mai) Inferior to Lu 1	

Sp 21 — Great Enveloping
Exit Point. General Connecting Point.

This point is considered the Junction Point of all Junction Points. It brings all-round harmony, uniting all the meridians. Can be combined with Sp 4 (Opening Point of the Chong Mai), thus connecting with all three Jiao. The use of this point can help a patient feel enveloped by Mother Earth's attributes of care, support and nourishment, especially if these are lacking in their life. Connects to Ht 1.

⊥	Δ		Location
3	3-7	In the 6th **IC Space** (occasionally in the 7th **IC Space)** On the mid-axillary line	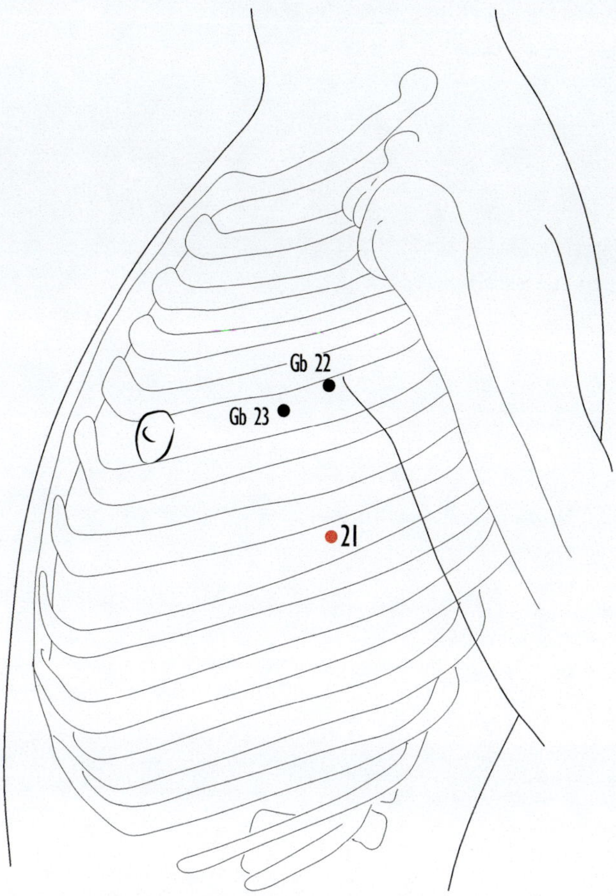

Ren Mai Conception Vessel

- **Ren Mai 'masters the uterus'. Sea of Yin energy**
- **Forms a closed energetic circuit flowing up the Du Mai and then down the Ren Mai**

Ren Mai Conception Vessel

Ren 1 — <u>Meeting of Yin</u> (Sea Bed)
Entry Point. General Junction Point. Ghost Point. Crossing Point of Ren Mai, Du Mai and Chong Mai. "Master Point of the Whole Body". First Aid: near-drowning.

This point resuscitates and tonifies the patient, particularly if work on the other Officials hasn't brought about the change you expect. Rarely, if ever, sedated. For people who are drowning spiritually when overwhelmed by life. It calms the Spirit. Ren 1 is like a last resort before a person 'gives up the ghost'. It is anatomically opposite to Du 20 (One Hundred Meetings), the meeting of all Yang meridians. Helpful for haemorrhoids and painful disorders of the vagina or penis. Regulates menstruation. An energy block may occur here after giving birth. Because of its location this point is commonly under-used.

Ren 2 — <u>Crooked Bone</u> (Bent Bone)
Crossing Point of Ren Mai and Liv

This point can do all that Ren 1 can do, except resuscitation. Consider for problems with conception or lack of virility (these two can also be helped by using Ren 3–7). Brings the influence of Liver to the Ren Mai — hope, birth, spring, new beginnings, or when a person has become stuck in their life. Consider using moxa here for cold in the lower jiao, uterus or bladder.

Ren 3 — <u>Utmost Middle</u> (Central Pole)
Alarm Point of Bl. Crossing Point of Ren Mai, Liv, Sp and Kid. Affects the endocrine system along with Ren 4–6.

Consider this crossing point if the three Yin Officials (Liv, Sp, Kid) are all in one pattern — either up or down. Has a grounding and stabilising effect on the lower jiao. For chronic or acute bladder or urinary problems, difficult menstruation, infertility, impotence, or where the body is generally weak and fatigued. Energises the patient's Yin aspect at a deep level. Said to be a point to consider after childbirth if the placenta is retained, and also for strengthening the mother's energy at this time. It lies at the very centre of a person, just as the 'Central Pole' (or Pole Star) lies at the centre of the sky in Chinese astrology, around which the other stars revolve.

⊥	Δ		Location
10	X	On the perineum Midway between the anus and the scrotum (in men) Midway betwwen the anus and the posterior commissure of the vagina (in women)	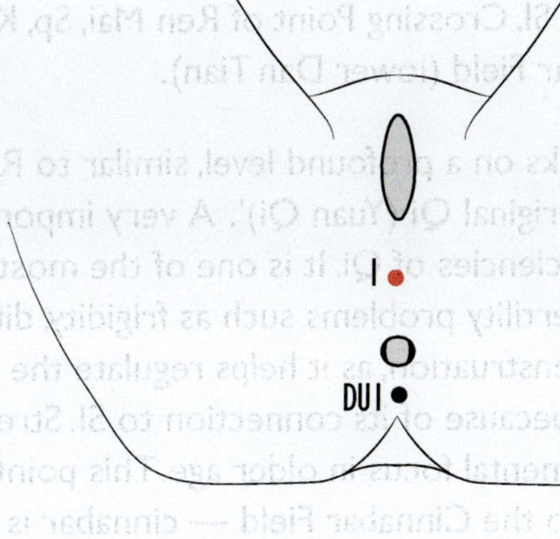
5	7	On the anterior median line **Just** superior to the superior border of symphysis pubis	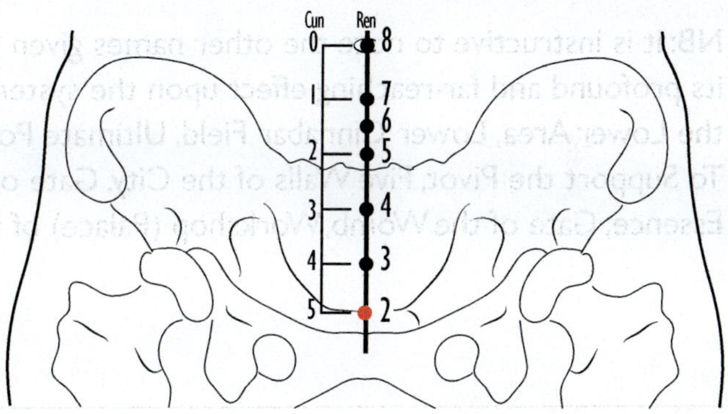
8	5-15	On the anterior median line **1 cun** superior to the superior border of symphysis pubis	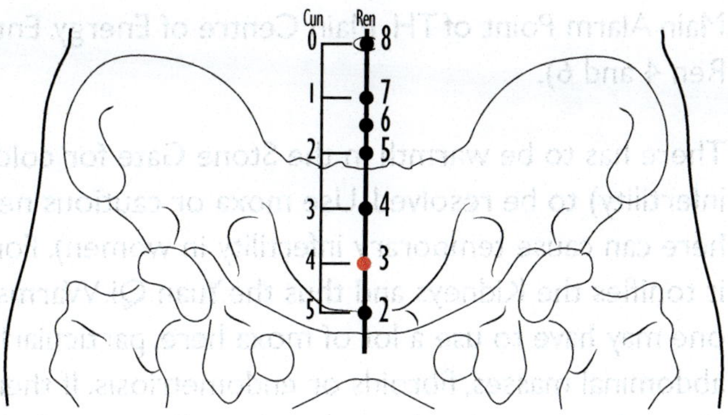

Ren Mai Conception Vessel

Ren 4 — <u>First Gate</u> (Origin Gate, Gate to the Original Qi)
Alarm Point of SI. Crossing Point of Ren Mai, Sp, Kid, Liv. "Elixir of Long Life". Entrance to the Lower Cinnabar Field (lower Dan Tian).

This point works on a profound level, similar to Ren 3 except deeper as it connects to Kidney Jing and our 'Original Qi (Yuan Qi)'. A very important point: it treats nutritional, respiratory and hereditary deficiencies of Qi. It is one of the most powerful points for Qi deficiency in the BMS. Consider for fertility problems such as frigidity, difficulty conceiving, impotence, poor sperm quality, or irregular menstruation, as it helps regulate the functioning of the uterus. Helpful for sorting out problems because of its connection to SI. Strengthens the whole system — especially good for enhancing mental focus in older age. This point can have excellent results when used with moxa. Refers to the Cinnabar Field — cinnabar is said to be exceptionally well-balanced in terms of Yin/Yang and, when heated, transforms from a solid state into a fluid one; it is thus an area of transformation. When used with Ren 14, Ren 4 can help re-establish the Jing-Shen (Heart-Kidney) link when this has been disturbed by severe shock or emotional turmoil.

NB: it is instructive to note the other names given to this point — an indication of the depth of its profound and far-reaching effect upon the system: The First Fortified Gate, Regulator, Gate of the Lower Area, Lower Cinnabar Field, Ultimate Point, Great Middle, Great Sea, Kun Lun Mountain, To Support the Pivot, Five Walls of the City, Gate of Children, Resting Place of the Son, House of Essence, Gate of the Womb, Workshop (Palace) of the Son, Gate of Destiny, Door of the Son.

Ren 5 — <u>Stone Gate</u> (Cinnabar Field, Life Gate)
Main Alarm Point of TH. Main Centre of Energy. Entrance to the Lower Cinnabar Field (along with Ren 4 and 6).

There has to be warmth in the Stone Gate for cold or empty conditions (e.g. weakness, inertia or infertility) to be resolved. Use moxa or cautious needle stimulation (as some texts say needling here can cause temporary infertility in women). For a chronic lack of vitality, lack of energy — it tonifies the Kidneys and thus the Yuan Qi. Warms the Three Jiao (especially the lower Jiao); one may have to use a lot of moxa here, particularly so if this area is stone cold. Consider for abdominal masses, fibroids or endometriosis. If there is a lack of response from using Kidney channel command points, come here (it opens the Water Passages). Regulates and eases pain during menstruation.

⊥	Δ		Location
10-15	7-15	On the anterior median line **2 cun** superior to the superior border of symphysis pubis	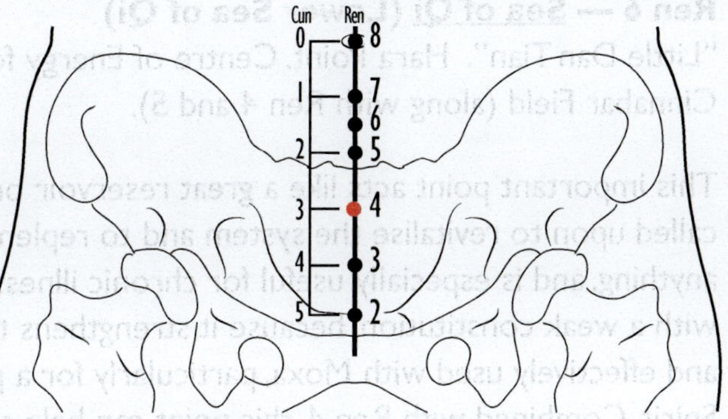
7-8	7-15	On the anterior median line **3 cun** superior to the superior border of symphysis pubis	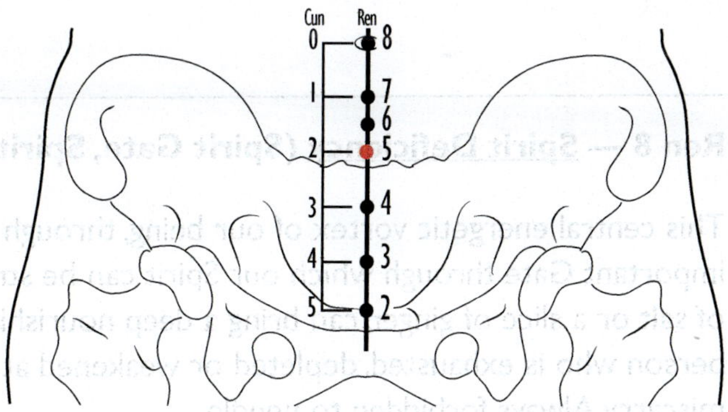

Ren Mai Conception Vessel

Ren 6 — <u>Sea of Qi</u> (Lower Sea of Qi)
"Little Dan Tian". Hara Point. Centre of Energy for the whole BMS. Entrance to the Lower Cinnabar Field (along with Ren 4 and 5).

This important point acts like a great reservoir or sea of energy for the whole Kingdom. It can be called upon to revitalise the system and to replenish depleted Qi energy. For a complete lack of anything, and is especially useful for chronic illness, lack of will, complete exhaustion, or for those with a weak constitution, because it strengthens the Kidneys and thus are Original Qi. Is commonly and effectively used with Moxa, particularly for a person who is cold or resigned in Body, Mind or Spirit. Combined with Ren 4, this point can help strengthen the male libido. Consider for prolapse or if the patient has a history of miscarriage.

Ren 7 —<u>Yin Crossing</u> (Cinnabar Field, Crossroads of the Yin Forces)
Crossing Point of Ren Mai, Chong Mai, TH, Pc and Kid. Alarm Point for the TH in the Lower Jiao.

This is a potent point on the Ren Mai for male sexual difficulties such as impotence or premature ejaculation. It can also help women with infertility and menstrual disorders because of its connection with the uterus, Ren Mai and Chong Mai. Beneficial for menopausal hot flushes; sometimes used with Ht 6 for this. Consider combining Ren 7 with Ht 6 and Ren 15 for calming and centring during the menopause. Provides stability and acts as an anchor for the Mind and Spirit.

Ren 8 — <u>Spirit Deficiency</u> (Spirit Gate, Spirit Palace Gate)

This central energetic vortex of our being, through which we were all sustained, remains an important Gate through which our Spirit can be strongly affected. Moxa used here, on a bed of salt or a slice of ginger, can bring a deep nourishing and revitalising warmth to the Spirit of a person who is exhausted, depleted or weakened at a deep level. Consider if there is a tendency to miscarry. Always forbidden to needle.

⊥	Δ		Location
8	7-15	On the anterior median line **3.5 cun** superior to the superior border of symphysis pubis	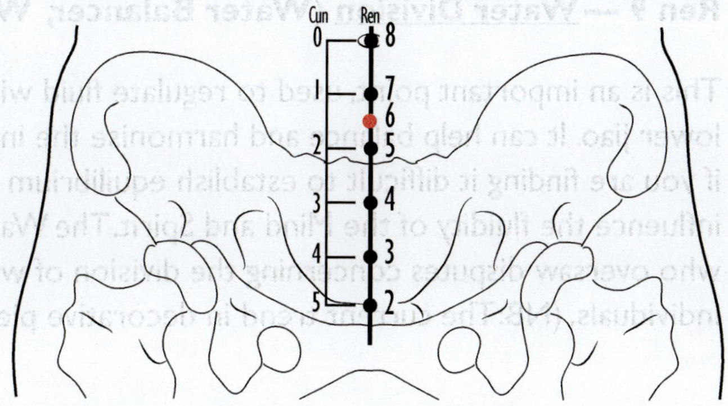
8	7	On the anterior median line **4 cun** superior to the superior border of symphysis pubis	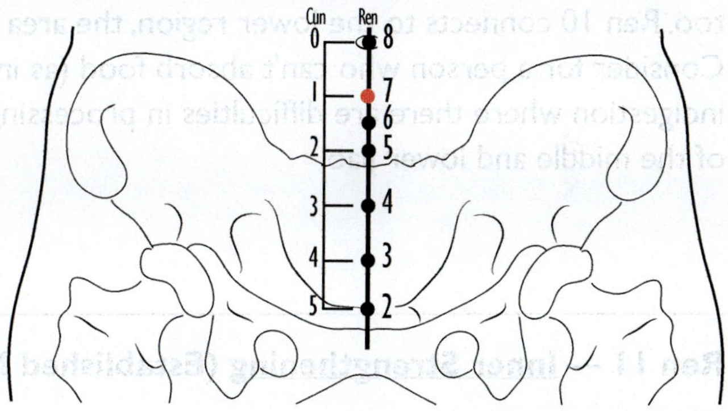
X	3-30	On the anterior median line **In the centre** of the umbilicus	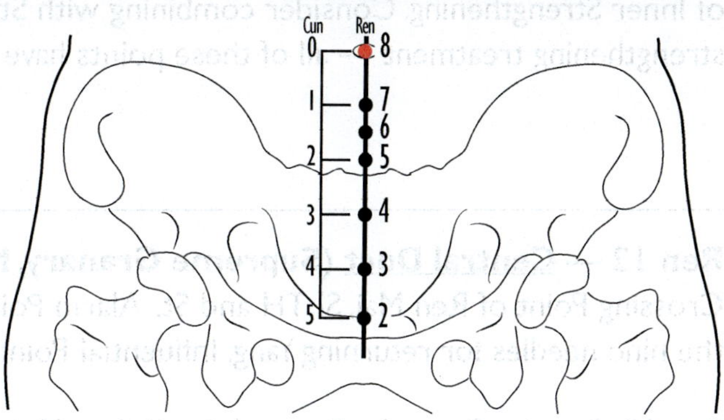

Ren Mai Conception Vessel

Ren 9 — Water Division (Water Balancer, Water Separation)

This is an important point, used to regulate fluid within the body, particularly in the middle and lower jiao. It can help balance and harmonise the internal secretions. Consider using this point if you are finding it difficult to establish equilibrium between the Water Officials. It can also help influence the fluidity of the Mind and Spirit. The Water Balancer was the name given to the Official who oversaw disputes concerning the division of water between neighbouring provinces, towns or individuals. (NB: The current trend in decorative piercings here can cause cystitis in some people).

Ren 10 — Lower Duct (Lower Portion of the Stomach)
Crossing Point of Ren Mai and Sp

Ren 10, 11, 12 and 13 all affect the Stomach to some degree and, in turn, can influence the Spleen too. Ren 10 connects to the lower region, the area responsible for moving food into the intestines. Consider for a person who can't absorb food (as in indigestion or anorexia), or for mental indigestion where there are difficulties in processing information. Helps harmonise the functioning of the middle and lower jiao.

Ren 11 — Inner Strengthening (Established Mile)

Helps strengthen the Stomach, Small Intestine and Spleen (the digestive organs). Aids the Body and Mind in extracting nourishment from food or information if a person is struggling with physical or mental indigestion. Strengthens the Earth Officials and the middle Jiao, hence its name of Inner Strengthening. Consider combining with St 36 and LI 10 for a particularly supportive and strengthening treatment — all of these points have 'Mile' in their names.

Ren 12 — Central Duct (Supreme Granary, Middle Portion of the Stomach)
Crossing Point of Ren Mai, SI, TH and St. Alarm Point of Stomach and TH in the Middle Jiao. One of the nine needles for returning Yang. Influential Point of the Yang Officials.

Ren 12 directly affects the Stomach itself. Ren 12 is somewhat like St 36 in that it treats all sorts of Stomach problems such as nausea, and problems with the assimilation or distribution of food. It can also be effective for mental problems associated with digestion such as chronic worry, overthinking, poor memory, or difficulties in processing information. Excellent point to strengthen the Earth. Good with moxa for cold symptoms associated with the Earth. Consider in cases where relationship problems such as lovesickness affect the appetite. Can be used early on in treatment.

⊥	Δ		Location
5	5-15	On the anterior median line **1 cun** superior to the level of the centre of the umbilicus	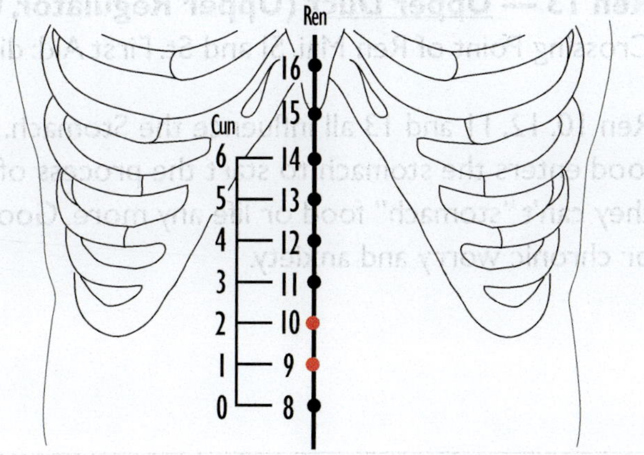
8	7-15	On the anterior median line **2 cun** superior to the level of the centre of the umbilicus	
5-8	5-15	On the anterior median line **3 cun** superior to the level of the centre of the umbilicus	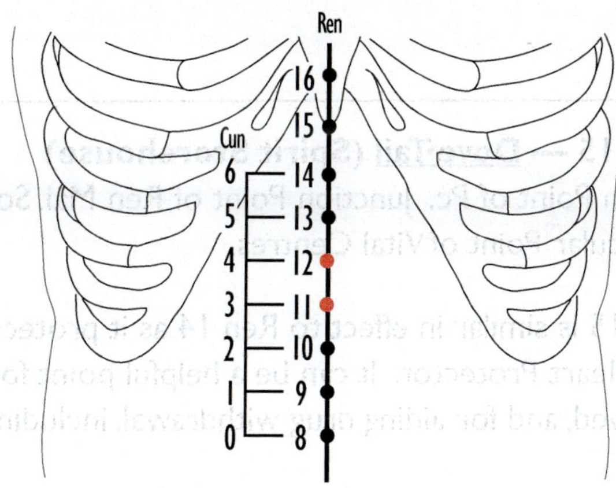
3-8	7-15	On the anterior median line **4 cun** superior to the level of the centre of the umbilicus **4 cun** inferior to the level of the xiphisternal joint	

Ren Mai Conception Vessel

Ren 13 — <u>Upper Duct</u> (Upper Regulator, Upper Portion of the Stomach)
Crossing Point of Ren Mai, SI and St. First Aid: difficulty in swallowing.

Ren 10, 12, 11 and 13 all influence the Stomach. Ren 13 controls the upper part, the region where food enters the stomach to start the process of rotting and ripening. Consider when a person feels they can't "stomach" food or life any more. Good for nausea, hiatus hernia, belching, reflux, hiccups, or chronic worry and anxiety.

Ren 14 — <u>Great Deficiency</u> (Greatest Palace Gate)
Alarm Point of Ht. First Aid: motion sickness, angina pectoris.

Protects, calms and supports the Supreme Controller (is connected to its deep pathway) particularly if a patient is lacking in inner joy and tranquillity. The effect can sometimes be immediate. For chest pain, palpitations, angina (consider using together with Pc 4), hiccups, or for those who feel out of control or agitated at a deep level. When used with Ren 4, Ren 14 can help re-establish the Jing-Shen (Heart-Kidney) link when this has been disturbed by emotional turmoil. Can be used after Ren 8 to further support the Heart if the patient's Spirit is still deficient.

Ren 15 — <u>Dove Tail</u> (Spirit Storehouse)
Alarm Point of Pc. Junction Point of Ren Mai. Source Point of 5 Yin Officials. Centre Reunion Particular Point of Vital Centres.

Ren 15 is similar in effect to Ren 14 as it protects and supports both the Supreme Controller and the Heart Protector. It can be a helpful point for panic attacks, particularly when loved ones are involved, and for aiding drug withdrawal, including tobacco.

⊥	Δ		**Location**
5-8	7-15	On the anterior median line **5 cun** superior to the level of the centre of the umbilicus **3 cun** inferior to the level of the xiphisternal joint	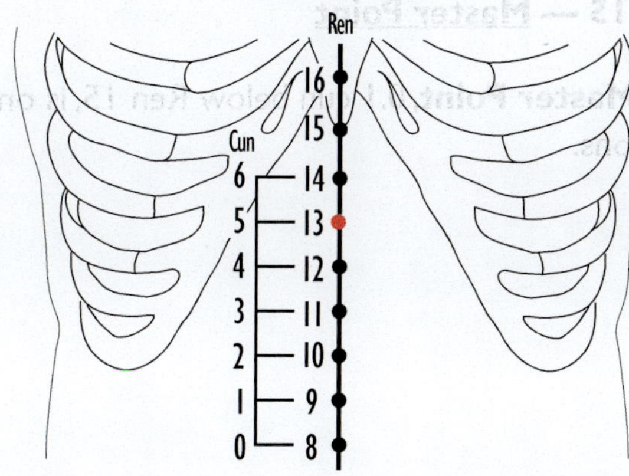
6	7-15	On the anterior median line **6 cun** superior to the level of the centre of the umbilicus **2 cun** inferior to the level of the xiphisternal joint	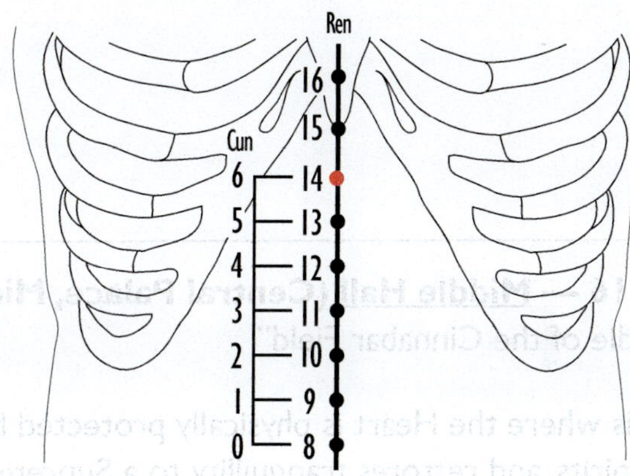
3-5	3-5	On the anterior median line At the tip of the Xiphoid Process **7 cun** superior to the level of the centre of the umbilicus **1 cun** inferior to the level of the xiphisternal joint	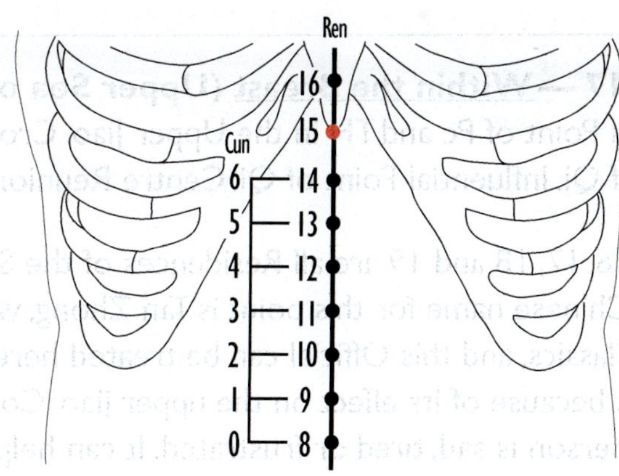

Ren 15 — Master Point

The **Master Point**, 0.1 cun below Ren 15, is one of the points used to release the Internal Dragons.

Ren 16 — Middle Hall (Central Palace, Middle Courtyard)
"Middle of the Cinnabar Field"

This is where the Heart is physically protected by the ribcage and sternum. This point Supports the Spirits, and restores tranquillity to a Supreme Controller and its Protector if they are in emotional turmoil or when severely depleted. Lies in the middle of the Dan Tian.

Ren 17 — Within the Breast (Upper Sea of Qi, Centre of the Chest, Central Hall)
Alarm Point of Pc and TH in the Upper Jiao. Crossing Point of Ren Mai, Sp, Kid, SI and Liv. Point of Sea of Qi. Influential Point of Qi. Centre Reunion Point of Breath. "Anti-smoking Point".

Ren 16, 17, 18 and 19 are all Residences of the Supreme Controller, and are powerful Spirit points. The Chinese name for this point is Tan Zhong, which is also the name of the Heart Protector in the Classics, and this Official can be treated here. It brings support and vitality to the Heart and Lungs because of its effect on the upper jiao. Consider this point when all the Seas are depleted or a person is sad, tired or frustrated. It can help the patient to respond more effectively to the Command Points. It relaxes and opens the Chest if there is Lu Qi or Ht Qi deficiency. The point can be used for a chronic cough, or to help with withdrawal from tobacco addiction. It is rarely needled because of its location on the breast bone. Moxa is commonly used here.

⊥	Δ		**Location**
3	X	Hangs like a raindrop **0.1 cun** below Ren 15	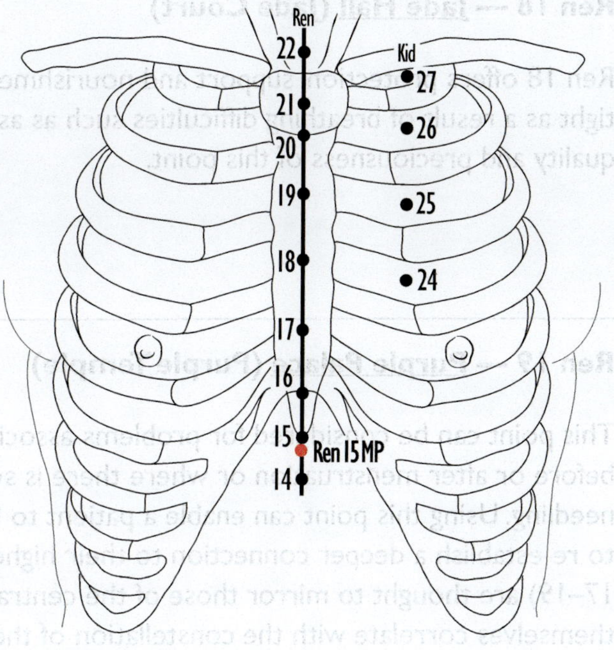
3	5	On the anterior median line At the inferior edge of the sternum At the xiphisternal joint At the level of the **5th IC Space**	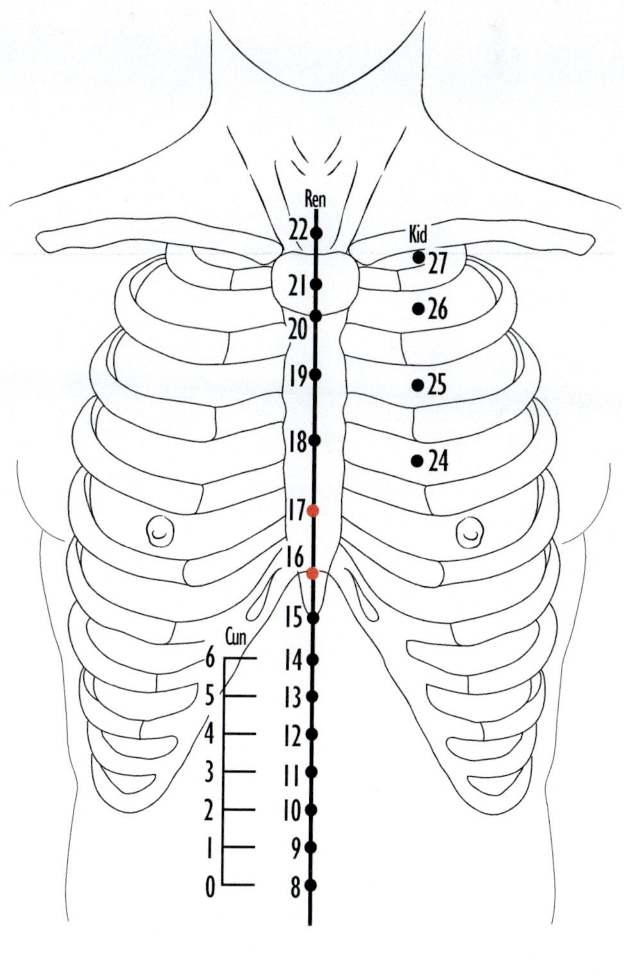
X	3	On the anterior median line On the body of the sternum At the level of the **4th IC Space** Midway between the nipples	

Ren Mai Conception Vessel

Ren 18 — Jade Hall (Jade Court)

Ren 18 offers protection, support and nourishment for the Heart. It can help when the chest is tight as a result of breathing difficulties such as asthma or bronchitis. Jade in its name reflects the quality and preciousness of this point.

Ren 19 — Purple Palace (Purple Temple)

This point can be considered for problems associated with the female breast — if they are tender before or after menstruation or where there is swelling, abscesses or mastitis. Apply caution when needling. Using this point can enable a patient to be more receptive to treatment, allowing them to re-establish a deeper connection to their higher self. These 'Imperial Residence' points (Ren 17–19) are thought to mirror those of the central palaces of the (Purple) Forbidden City, which themselves correlate with the constellation of the The Plough/Big Dipper.

⊥	Δ		**Location**
3	5	On the anterior median line On the body of the sternum At the level of the **3rd IC Space**	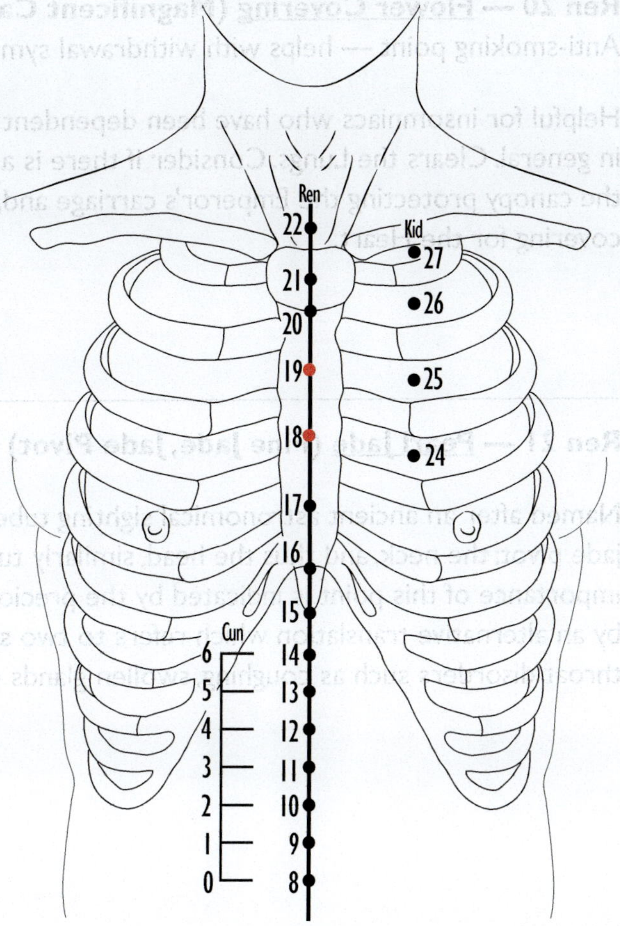
3	5	On the anterior median line On the body of the sternum At the level of the **2nd IC Space**	

Ren 20 — <u>Flower Covering</u> (Magnificent Canopy)
Anti-smoking point — helps with withdrawal symptoms

Helpful for insomniacs who have been dependent on drugs for a long time, or for drug addiction in general. Clears the Lungs. Consider if there is a lack of a sense of smell. The name refers to the canopy protecting the Emperor's carriage and, by extension, to the Lung's role as a protective covering for the Heart.

Ren 21 — <u>Pearl Jade</u> (Fine Jade, Jade Pivot)

Named after an ancient astronomical sighting tube (for viewing the Big Dipper) which turned on a jade pivot; the neck, and thus the head, similarly turns on a pivot — the clavicle and sternum. The importance of this point is indicated by the preciousness and rarity of pearl-coloured jade, and also by an alternative translation which refers to two stars in the Big Dipper constellation. Consider for throat disorders such as coughing, swollen glands or difficulty in swallowing.

Ren 22 — <u>Heaven Rushing Out</u> (Celestial Chimney, Heavenly Process)
Window of the Sky. Crossing Point of Yin Wei Mai (Linking Vessel) and Ren Mai.

This point can open up a new and refreshing perspective on life, for those living under a continual dark cloud. For drug addiction where the patient is living in a self-imposed prison. Consider when a person doesn't want to converse or can't express their feelings or, conversely, are 'spaced out' through drug use. Can be helpful for throat and speech difficulties. Before needling, caress this point with gentle massage. This is a Window of the Sky point, but the practitioner may wish to consider using a Window point on the patient's CF first to gauge the response.

⊥	△		Location
3	3	On the anterior median line At the superior edge of the crest of the sternal angle At the level of the **1st IC Space**	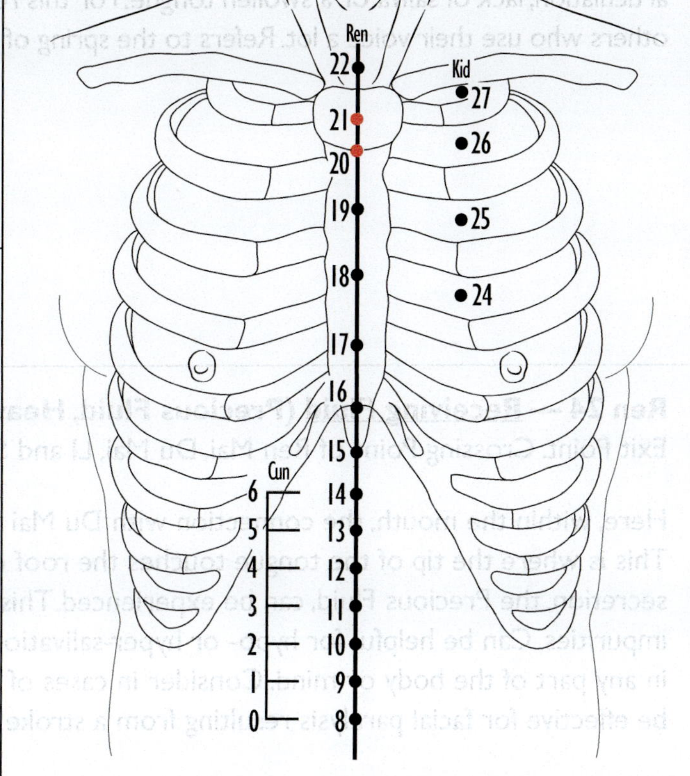
3	5	On the anterior median line At the centre of the sternal manubrium Level with the **articulation of the 1st rib** **1 cun** inferior to Ren 22	
3	3-7	**Five Element Acupuncture Location** On the anterior aspect of the neck On the pharynx Directly inferior to the cricoid cartilage On the anterior median line **TCM location** On the anterior median line In the centre of the suprasternal fossa **0.5 cun** superior to the suprasternal notch	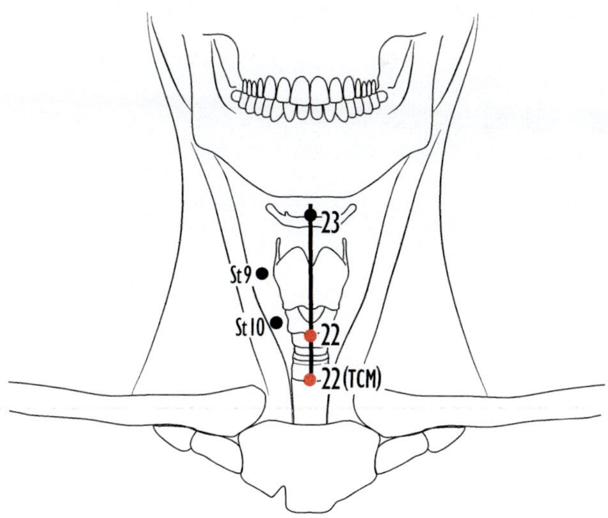

Ren Mai Conception Vessel

Ren 23 — <u>Angle Spring</u> (Pure Spring)
Crossing Point of Yin Wei Mai (Linking Vessel) and Ren Mai

Because of its connection with the tongue, this point is said to be helpful with difficulties of speech and articulation, lack of saliva or a swollen tongue. For this reason it can be helpful for teachers, singers and others who use their voice a lot. Refers to the spring of saliva which lies under the tongue.

Ren 24 — <u>Receiving Fluid</u> (Precious Fluid, Heavenly Pond)
Exit Point. Crossing Point of Ren Mai, Du Mai, LI and St. Ghost Point.

Here, within the mouth, the connection with Du Mai is made, thus linking the Yin with the Yang. This is where the tip of the tongue touches the roof of the mouth, and from which an inner secretion, the Precious Fluid, can be experienced. This fluid cleanses, bathes and washes away impurities. Can be helpful for hypo- or hyper-salivation. Lack of coordination is a key factor here — in any part of the body or mind. Consider in cases of dumbness and insanity, fear and anxiety. Can be effective for facial paralysis resulting from a stroke, or in cases of Bell's Palsy.

⊥	Δ		Location
3	3-7	In the depression at the superior border of the hyoid bone	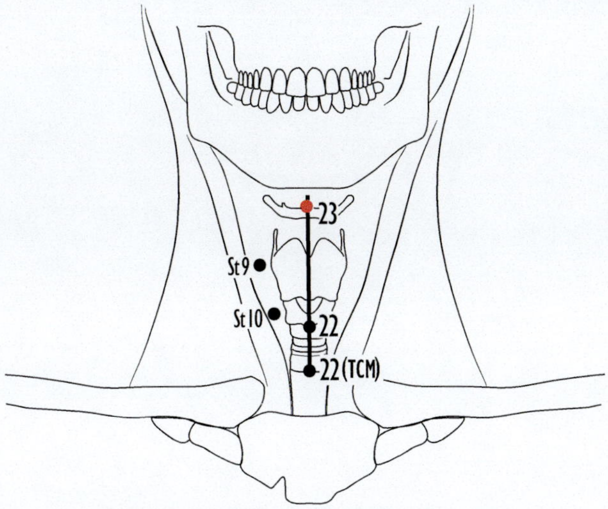
1-3	3-7	In the middle of the mentolabial groove Directly superior to the mental shelf At the inferior border of the orbicularis oris muscle	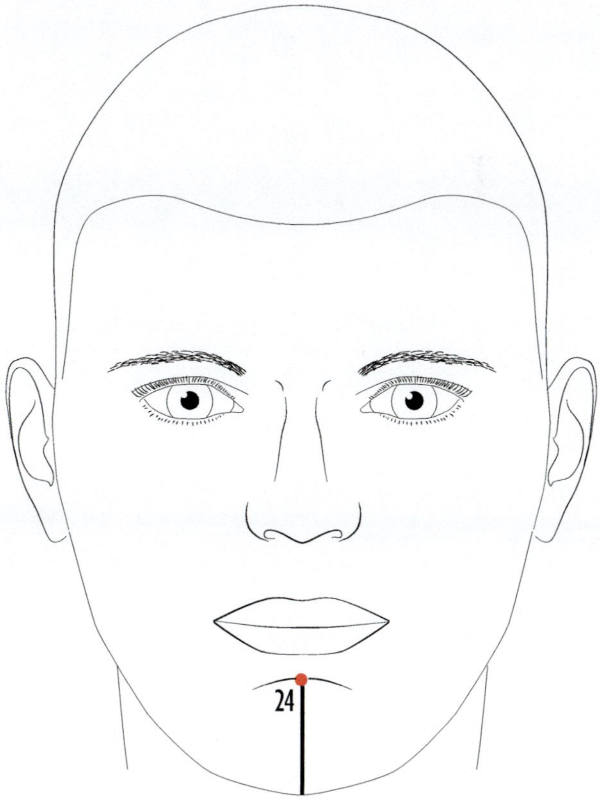

Du Mai Governor Vessel

- **Sea of Yang Energy**
- **Guards the Yang within**

Du Mai Governor Vessel

Du 1 — <u>Long Strength</u> (Long and Strong)
Entry Point. Junction Point of Du Mai. Crossing Point of Du Mai, Ren Mai, Kid and Gb.

As the Entry Point, it brings in the Yang influence with its attributes of strength, clarity and flexibility. Connects to the brain and our heavenly aspect. As a Junction Point, it regulates, connects and re-establishes communication between our internal Yin and Yang. Consider for emotional instability, lack of coordination, lack of cooperation, or where a person is completely distraught; this point brings much strength to the Body, Mind and Spirit. Can strengthen the 'backbone' of a person. Consider for lower back pain, haemorrhoids, vaginal or anal prolapse.

Du 2 — <u>Loins Correspondence</u> (Lumbar Door)
Associated Effect Point of the Loins Area

For problems in the area of the loins such as back pain, stiffness, chronic sacral pain or general aching in the loins. Consider for irregular menstruation, or where a person is extremely irritable, rather than depressed, at the start of menstruation. For paralysis of the legs and feet.

Du 3 — <u>Loins Yang Passageway</u> (Loins Yang Border, Yang Gate, Lumbar Yang Gate)

This is a passageway from the loins through the Gate of Life, and eventually to the head and brain. Tonifies the Kidneys. Helps bring strength and flexibility to the spine, and can be considered for lower back pain. Also useful if the patient can't bend from the knees, has arthritis or rheumatism in the lower limbs, or for cold feet. Moxa used here warms through to the abdomen and the lower jiao, and is helpful for fear around sexual intimacy or for male sexual weakness.

⊥	Δ		Location
3	5-15	At the tip of the coccyx	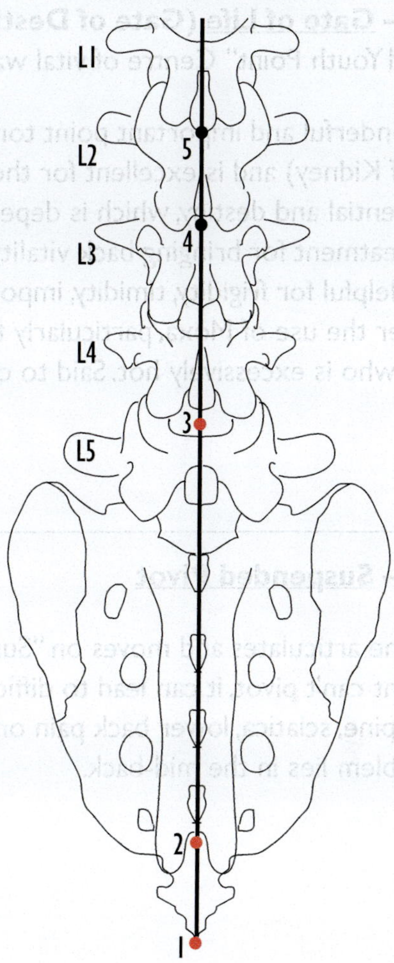
3-5	5-15	In the sacro-coccygeal articulation At the sacral hiatus	
3-5	5-15	On the posterior median line Between the **4th and 5th Lumbar vertebrae**	

Du Mai Governor Vessel

Du 4 — <u>Gate of Life</u> (Gate of Destiny, Palace of Jing/Essence)
"Second Youth Point" Centre of vital warmth

This wonderful and important point tonifies the Kidneys and thus the Jing (it lies between the AEP's of Kidney) and is excellent for those with a weak constitution. Du 4 has to do with fulfilling our potential and destiny, which is dependent on access to this Jing. Consider using this point early on in treatment for bringing back vitality and energy to a person who is lifeless, cold, with no joy in life. Helpful for frigidity, timidity, impotence, infertility, menstrual pain or menstrual disorders. Consider the use of Moxa, particularly for cold-related problems, taking care not to overheat a person who is excessively hot. Said to correlate with the Hall of Union in the Forbidden City.

Du 5 — <u>Suspended Pivot</u>

The spine articulates and moves on "Suspended Pivot", and this point is to do with its flexibility. If this point can't pivot, it can lead to difficulties in movement giving rise to problems such as: rigidity of the spine, sciatica, lower back pain or aching in the back. It is sometimes combined with Du 7 if the problem lies in the mid-back.

Du 6 — <u>Middle of the Spine</u> (Spiritual Ancestor)
Said to affect the whole endocrine system

This point can also be used to strengthen the spine and aid its flexibility. It has additional benefits on the mental level: consider its use for anxiety, overthinking or difficulty processing thoughts. It is said to help in cases of hysteria and insanity, epilepsy or depression. Moxa is usually forbidden.

Du 7 — <u>Middle Pivot</u> (Central Pivot)

This point, together with Du 5 and Du 6, can be used for stiffness (inflexibility) of the spine. Moxa is usually forbidden.

⊥	Δ		Location
3	7-15	On the posterior median line Between the **2nd and 3rd Lumbar vertebrae**	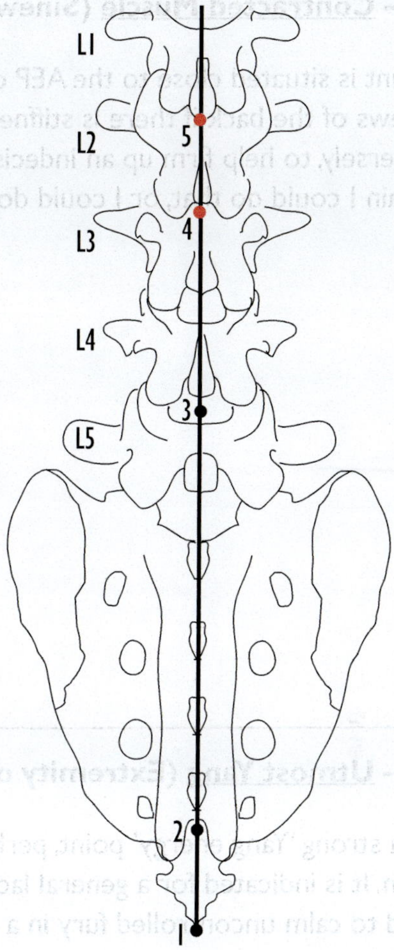
3	7-15	On the posterior median line Between the **1st and 2nd Lumbar vertebrae**	
3	X	On the posterior median line Between the **11th and 12th Thoracic vertebrae**	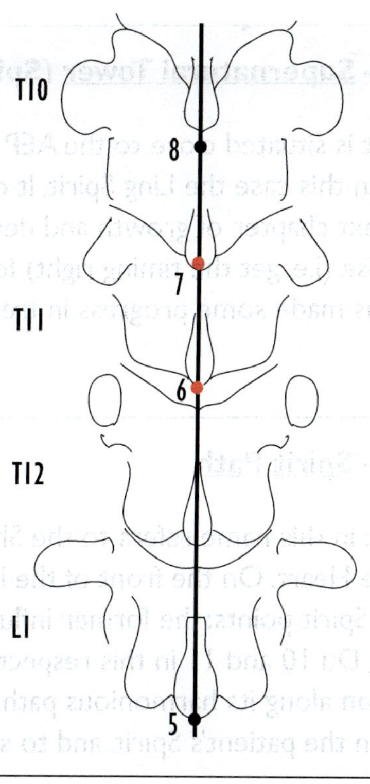
X	X	On the posterior median line Between the **10th and 11th Thoracic vertebrae** Some texts permit needling.	

Du 8 — <u>Contracted Muscle</u> (Sinew Binder)

This point is situated close to the AEP of the Liver, and is commonly sedated to relax the muscles and sinews of the back if there is stiffness, tension or spasm there. Consider also for mental rigidity or, conversely, to help firm up an indecisive person, e.g. someone who says "well I could do this, then again I could do that, or I could do both" — a common Gallbladder dilemma.

Du 9 — <u>Utmost Yang</u> (Extremity of Yang)

This is a strong 'Yang energy' point, perhaps the most Yang point on this predominantly Yang meridian. It is indicated for a general lack of vitality and weariness of the Body, Mind and Spirit. It is also said to calm uncontrolled fury in a person.

Du 10 — <u>Supernatural Tower</u> (Spirit Tower, Temple of the Soul)

This point is situated close to the AEP of the Heart, and can be used to strengthen a person's Spirit — in this case the Ling Spirit. It can help bring perspective to a patient, and prepare them for the next chapter of growth and development in their life. In this respect it is important to synchronise (i.e. get the timing right) for its full effect to be achieved, so consider its use after the patient has made some progress in treatment, particularly at a deeper level.

Du 11 — <u>Spirit Path</u>

The Spirit in this name refers to the Shen Spirit, and this point is situated at the level of the Back Shu of the Heart. On the front of the body, at a similar level, lie Kid 24 and Kid 25, two other powerful Spirit points; the former influencing the Ling whilst the latter nourishes the Shen, thus mirroring Du 10 and 11 in this respect. After awakening the Spirit at Du 10, we need to ensure its progression along its harmonious path. For this reason, it is often combined with Du 10 in order to strengthen the patient's Spirit, and to support their own deeper personal development.

⊥	Δ		Location
4	3	On the posterior median line Between the **9th and 10th Thoracic vertebrae**	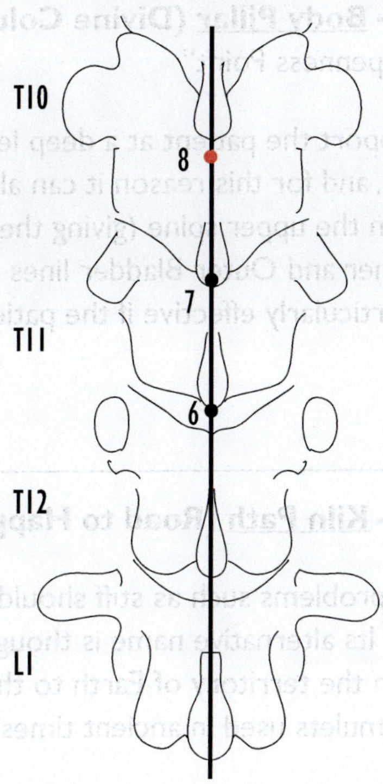
5	7	On the posterior median line Between the **7th and 8th Thoracic vertebrae**	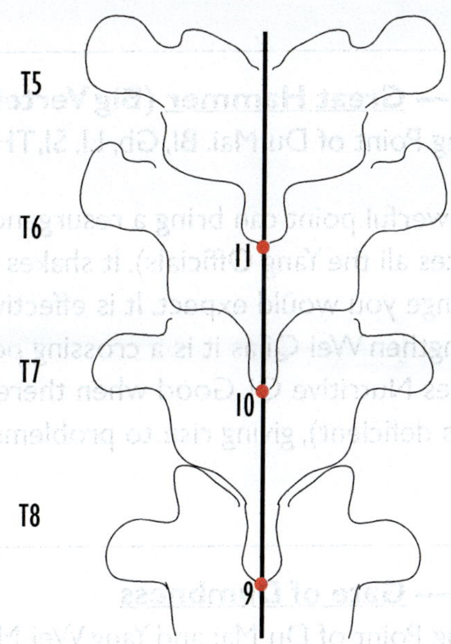
X	3-7	On the posterior median line Between the **6th and 7th Thoracic vertebrae** Some texts permit needling.	
X	3-5	On the posterior median line Between the **5th and 6th Thoracic vertebrae** Some texts permit needling.	

Du Mai Governor Vessel

Du 12 — <u>Body Pillar</u> (Divine Column, Body Support)
"Social Openness Point"

Helps support the patient at a deep level; it's like a pillar for the Spirit. It can augment treatment on the Lungs, and for this reason it can also be helpful for long-term grief and sadness. This point can strengthen the upper spine (giving the patient 'backbone'), and can be combined with other points on the Inner and Outer Bladder lines to reinforce this. Du 12 can be used with a lot of Moxa, and can be particularly effective if the patient is cold, weak or inert. Connects, via a deep pathway, to Bl 12.

Du 13 — <u>Kiln Path</u> (Road to Happiness)

For local problems such as stiff shoulders and neck pain, or an inability to raise the arms. It calms the Spirit. Its alternative name is thought to arise from the upward energetic movement, from its location in the territory of Earth to that of Heaven. Strengthens Wei Qi. Kiln is said to refer to the ceramic amulets used in ancient times to ward off evil spirits. Here the Bl meridian connects to Du Mai.

Du 14 — <u>Great Hammer</u> (Big Vertebrae)
Crossing Point of Du Mai, Bl, Gb, LI, SI, TH and St. Point of Sea of Qi. Influential Point of Yang.

This powerful point can bring a resurgence of strength and vitality to a person's energy system (it influences all the Yang Officials). It shakes up these Officials. Consider if treatment is not generating the change you would expect. It is effective for chronic illness. Consider Moxa here. Can be used to strengthen Wei Qi as it is a crossing point of St, Bl, and Gb as well as being a Sea of Qi point. Regulates Nutritive Qi. Good when there is distress of the Mind and Spirit (particularly if the Heart is deficient), giving rise to problems such as depression, sadness or insomnia.

Du 15 — <u>Gate of Dumbness</u>
Crossing Point of Du Mai and Yang Wei Mai (Linking Vessel). Point of Sea of Marrow. One of the nine needles for returning Yang. Some texts classify it as a Sea of Qi Point.

This point can treat speech and voice disorders, as it connects to the tongue which itself is linked to the Ht and speech. Consider for children with speech difficulties, or for speech difficulties in adults after Wind Stroke. For sudden loss of voice. Needle with care. Moxa usually forbidden. Useful for anger, headache, dizziness or seizures which arise from interior invasion of Wind. As a Sea of Marrow Point, in combination with Du 16, 19 and 20, this point can nourish the brain and the senses, and aid in the integration of the three levels of Body, Mind and Spirit.

⊥	△		Location
4	5-30	On the posterior median line Between **the 3rd and 4th Thoracic vertebrae**	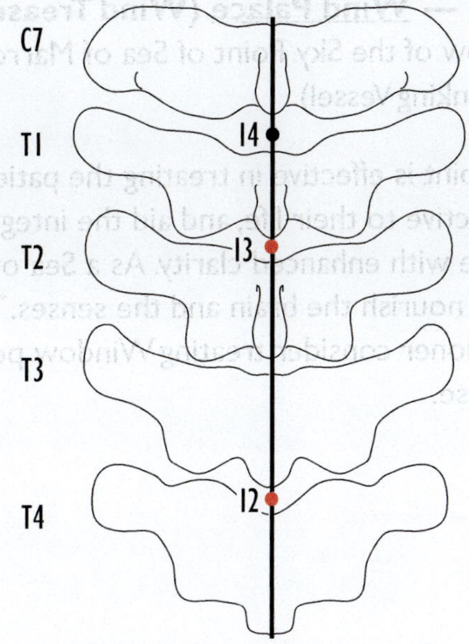
4	5-10	On the posterior median line Between the **1st and 2nd Thoracic vertebrae**	
4	5-15	On the posterior median line Between the **7th Cervical** and **1st Thoracic vertebrae**	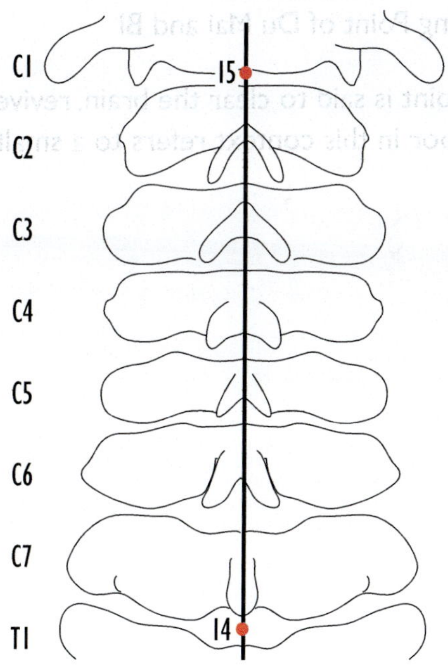
3	X	Shallow needling only On the posterior median line Between the **1st and 2nd Cervical vertebrae** **0.5 cun** superior to the natural posterior hairline **0.5 cun** inferior to Du 16 Level with Bl 10	

Du Mai Governor Vessel

Du 16 — <u>Wind Palace</u> (Wind Treasury)
Window of the Sky. Point of Sea of Marrow. Ghost point. Crossing Point of Du Mai and Yang Wei Mai (Linking Vessel).

This point is effective in treating the patient at the Spirit level. It can clear the head and bring perspective to their life, and aid the integration of Body Mind and Spirit. Helps the patient to hear and see with enhanced clarity. As a Sea of Marrow Point, in combination with Du 15, 19 and 20, Du 16 can nourish the brain and the senses. This is a Window of the Sky point; it is suggested that the practitioner consider treating Window points on the CF first before using this point to gauge its response.

Du 17 — <u>Brain Door</u>
Crossing Point of Du Mai and Bl

This point is said to clear the brain, revive consciousness, treat epilepsy and stimulate the senses. The door in this context refers to a small important opening into a specific area — in this case the brain.

<table>
<tr><th>⊥</th><th>Δ</th><th></th><th>Location</th></tr>
<tr><td>3</td><td>X</td><td>On the posterior torso at the nape of the neck — junction of head and neck
On the posterior median line
Between the attachments of the trapezius muscles
Just inferior to the base of the external occipital protuberance of the occipital bone
1 cun superior to the natural posterior hairline
0.5 cun superior to Du 15</td><td>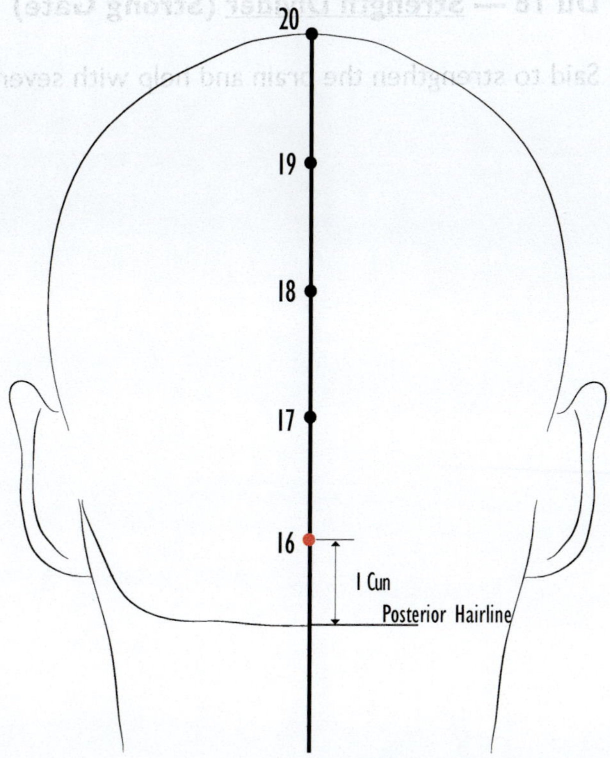
</td></tr>
<tr><td>X</td><td>X</td><td>On the occipital bone
On the level of the superior border of the external occipital bone and Bl 9
1.5 cun superior to Du 16
2.5 cun superior to the natural posterior hair line
Some texts permit needling.</td><td>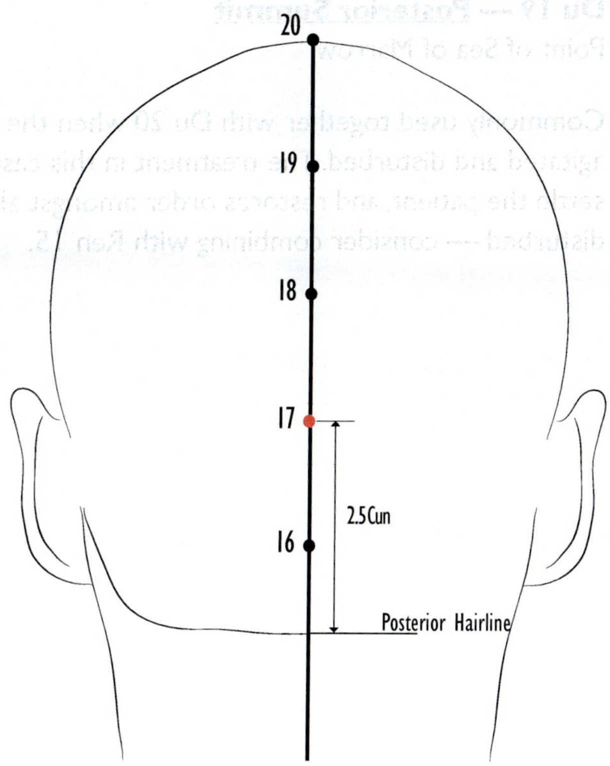
</td></tr>
</table>

Du 18 — Strength Divider (Strong Gate)

Said to strengthen the brain and help with severe headaches.

Du 19 — Posterior Summit
Point of Sea of Marrow

Commonly used together with Du 20 when the pulse picture is chaotic, and the patient is severely agitated and disturbed. The treatment in this case is usually sedation. This point helps calm and settle the patient, and restores order amongst all the Officials. For anxiety when the (Shen) Spirit is disturbed — consider combining with Ren 15.

⊥	Δ		Location
2	X	At the junction of the sagittal and lambdoid sutures **1.5 cun** superior to Du 17 **4 cun** superior to the natural posterior hair line	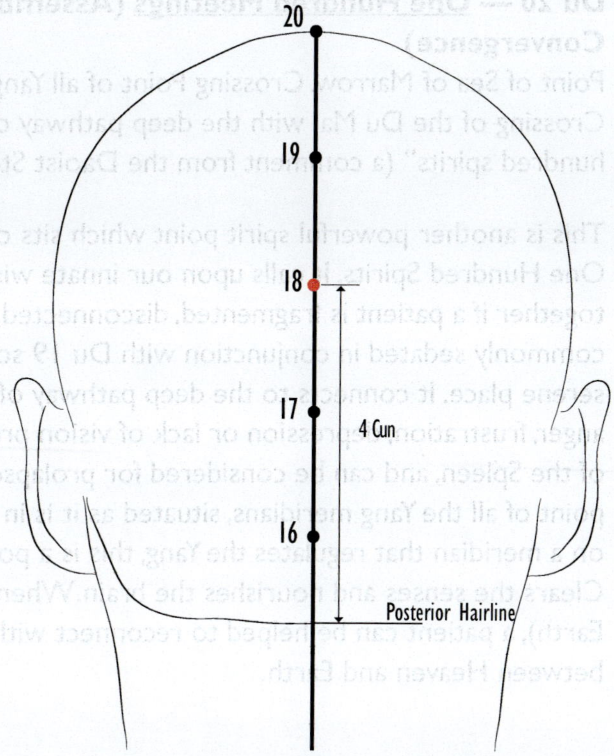
3	7	**1.5 cun** superior to Du 18 **5.5 cun** superior to the natural posterior hairline	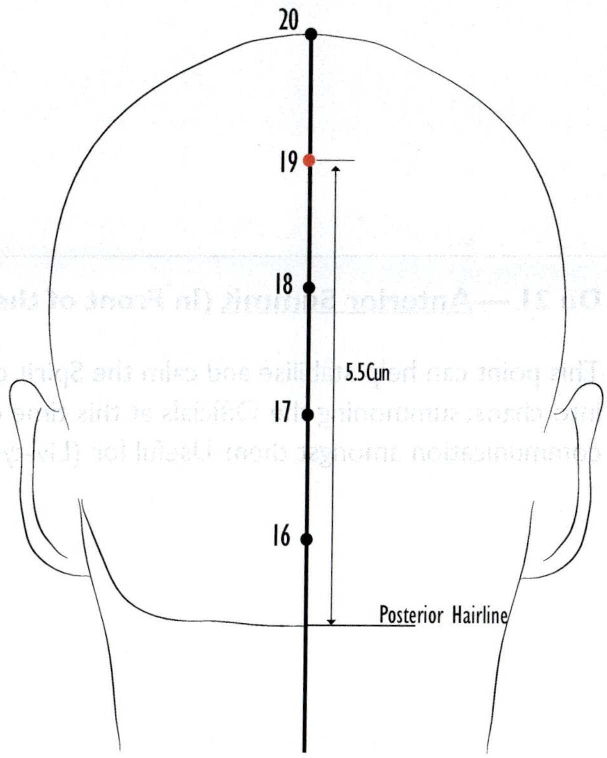

Du 20 — <u>One Hundred Meetings</u> (Assembly of the One Hundred, Hundred Convergence)

Point of Sea of Marrow. Crossing Point of all Yang Meridians. Point to release the External Dragons. Crossing of the Du Mai with the deep pathway of the Liver. "The head is the meeting place of the hundred spirits" (a comment from the Daoist Storehouse text).

This is another powerful spirit point which sits on top of the head — the meeting place of the One Hundred Spirits. It calls upon our innate wisdom and knowledge, and can bring everything together if a patient is fragmented, disconnected, chaotic or severely agitated. In these cases, it is commonly sedated in conjunction with Du 19 so that the patient may be returned to a calm and serene place. It connects to the deep pathway of the Liver, and thus can be effective in cases where anger, frustration, depression or lack of vision predominate. It strengthens the ascending function of the Spleen, and can be considered for prolapse of the anus, vagina or uterus. As the crossing point of all the Yang meridians, situated as it is in a prime position to receive the heavenly influxes, on a meridian that regulates the Yang, this is a point that strongly influences this aspect of a person. Clears the senses and nourishes the brain. When combined with Kid 1 (the point closest to the Earth), a patient can be helped to reconnect with their authentic self and their rightful position between Heaven and Earth.

Du 21 — <u>Anterior Summit</u> (In Front of the Summit)

This point can help stabilise and calm the Spirit of the patient. Use before things have descended into chaos; summoning the Officials at this time can prevent disaster by ensuring there is free communication amongst them. Useful for (Liv-type) headaches at the top of the head.

⊥	△		Location
3	7	On the top of the Head — On the parietal bone **1.5 cun** superior to Du 19 **7 cun** superior to the natural posterior hairline **5 cun** posterior to the natural anterior hair line	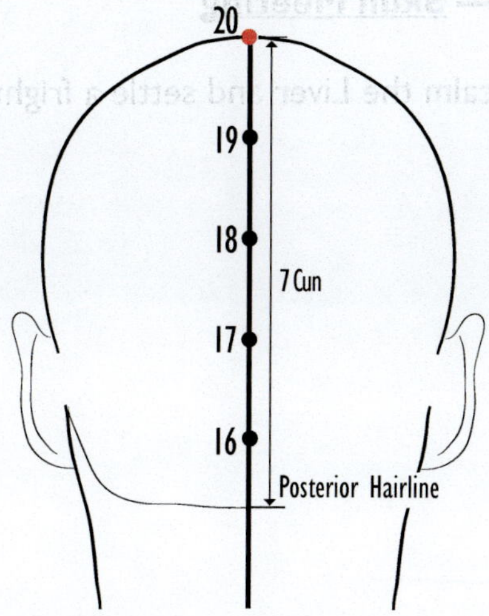
			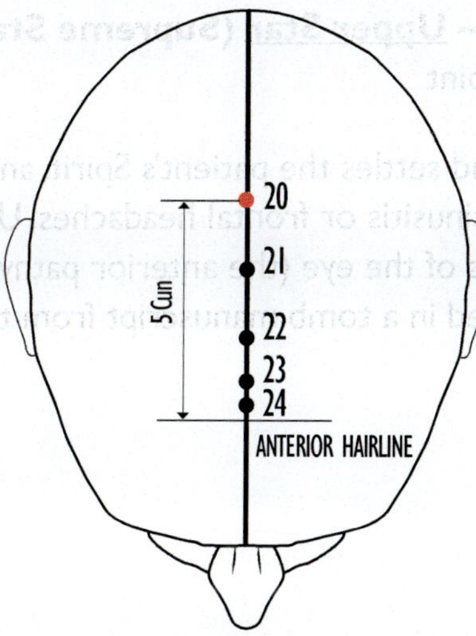
2	3-7	**1.5 cun** anterior to Du 20 **3.5 cun** posterior to the natural anterior hairline	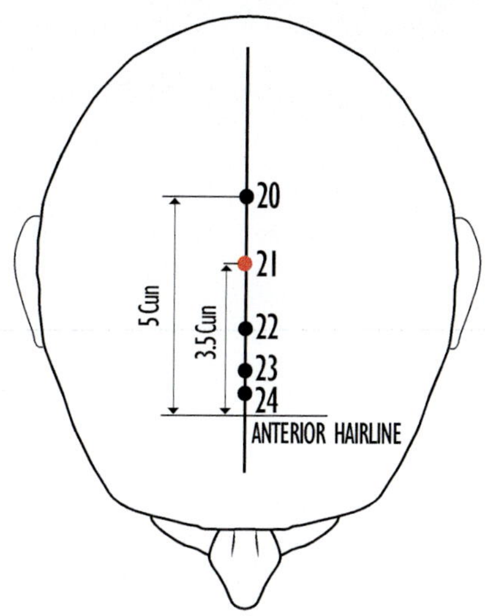

Du 22 — Skull Meeting

Said to calm the Liver and settle a frightened person. Consider for insomnia.

Du 23 — Upper Star (Supreme Star)
Ghost Point

Calms and settles the patient's Spirit, and is said to clear past traumas from the mind. Helpful for chronic sinusitis or frontal headaches. Used for chronic allergic rhinitis or nasal polyps. Treats disorders of the eye (the anterior pathway of the Du Mai passes between the eyes). Its name is mentioned in a tomb manuscript from the 1st century BCE.

⊥	Δ		Location
1	3	At the junction of the coronal and sagittal suture **2 cun** posterior to the natural anterior hair line **3 cun** anterior to Du 20	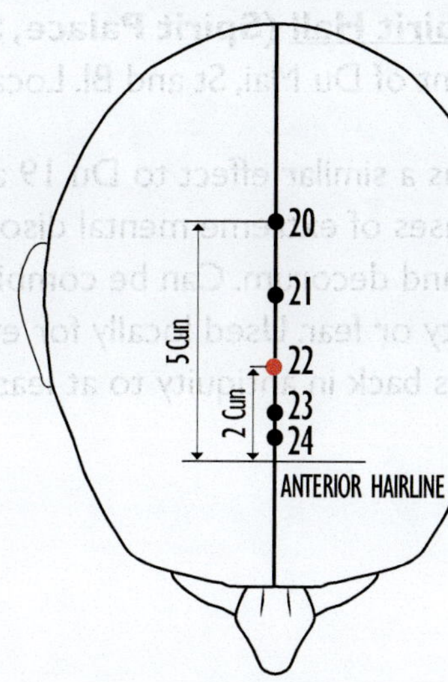
2	5	**1 cun** posterior to the natural anterior hairline **1 cun** anterior to Du 22 **4 cun** anterior to Du 20	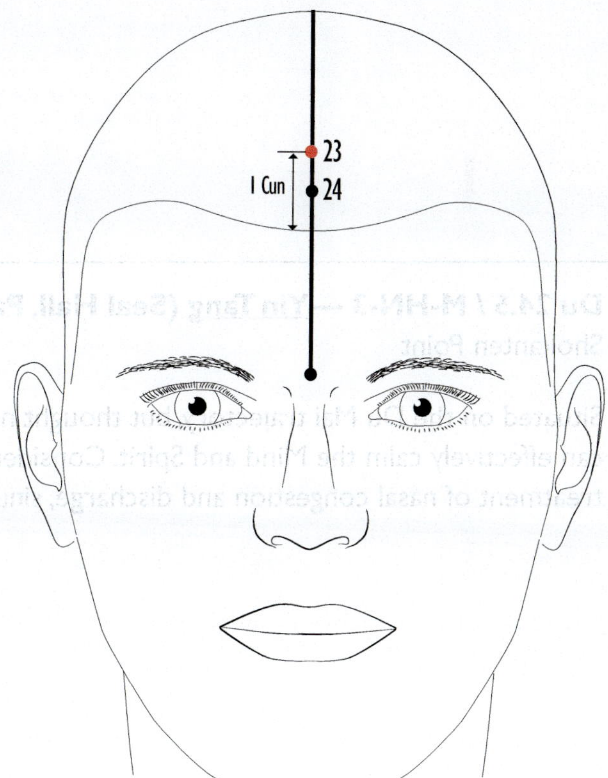

Du Mai Governor Vessel

Du 24 — <u>Spirit Hall</u> (Spirit Palace, Spirit Courtyard)
Crossing Point of Du Mai, St and Bl. Located in the upper Dan Tian.

This point has a similar effect to Du 19 and 20. It calms the Mind and Spirit in a powerful way. Can be used in cases of extreme mental disorders, e.g. schizophrenia, obsessive thinking patterns, loss of uprightness and decorum. Can be combined with Gb 13 or Yin Tang to augment its effect in calming severe anxiety or fear. Used locally for eye pain, redness or swelling of the eyes, rhinitis or sinusitis. Its name goes back in antiquity to at least the 1st century BCE.

Du 24.5 / M-HN-3 — <u>Yin Tang</u> (Seal Hall, Palace of Impression)
Shokanten Point

Situated on the Du Mai trajectory, but thought not to be a part of it. This is an extra point that can effectively calm the Mind and Spirit. Consider for frontal headache. Benefits the nose in the treatment of nasal congestion and discharge, sinus pain, rhinitis and nosebleed.

⊥	Δ		Location
X	5	**0.5 cun** posterior to the natural anterior hairline **0.5 cun** anterior to Du 23 Some texts permit needling.	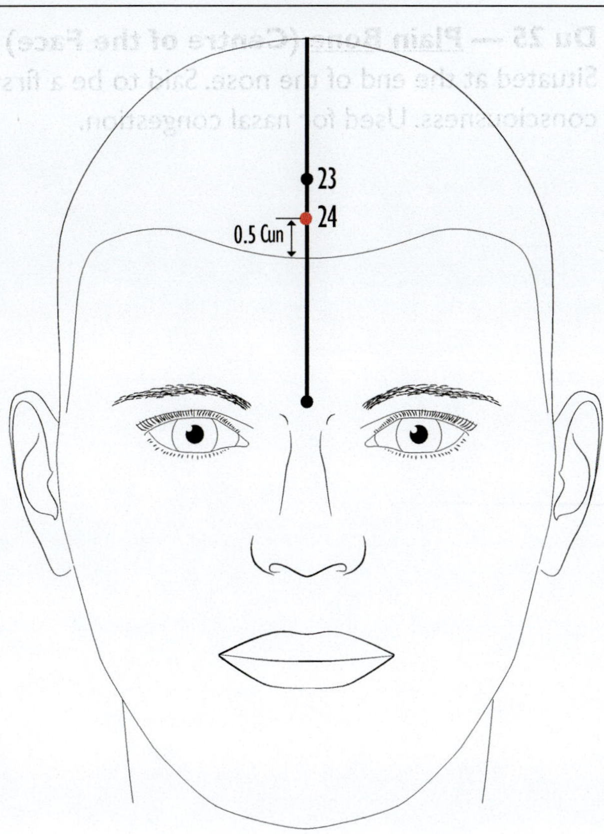
1-3	3-5	At the glabella, at the midpoint between the medial extremities of the eyebrows	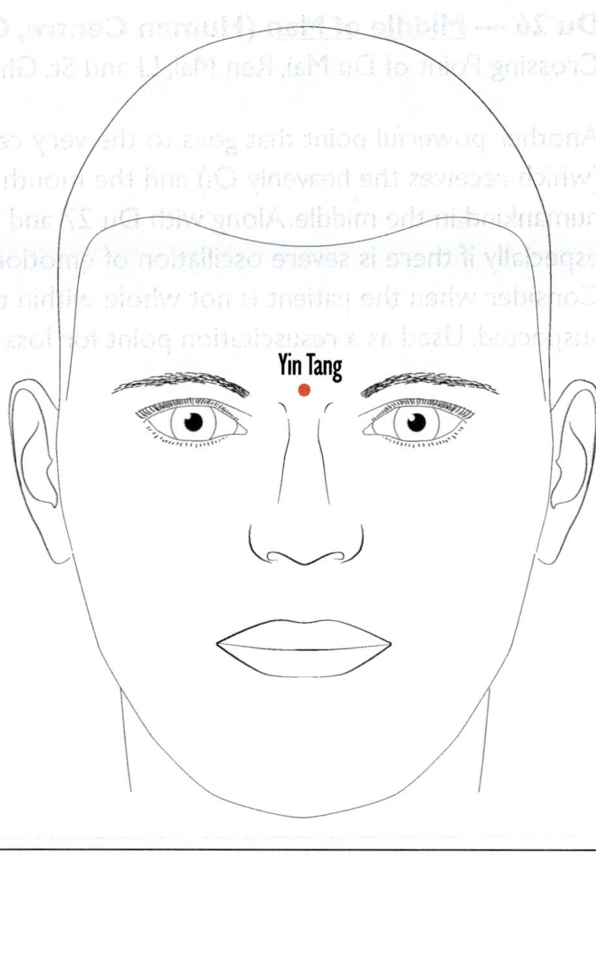

Du 25 — <u>Plain Bone</u> (Centre of the Face)
Situated at the end of the nose. Said to be a first aid point for drunkenness. Restores consciousness. Used for nasal congestion.

Du 26 — <u>Middle of Man</u> (Human Centre, Ghost Palace)
Crossing Point of Du Mai, Ren Mai, LI and St. Ghost Point

Another powerful point that goes to the very centre of our being, as it sits between the nose (which receives the heavenly Qi) and the mouth (which receives the potential for earthly Qi), with humankind in the middle. Along with Du 27 and 28, it helps regulate the Yin/Yang balance within, especially if there is severe oscillation of emotion or mood (such as bipolar disorder or mania). Consider when the patient is not whole within their Spirit, or when a degree of Possession is suspected. Used as a resuscitation point for loss of consciousness.

⊥	Δ		Location
1-2	X	At the tip of the nose At the apex of the cartilage of the septum of the nose	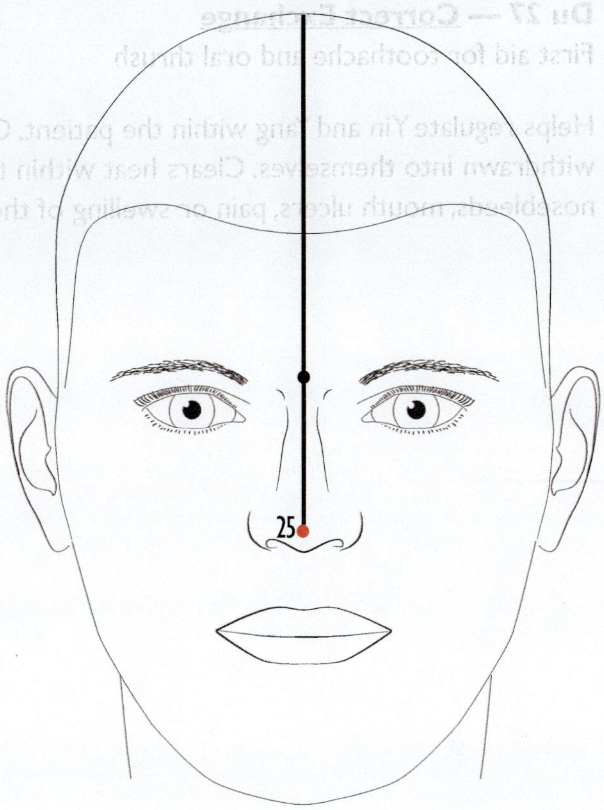
2	3	On the philtrum below the nose One third the distance from the root of the nasal spine to the vermilion border of the upper lip	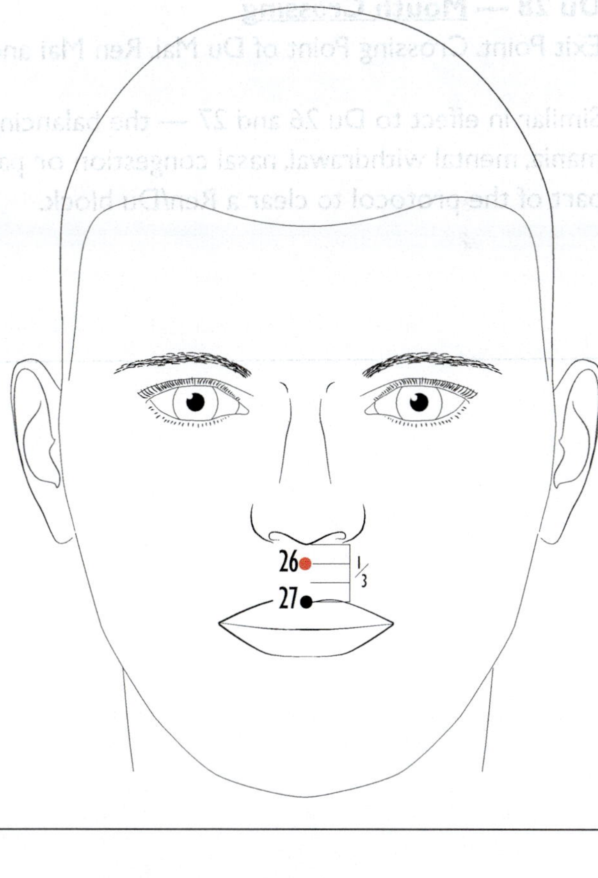

Du Mai Governor Vessel

Du 27 — Correct Exchange
First aid for toothache and oral thrush

Helps regulate Yin and Yang within the patient. Consider for mania, or where a person has withdrawn into themselves. Clears heat within the system, and thus can be effective in treating nosebleeds, mouth ulcers, pain or swelling of the gums.

Du 28 — Mouth Crossing
Exit Point. Crossing Point of Du Mai, Ren Mai and St.

Similar in effect to Du 26 and 27 — the balancing of Yin and Yang within the patient. Consider for mania, mental withdrawal, nasal congestion or pain in the centre of the face. Most often used as part of the protocol to clear a Ren/Du block.

⊥	△		Location
2	2	On the philtrum below the nose At the junction of the philtrum and the vermilion border of the upper lip	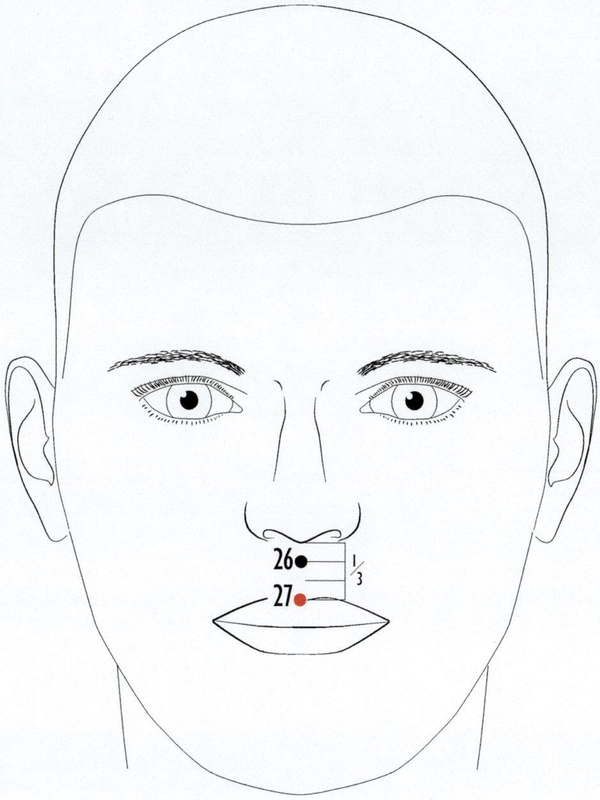
2	X	In the mouth At the junction of the frenulum of the upper lip and the upper gum	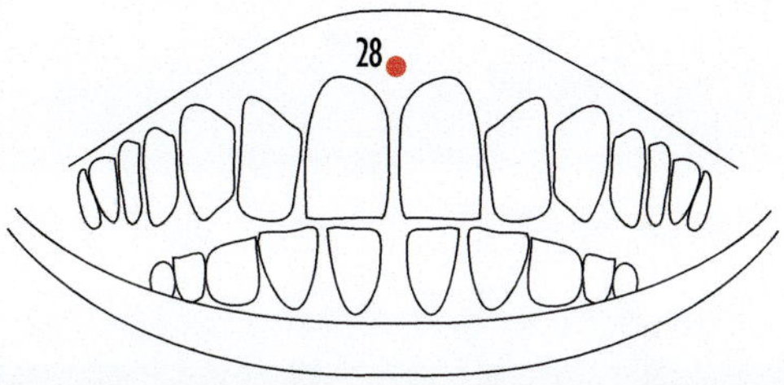

Appendix 1: Point Groupings, Categories and Cun (ACI) Measurements

Point Categories

	Source Point	Junction Point	Accumulation Point	Entry Point	Exit Point	Tonification Point	Sedation Point
Lung	Lu 9	Lu 7	Lu 6	Lu 1	Lu 7	Lu 9	Lu 5
Large Intestine	LI 4	LI 6	LI 7	LI 4	LI 20	LI 11	LI 2
Stomach	St 42	St 40	St 34	St 1	St 42	St 41	St 45
Spleen	Sp 3	Sp 4	Sp 8	Sp 1	Sp 21	Sp 2	Sp 5
Heart	Ht 7	Ht 5	Ht 6	Ht 1	Ht 9	Ht 9	Ht 7
Small Intestine	SI 4	SI 7	SI 6	SI 1	SI 19	SI 3	SI 8
Bladder	Bl 64	Bl 58	Bl 63	Bl 1	Bl 67	Bl 67	Bl 65
Kidney	Kid 3	Kid 4	Kid 5	Kid 1	Kid 22	Kid 7	Kid 1
Pericardium	Pc 7	Pc 6	Pc 4	Pc 1 (males) Pc 2 (females)	Pc 8	Pc 9	Pc 7
Triple Heater	TH 4	TH 5	TH 7	TH 1	TH 22	TH 3	TH 10
Gallbladder	Gb 40	Gb 37	Gb 36	Gb 1	Gb 41	Gb 43	Gb 38
Liver	Liv 3	Liv 5	Liv 6	Liv 1	Liv 14	Liv 8	Liv 2

	Horary Point	Seasonal Horary	Back Shu Point	Alarm Point	Windows of the Sky
Lung	Lu 8	Autumn	Bl 13	Lu 1	Lu 3
Large Intestine	LI 1	Autumn	Bl 25	St 25	LI 18
Stomach	St 36	Late Summer	Bl 21	Ren 12	St 9
Spleen	Sp 3	Late Summer	Bl 20	Liv 13	—
Heart	Ht 8	Summer	Bl 15	Ren 14	—
Small Intestine	SI 5	Summer	Bl 27	Ren 4	SI 16 SI 17
Bladder	Bl 66	Winter	Bl 28	Ren 3	Bl 10
Kidney	Kid 10	Winter	Bl 23	Gb 25	—
Pericardium	Pc 8	Summer	Bl 14	Ren 17, 15	Pc 1 (males) Pc 2 (females)
Triple Heater	TH 6	Summer	Bl 22	Ren 5	TH 16
Gallbladder	Gb 41	Spring	Bl 19	Gb 24, 23	—
Liver	Liv 1	Spring	Bl 18	Liv 14	—

Windows of the Sky Points also include Ren 22 and Du16

Transporting Points/Antique Points

Yin Meridians	Jing-Well/ Winter	Ying-Spring/ Spring	Shu-Stream/ Summer	Jing-River/ Late-Summer	He-Sea/ Autumn
Lung	Lu 11	Lu 10	Lu 9	Lu 8	Lu 5
Pericardium	Pc 9	Pc 8	Pc 7	Pc 5	Pc 3
Heart	Ht 9	Ht 8	Ht 7	Ht 4	Ht 3
Spleen	Sp 1	Sp 2	Sp 3	Sp 5	Sp 9
Liver	Liv 1	Liv 2	Liv 3	Liv 4	Liv 8
Kidney	Kid 1	Kid 2	Kid 3	Kid 7	Kid 10
Yang Meridians	**Jing-Well/ Winter**	**Ying-Spring/ Spring**	**Shu-Stream/ Summer**	**Jing-River/ Late-Summer**	**He-Sea/ Autumn**
Large Intestine	LI 1	LI 2	LI 3	LI 5	LI 11
Triple Heater	TH 1	TH 2	TH 3	TH 6	TH 10
Small Intestine	SI 1	SI 2	SI 3	SI 5	SI 8
Stomach	St 45	St 44	St 43	St 41	St 36
Gallbladder	Gb 44	Gb 43	Gb 41	Gb 38	Gb 34
Bladder	Bl 67	Bl 66	Bl 65	Bl 60	Bl 40

Element Points

Yin Meridians	Wood	Fire	Earth	Metal	Water
Lung	Lu 11	Lu 10	Lu 9	Lu 8	Lu 5
Pericardium	Pc 9	Pc 8	Pc 7	Pc 5	Pc 3
Heart	Ht 9	Ht 8	Ht 7	Ht 4	Ht 3
Spleen	Sp 1	Sp 2	Sp 3	Sp 5	Sp 9
Liver	Liv 1	Liv 2	Liv 3	Liv 4	Liv 8
Kidney	Kid 1	Kid 2	Kid 3	Kid 7	Kid 10
Yang Meridians	**Wood**	**Fire**	**Earth**	**Metal**	**Water**
Large Intestine	LI 3	LI 5	LI 11	LI 1	LI 2
Triple Heater	TH 3	TH 6	TH 10	TH 1	TH 2
Small Intestine	SI 3	SI 5	SI 8	SI 1	SI 2
Stomach	St 43	St 41	St 36	St 45	St 44
Gallbladder	Gb 41	Gb 38	Gb 34	Gb 44	Gb 43
Bladder	Bl 65	Bl 60	Bl 40	Bl 67	Bl 66

Eight Influential Points (Hui-Meeting/ Gathering/Assembling Points)

Point	Region
Liv 13	Yin Officials (Zang)
Ren 12	Yang Officials (Fu)
Ren 17	Qi
Bl 17	Blood
Gb 34	Sinews, Muscles, Tendons
Lu 9	Blood Vessels
Bl 11	Bones
Gb 39	Marrow

Greater Influential Points (Greater Gathering/Greater Assembling Points)

Point	Region
SI 7	Head and neck
LI 4	Face and Mouth
St 36	Stomach and Abdomen
Bl 40	Back and Vertebrae

Sea Points

	Points
Sea of Qi	St 9, Bl 10 (or Du 14 & Du 15), Ren 17
Sea of Marrow	Du 15, Du 16, Du 19, Du 20
Sea of Nourishment	St 30, St 36
Sea of Blood	Upper Body: Bl 11 Lower Body: St 37, St 39
Lower He-Sea	LI — St 37 Bl — Bl 40 St — St 36 TH — Bl 39 SI — St 39 Gb — Gb 34

Eight Extraordinary Meridians

	Master/ Confluent Point	Coupled point	Junction Point	Accumulation Point
Ren Mai (Conception Vessel)	Lu 7	Kid 6	Ren 15	—
Du Mai (Governor Vessel)	SI 3	Bl 62	Du 1	—
Chong Mai (Penetrating Vessel)	Sp 4	Pc 6	—	—
Dai Mai (Girdle Vessel)	Gb 41	TH 5	—	—
Yin Qiao Mai (Heel Vessel/Motility Vessel)	Kid 6	Lu 7	—	Kid 8
Yang Qiao Mai (Heel Vessel/Motility Vessel)	Bl 62	SI 3	—	Bl 59
Yin Wei Mai (Linking Vessel)	Pc 6	Sp 4	—	Kid 9
Yang Wei Mai (Linking Vessel)	TH 5	Gb 41	—	Gb 35

Nine Needles to Return Yang — Used in cases of extreme Yang deficiency

	Points
Loss of Yang Rooted in Kidneys	Kid 1, Kid 3
Loss of Yang from Dampness and/or Cold	Sp 6, St 36, Ren 12
Loss of Yang from Exuberant Heat with Wind	Du 15, LI 4
Loss of Yang from Heart	Pc 6
Loss of Yang due to Bi-Obstruction in the Limbs	Gb 30

Points to Release the Internal Dragons (commonly used)
Ren 15 (Master Point)
St 25
St 32
St 41

Points to Release the Internal Dragons — With Depression (rarely used)
Ren 15 (Master Point)
St 25
St 32
St 36.5 (M-LE-13)
St 41

Points to Release the External Dragons
Du 20
Bl 11
Bl 23
Bl 61

Points to treat Husband–Wife Block
Bl 67
Kid 3
Kid 7
Liv 4
Tonification of Ht 7 and SI 4 is also recommended

Ghost Points

Point	Ghost Point Name
Du 26	Ghost Palace (Ghost Reception Room)
Du 23	Ghost Hall
Du 16	Ghost Pillow, Ghost Hole
Ren 24	Ghost Market
Lu 11	Ghost Faith
LI 11	Ghost Leg, Ghost Minister
Pc 7	Ghost Heart
Pc 8	Ghost Cave (Pc 5 is an alternative to Pc 8)
Pc 5	Ghost in the Cave, Ghost Road (Pc 8 is an alternative to Pc 5)
St 6	Ghost's Bed, Ghost Forest
Sp 1	Ghost Fortress, Ghost Pile, Ghost Eye
Bl 62	Ghost Path
M-HN-37 Guifeng Extra Point on the underside of the tongue, one cun from the tip of the midline	Ghost Seal
Ren 1 originally described as Yumentou (Extra Point — Women) Yinxiafeng (Extra Point — Men)	Ghost Store, Ghost in the Hidden Place

Ma Danyang Heavenly Star Points

Lu 7	Bl 40
LI 4	Bl 57
LI 11	Bl 60
St 36	Gb 30
St 44	Gb 34
Ht 5	Liv 3

Shokanten Points

Lu 9	Kid 16
Ht 7	Kid 19
TH 21	Kid 21
LI 4	St 2
Liv 3	St 25
Liv 13	St 27
Liv 14	St 42
Kid 12	Tai Yang (extra point)

Cun (ACI) Measurements

Anterior Torso	
Anterior median line to tip of acromion process	8 cun
Anterior median line to Medial border of the anterior superior iliac spine	4 cun
Superior border of symphysis pubis bone (at Ren 2) to Centre of the Umbilicus (navel)	5 cun
Centre of the Umbilicus (navel) to Xiphisternal joint (at Ren 16)	8 cun
Arm	
Anterior end of axillary fold (where the upper arm joins the torso) to Flexure of the elbow (transverse crease/elbow crease)	9 cun
Flexure of the elbow (transverse crease/elbow crease) to Wrist flexure	12 cun
Leg	
Inferior border of symphysis pubis to Popliteal crease	14 cun
Gluteal crease to Popliteal crease	14 cun
Popliteal crease on lateral side of knee flexure to Prominence of the lateral malleolus	16 cun
Popliteal crease on medial side of knee flexure to Prominence of the medial malleolus	15 cun
Head	
Natural anterior hairline to Natural posterior hairline	12 cun
Between two corners of the head (at St 9)	9 cun
Posterior Torso	
Posterior median line to Medial border of the scapula at the level of T3	3 cun

Glossary

Accumulation Points
These are synonymous with Xi-cleft Points.

Aggressive Energy (AE)
This is synonymous with Perverse, Evil or Xie Qi.

Akabane(i) Test
This test assesses the bilateral balance within a meridian using heat sensitivity on the terminal nail points of the fingers and toes.

Alarm Points
These are synonymous with Front connecting or Mo (u) Points.

Back Shu Points
These are synonymous with Associated Effect Points (AEP).

Causative Factor.
The term Causative Factor (CF), or constitutional imbalance, indicates the one Element of the Five most in need of supportive treatment.

Crossing Point
The words "Crossing Point" are used in order to standardise the term which in other traditions can be translated as "Reunion", "Coalescing" or "Meeting" Points.

"Cun".
This term is synonymous with Anatomical Chinese Inch (ACI). Please see Appendix I.

Dragons.
This term refers to the Point combinations used in the treatment of demonic possession due to either Internal or External devils.

Husband Wife Imbalance
This protocol aims to re-establish harmony that has been severely compromised between the pulses on the left hand side and those on the right.

Influential Points
These are synonymous with Assembling, Hui — Meeting or Gathering Points.

Junction Points
These are synonymous with Luo, Connecting or Passage Points.

Needle Depth
This is given in "fen".

Officials (The)
The 12 Officials are the personification of the organs (the Zang Fu) whose functions and responsibilities are described in Su Wen chapter 8 in which is emphasised the importance of their mutual support and cooperation so that peace and harmony may prevail within the kingdom of the human body.

Spirit of the Points.
This term refers to the inherent quality unique to each Point which bestows the ability to initiate positive change in a patient's life. However, for this latent potential to be fully realised, it is incumbent upon the practitioner that their inner state be in harmony so that their own virtuosity and compassionate intention is present at the time of needling. This is relevant for any Point but essential when addressing those on the spirit level.

Window of the Sky Points
These are synonymous with Window of Heaven Points.

Notes

Names

The first name given to each Point is generally considered to be the most significant translation from the Chinese although some of these are debateable. Additional translations which follow certain Points are taken from various sources and are included so that they may bestow a further understanding from, and a flavour of the ancient Chinese characters.

Within quotation marks are short descriptive phrases given to certain Points which are attributed to Roger de la Fuÿe (de la Filye).

Needle (⊥) and Moxa (Δ)

The common needle depth for each point is given in fen together with the common number of moxas.

Forbidden points are marked with an X. However all three can vary depending on the College attended/Tradition studied.

Variant Point Location

Some practitioners use a variant location of certain Points to those in this book, particularly on the Yin meridians of the leg which can vary by one cun (one ACI). Furthermore the physiological differences between individuals means that the points can vary slightly and should therefore be palpated for their precise location.

Bibliography

Bertschinger, Richard. 1991. "The Golden Needle" and Other Odes of Traditional Acupuncture. Churchill Livingstone, Edinburgh.

College of Traditional Acupuncture. "The Jing Luo: The Definitive Guide to Point Location". (Dean Lander). Leamington Spa (1996) UK.

College of Traditional Acupuncture. "Acupuncture Point Compendium". (Claire-Louise Hatton). Leamington Spa, UK (2000).

Deadman, Peter *et al.*, 1998. "A Manual of Acupuncture". JCM Publications, Hove, UK.

Eckman, Peter. "In The Footsteps of the Yellow Emperor". Long River Press, San Francisco, USA, 2007.

Ellis, A., Wiseman, N., Boss, K. 1989. "Grasping the Wind". Brookline, MA: Paradigm Publications USA.

Hicks, Angela, Hicks, John & Mole, Peter. "Five Element Constitutional Acupuncture", 2004, Elsevier Limited, UK.

Hicks, Sara. "Catalogue of Acupuncture Point Translations", 1985, privately published.

Kaptchuk, Ted. "The Web That Has No Weaver". Congdon and Weed. NY 1983, USA.

Lade, A. "Acupuncture Points: Images and Functions". Seattle, WA. Eastland Press, USA.

Larre, Claude, Schatz, J, & Rochat de la Vallee Elizabeth. 1986. "Survey of Traditional Chinese Medicine". Institut Ricci, Paris, France.

Larre, Claude & Rochat, Elizabeth. 1992. "The Secret Treatise of the Spiritual Orchid". Monkey Press, Cambridge, UK.

Larre, Claude. 1994. "The Way of Heaven". Monkey Press, Cambridge, UK.

Larre, Claude & Rochat, Elizabeth. 1995. "Rooted In Spirit". Station Hill Press, New York, USA.

Larre, Claude & Rochat, Elizabeth. 1996. "The Seven Emotions". Monkey a Press, Cambridge, Uk.

Larre, Claude & Rochat, Elizabeth. 1997. "The Eight Extraordinary Meridians". Monkey Press, Cambridge, UK.

Larre, Claude & Rochat, Elizabeth. 1999. "Essence, Spirit, Blood and Qi". Monkey Press, Cambridge, UK.

Larre, Claude & Rochat, Elizabeth. 2001. "The Lung". Monkey Press, Cambridge, UK.

Larre, Claude & Rochat, Elizabeth. 2003. "The Extraordinary Fu". Monkey Press, Cambridge, UK.

Lavier, Jacqes. "Histoire, doctrine et practique de l'acupuncture chinoise." Tchou. Paris. 1996.

Lightbody, Stuart. "The 1984 China Study Tour". Privately published.

Lightbody, Stuart. "The Forbidden City and it's Correlation with Classical Acupuncture and the Human Body". EJOM. Vol. 8. No. 6. 2017.

Maciocia, Giovanni. 1989. "The Foundations of Chinese Medicine". Churchill Livingstone, Edinburgh, UK.

Mann, Felix. "The Treatment of Disease by Acupuncture". Heinemann. London. 1963.

Mann, Felix. "Acupuncture: The Ancient Chinese Art of Healing". Heinemann. London. 1971.

Pirog, J. 1996. "Practical Application of Meridian Style Acupuncture". Pacific View Press. Berkeley. USA.

Ross, J. 1995. "Acupuncture Point Combinations". Churchill Livingstone, Edinburgh, UK.

Turner & Low, 1981. "The Principles and Practice of Moxibustion". Thornsons. Northants, UK.

Unschuld, Paul. 1986. "Nan Ching: Classic of Difficult Issues". University of California Press, USA.

Veith, Ilza. 1972. "The Yellow Emperor's Classic of Internal Medicine". University of California Press, Berkeley, CA, USA.

Venn, Lois. 1994. "Spirits and Functions". College of Traditional Acupuncture, Leamington Spa, UK.

Worsley, J.R. 1975. "Acupuncturists' Therapeutic Pocket Book". The Centre for Traditional Acupuncture, Inc. American City Building. Columbia. Maryland, USA.

Worsley, J.R. 1979. "The Meridians of Ch'i Energy: Point Reference Guide". Tai Sophia Institute, Laurel, MD, USA.
Worsley, J.R. 1982. "Traditional Chinese Acupuncture, Volume 1, Meridians and Points". Element Books, Tisbury, UK.
Wu Wei-P'ing. 1962. "Chinese Acupuncture". J Lavier (trans from Chinese) and P. Chancellor (trans from French). Health Science Press, Denington Estate, USA.
Yang, Ji-Zhou. 1601ce. "Zhen Jiu Da Chang — Great Compendium of Acupuncture and Moxibustion". In Chinese.

Index of Point Names

Heart

HT 1 — Utmost Source (Extreme Source, Utmost Spring, Supreme Spring)

HT 2 — Blue Green Spirit (Green Spirit)

HT 3 — Lesser Sea (Little Sea, Yellow Sea, Lesser Yin Sea)

HT 4 — Spirit Path (Route of the Spirit, Spirit Way)

HT 5 — Penetrating Inside (Communication with the Interior)

HT 6 — Yin Mound (Yin Reserve, Stone Palace, Yin Cleft)

HT 7 — Spirit Gate (Central Metropolis)

HT 8 — Lesser Palace (Palace of Weariness, Lesser Treasury, Little Storehouse)

HT 9 — Little Rushing In (Lesser Surge, Lesser Rushing)

Small Intestine

SI 1 — Lesser Marsh (Little Marsh)

SI 2 — Forward Valley (Front Valley)

SI 3 — Back Ravine (Back Stream)

SI 4 — Wrist Bone

SI 5 — Yang Valley

SI 6 — Nourishing the Old (Supporting the Old)

SI 7 — Upright Branch (Branch to the Upright)

SI 8 — Small Sea

SI 9 — Upright Shoulder (Shoulder Virtue, Shoulder Divination)

SI 10 — Shoulder Blade

SI 11 — Heavenly Ancestor (Celestial Ancestor, Celestial Gathering)

SI 12 — Grasping the Wind (sometimes known as 'Clutching at Straws')

SI 13 — Crooked Wall (Bend Wall, Curved Wall)

SI 14 — Outside Shoulder Correspondence

SI 15 — Middle of Shoulder Correspondence

SI 16 — Heavenly Window (Celestial Window)

SI 17 — Heavenly Appearance (Celestial Countenance)

SI18 — Cheek Bone.

SI 19 — Listening Palace (Auditory Palace, Temple of Understanding)

Bladder

Bl 1 — Eyes Bright (Eyes Clarity)

Bl 2 — Collect Bamboo (Bamboo Gathering, Beginning of Light)

Bl 3 — Eyebrows Rushing (Eyebrow Ascension)

Bl 4 — Crooked Servant (Nose Thoroughfare)

Bl 5 — Five Places (Fifth Place, Five Dwelling)

Bl 6 — Receive Light (Guarding the Light)

Bl 7 — Penetrate Heaven (Celestial Connection, Celestial White)

Bl 8 — Strong Yang (Brain Cover, Connecting Cleft)

Bl 9 — Jade Pillow

Bl 10 — Heavenly Pillar (Celestial Pillar)

Bl 11 — Great Shuttle

Bl 12 — Wind Gate (Heat Palace, Wind Door)

Bl 13 — Lungs Correspondence

Bl 14 — Circulation/Sex Correspondence

Bl 15 — Heart Correspondence

Bl 16 — Governor Vessel Correspondence

Bl 17 — Diaphragm Correspondence

Bl 18 — Liver Correspondence

Bl 19 — Gallbladder Correspondence

Bl 20 — Spleen Correspondence

Bl 21 — Stomach Correspondence

Bl 22 — Three Heater Correspondence

Bl 23 — Kidney Correspondence

Bl 24 — Sea of Qi Correspondence

Bl 25 — Large Intestine Correspondence

Bl 26 — First Gate Correspondence (Origin Pass)

Bl 27 — Small Intestine Correspondence

Bl 28 — Bladder Correspondence

Bl 29 — Middle of the Backbone Correspondence (Central Spine)

Bl 30 — White Ring Correspondence

Bl 31 — Upper Sacral Bone

Bl 32 — Second Sacral Bone

Bl 33 — Middle Sacral Bone

Bl 34 — Lower Sacral Bone

Bl 35 — Meeting of Yang

Bl 36 (Bl 50) — Receive and Support (Bearing Support, Prop up and Hold)

Bl 37 (Bl 51) — Prosperous Gate

Bl 38 (Bl 52) — Floating Reserve

Bl 39 (Bl 53) — Equilibrium Yang
Bl 40 (Bl 54) — Equilibrium Middle (Bending Centre, Perfect Equilibrium, Supporting the Middle)
Bl 41 (Bl 36) — Near Division
Bl 42 (Bl 37) — Soul Door (Animal Soul Door, Door of the P'o [the Corporeal Soul])
Bl 43 (Bl 38) — Rich for the Vitals (Chronic Illness Point)
Bl 44 (Bl 39) — Spirit Hall (Meeting Place for the Spirit)
Bl 45 (Bl 40) — Wail of Grief (Cry of Pain)
Bl 46 (Bl 41) — Diaphragm Border (Diaphragm Gate)
Bl 47 (Bl 42) — Spiritual Soul Gate (Soul Gate, Gate of the Hun)
Bl 48 (Bl 43) — Yang Net
Bl 49 (Bl 44) — Thought Dwelling (Reflection Abode, Intelligence Lodge, Residence of an Idea)
Bl 50 (Bl 45) — Stomach Granary
Bl 51 (Bl 46) — Diaphragm Gate of Vitality (Vitals Gate)
Bl 52 (Bl 47) — Ambition Room (Determination House, Will Dwelling)
Bl 53 (Bl 48) — Womb and Heart Diaphragm (Bladder Vitals)
Bl 54 (Bl 49) — Orderly Frontier (Ordered Boundary)
Bl 55 — Harmonious Yang (Uniting Yang, Yang Union)
Bl 56 — Supporting Muscles (Sinew Support)
Bl 57 — Supporting Mountain (Mountain Receiving)
Bl 58 — Fly and Scatter (Taking Flight, Flying Yang)
Bl 59 — Foot Bone Yang (Instep Yang)
Bl 60 — Kun Lun Mountain
Bl 61 — Servants Reporting (Official's Aide, Servant's Respect, Set on the Calcaneum)
Bl 62 — Extended Meridian (Extended Vessel)
Bl 63 — Golden Gate
Bl 64 — Capital Bone (Citadel of the Bone)
Bl 65 — Bone Binder (Binding Bone)
Bl 66 — Penetrating Valley (Through the Valley, Passing Valley)
Bl 67 — Extremity of Yin (Arrival of Yin)

Kidney

Kid 1 — Bubbling Spring (Fountain of Life, Earth Surge)
Kid 2 — Blazing Valley (Dragon Spring)
Kid 3 — Greater Mountain Stream (Supreme Stream, Reflecting Sea, Great Torrent)
Kid 4 — Great Bell (Big Bell Clock, Great Cup)
Kid 5 — Water Spring (Water Source)
Kid 6 — Illuminated Sea (Shining Sea, Luminous Sea)
Kid 7 — Returning Current (Return Flow, Deeply White, Bearing White)
Kid 8 — Exchange Pledges (Exchange Trust, Faith Intersection)

Kid 9 — Building Guest (Strengthening the River Bank, Guest House)

Kid 10 — Yin Valley

Kid 11 — Transverse Bone

Kid 12 — Great Brightness (Great Manifestation, Yin Gate)

Kid 13 — Door of Infants (Gate of the Womb, Qi Cave)

Kid 14 — Four Full (Fourfold Fullness, Marrow Mansion)

Kid 15 — Middle Flowing Out (Central Flow)

Kid 16 — Vitals Correspondence

Kid 17 — Merchant Crooked (Shang Bend)

Kid 18 — Stone Border (Stone Pass, Stone Gate)

Kid 19 — Yin Capital (Yin Metropolis)

Kid 20 — Through the Valley (Upper Gate)

Kid 21 — Dark Gate (Secret Gate)

Kid 22 — Walking on the Verandah (Corridor Walk)

Kid 23 — Spirit Seal (Spirit's Altar, Altar Mound)

Kid 24 — Spirit Burial Ground (Empty Spirit, Spirit Ruins)

Kid 25 — Spirit Storehouse (Storing the Spirit)

Kid 26 — Amidst Elegance (Elegant Centre, Lively Centre)

Kid 27 — Storehouse (Treasury, Empty Treasury)

Pericardium. Heart Protector. Circulation Sex. Tan Zhong.

Pc 1 — Heavenly Pond (Celestial Pool)

Pc 2 — Heavenly Spring (Celestial Source, Heavenly Fountain)

Pc 3 — Crooked Marsh (Marsh at the Bend)

Pc 4 — Gate of Qi Reserve (Gate of the Meridian, Cleft Gate, Accumulation Door)

Pc 5 — The Intermediary (Mediating Messenger, Intermediate Emissary)

Pc 6 — Inner Frontier Gate (Inner Gate, Inner Pass)

Pc 7 — Great Mound

Pc 8 — Palace of Weariness (Suffering Palace, Labour Palace,Temple of Hard Work)

Pc 9 — Rushing into the Middle (Central Surge)

Triple Heater. Three Heater. Triple Burner. San Jiao.

TH 1 — Rushing the Frontier Gate (Thoroughfare Gate, Passage Hub)

TH 2 — Fluid Secretion Gate (Door of fluids)

TH 3 — Middle Islet (Central Islet, Middle of the Pond)

TH 4 — Yang Pond (Accumulation of Yang)

TH 5 — Outer Frontier Gate (External Gate, Conserver of Yang)

TH 6 — Branch Ditch (Flying Tiger)

TH 7 — Assembly of Ancestors (Ancestral Cooperation)

TH 8 — Three Yang Junction(Three Yang Connection)

TH 9 — Fourth Gutter (Four Ditches, Four Rivers)

TH 10 — Heavenly Well (Celestial Well)

TH 11 — Pure Cold Abyss (Clear Cold Abyss)

TH 12 — Relax and Joy (Dispersing Brilliance)

TH 13 — Shoulder Meeting (Shoulder Convergence)

TH 14 — Shoulder Bone (Shoulder Opening)

TH 15 — Heavenly Bone (Celestial Hearing, Heavenly Foramen)

TH 16 — Heavenly Window

TH 17 — Wind Screen

TH 18 — Feeding Meridians (Supporting Vessel)

TH 19 — Skull Breathing (Skull Rest)

TH 20 — Small Angle of Ear

TH 21 — Ear Gate (Ear Door)

TH 22 — Harmony Bone (Harmony Foramen)

TH 23 — Silk Bamboo Hollow

Gallbladder

Gb 1 — Orbit Bone (Pupil Crevice, Pupil Foramen)

Gb 2 — Hearing Assembly (Auditory Convergence)

Gb 3 — Upper Gate (Upper Pass, Upper Fortified Gate)

Gb 4 — Loathsome Jaws (Forehead Fullness)

Gb 5 — Suspended Skull

Gb 6 — Suspended Regulator (Suspended Tuft)

Gb 7 — Crooked Hair on the Temple (Temporal Hairline Curve)

Gb 8 — Flowing Valley

Gb 9 — Heaven Rushing (Penetrating Heaven, Celestial Crossroads, Celestial Surge)

Gb 10 — Floating White (Volatile White, Rising White)

Gb 11 — Head Hole Yin (Head Portal Yin, Penetration of Yin)

Gb 12 — Final Bone(Mastoid Process, Completed Bone)

Gb 13 — Root Spirit (Spirit Origin, Root of the Spirit)

Gb 14 — Yang White (Yang Brightness)

Gb 15 — Head Above Tears (On the Point of Weeping)

Gb 16 — Eye Window

Gb 17 — Upright Living (Correct Regulation)

Gb 18 — Receiving Spirit (Spirit Support)

Gb 19 — Brain Hollow

Gb 20 — Wind Pond (Wind Pool, Wind Mansion)

Gb 21 — Shoulder Well

Gb 22 — Armpit Abyss (Armpit Gate)

Gb 23 — Neglected Muscles (Sinew Seat)

Gb 24 — Sun and Moon (Spirit Light)

Gb 25 — Capital Gate (Palace Door)

Gb 26 — Girdle Vessel

Gb 27 — Five Pivots (Fifth Pivot)

Gb 28 — Binding Path (Linking Path)

Gb 29 — Dwelling in the Bone

Gb 30 — Jumping Circle

Gb 31 — Wind Market

Gb 32 — Central River (Middle Ditch)

Gb 33 — Knee Yang Border (Cold Mansion)

Gb 34 — Yang Mound Spring

Gb 35 — Yang Crossing (Yang Intersection)

Gb 36 — Outer Mound

Gb 37 — Bright and Clear (Bright Light)

Gb 38 — Yang Support (Yang Assistance)

Gb 39 — Hanging Cup (Marrow Convergence)

Gb 40 — Wilderness Mound

Gb 41 — Foot above Tears (On the Point of Weeping, Foot Overlooking Tears)

Gb 42 — Earth Five Meetings (Five Terrestrial Reunions)

Gb 43 — Valiant Stream (Narrow Ravine)

Gb 44 — Foot Hole Yin (Cavity of Yin, Foot Portal Yin, Foot Opening Yin)

Liver

Liv 1 — Great Esteem (Great Mound, Great Clarity)

Liv 2 — Walk Between (Moving Between, Walking Space)

Liv 3 — Supreme Rushing (Great Surge, Happy Calm)

Liv 4 — Middle Seal (Central Mound, Middle Border)

Liv 5 — Insect Ditch (Insect Gate, Wormwood Canal)

Liv 6 — Middle Capital (Central Metropolis)

Liv 7 — Knee Gate (Knee Border)

Liv 8 — Crooked Spring (Spring at the Bend)

Liv 9 — Yin Wrapping (Yin Bladder)

Liv 10 — Foot Five Miles (Five Miles)

Liv 11 — Yin Angle (Yin Corner)

Liv 12 — Hasty Pulse (Urgent Pulse, Anxious Pulse)

Liv 13 — Chapter Gate (Gate of Perfection, Camphorwood Gate)

Liv 14 — Gate of Hope (Period Door, Cycle Gate)

Lung

Lu 1 — Central Treasury (Central Storehouse, Middle Palace)

Lu 2 — Cloud Gate (Cloud door)

Lu 3 — Heavenly Palace (Celestial Storehouse, Heavenly Treasury, Heaven's Residence)

Lu 4 — Valiant White (Chivalry White, Pure White, Guarding White)

Lu 5 — Outside Marsh (Foot Marsh, Cubit Marsh)

Lu 6 — Greatest Hole

Lu 7 — Narrow Defile (Balancing Deficiencies, Broken Sequence)

Lu 8 — Meridian Gutter (Meridian Ditch, Regulating Drain, Flowing Gutter)

Lu 9 — Very Great Abyss (Great Abyss, Supreme Whirlpool, Corpse Reviver)

Lu 10 — Fish Region (Fish Border)

Lu 11 — Little Merchant (Scarce Trade, Young Musician)

Large Intestine

LI 1 — Merchant Yang (Metal Yang)

LI 2 — Second Interval (Second Section)

LI 3 — Third Interval (Third Section)

LI 4 — Joining of the Valleys (Great Eliminator, Harmonious Valleys, Meeting of the Valleys)

LI 5 — Yang Stream (Yang Ravine)

LI 6 — Side Passage (Deflected Passage, Page of History, Slanting Passage)

LI 7 — Warm Current (Warm Flow)

LI 8 — Lower Angle (Lower Aspect, Lower Ridge)

LI 9 — Upper Angle (Upper Aspect, Upper Ridge)

LI 10 — Arm Three Miles (Upper Three Miles)

LI 11 — Crooked Pond (Ghost Minister)

LI 12 — Elbow Bone

LI 13 — Arm Five Miles

LI 14 — Outer Bone of the Arm (Thoroughfare to the Head)

LI 15 — Shoulder Joint

LI 16 — Great Bone

LI 17 — Heavenly Vessel

LI 18 — Support and Rush Out (Supporting Process Support the Prominence)

LI 19 — Grain Bone

LI 20 — Welcome Fragrance (Receiving Fragrance)

Stomach

St 1 — Receive Tears (Containing Tears, Weeping Support)

St 2 — Four Whites (Grain Gate)

St 3 — Great Cheekbone

St 4 — Earth Granary (Stomach Link)

St 5 — Great Welcome (Great Reception)

St 6 — Mandible Wheel (Jaw Bone)

St 7 — Lower Passage (Lesser Gate, Lower Pass)

St 8 — Head Tied (Corner of the Head)

St 9 — People Welcome (Humankind Receiving)

St 10 — Water Rushing Out

St 11 — Qi Cottage (Qi Abode)

St 12 — Broken Bowl (Empty Basin, Celestial Cover)

St 13 — Qi Door

St 14 — Storehouse (Granary Building, Treasury Room)

St 15 — Room Screen (Roof)

St 16 — Breast Window

St 17 — Centre of the Breast

St 18 — Root of the Breast

St 19 — Not at Ease (Not Contained, Not Enduring)

St 20 — Receiving Fullness (To Receive Satisfaction)

St 21 — Bridge Gate (Connecting Gate. Beam Gate)

St 22 — Border Gate

St 23 — Great Oneness (Supreme Unity)

St 24 — Lubrication Food Gate

St 25 — Heavenly Pivot (Celestial Pivot, This point has at least nine other names)

St 26 — Outside Mound

St 27 — Great Might (Great Fullness)

St 28 — Water Path (Water Passage)

St 29 — The Return

St 30 — Qi Rushing (Surging Qi)

St 31 — Thigh Border

St 32 — Prostrate Hare (Crouching Rabbit)

St 33 — Yin Market

St 34 — Beam Mound (Hip Bone, Bridge Mound)

St 35 — Calf Nose (Knee Eye)

St 36 — Leg Three Miles (Lower Sea of Qi, Lower Three Miles)

St 37 — Upper Great Void (Upper Great Emptiness)

St 38 — Branch Opening (Narrow Opening)

St 39 — Lower Great Void (Lower Great Emptiness)

St 40 — Abundant Splendour. (Abundant Prosperity. Rich and Prosperous)

St 41 — Released Stream

St 42 — Rushing Yang (Surging Yang)

St 43 — Sinking Valley (Sunken Valley)

St 44 — Inner Courtyard

Spleen

Sp 1 — Hidden White (Mysterious White, Yin White)

Sp 2 — Great Capital (Great Metropolis)

Sp 3 — Supreme White (Greater White, Extreme Whiteness, Great Brightness)

Sp 4 — Prince's Grandson (Supreme Grandchild, Yellow Emperor, Ancestor and Descendant, Grandfather and Grandson)

Sp 5 — Merchant Mound (Shang Hill)

Sp 6 — Three Yin Crossing (Reunion of Three Yin)

Sp 7 — Leaky Valley

Sp 8 — Earth Motivator (Earth's Pivot, Earth's Crux)

Sp 9 — Yin Mound Spring

Sp 10 — Sea of Blood

Sp 11 — Basket Gate (Winnowing Gate)

Sp 12 — Rushing Gate (Penetrating Gate, Surging Gate)

Sp 13 — Official Residence. (Treasury Dwelling. Bowel Abode)

Sp 14 — Abdomen Knot (Contracted Belly)

Sp 15 — Great Horizontal

Sp 16 — Abdomen Sorrow (Abdominal Lament)

Sp 17 — Food Drain (Great Gate of the Will of Heaven)

Sp 18 — Heavenly Stream (Celestial Ravine)

Sp 19 — Chest Region (Neighbourhood of the Breast)

Sp 20 — Encircling Glory (Complete Glory)

Sp 21 — Great Enveloping

Ren Mai Conception Vessel

Ren 1 — Meeting Of Yin (Sea Bed)

Ren 2 — Crooked Bone (Bent Bone)

Ren 3 — Utmost Middle (Central Pole)

Ren 4 — First Gate (Origin Gate, Gate to the Original Qi)

Ren 5 — Stone Gate (Cinnabar Field, Life Gate)

Ren 6 — Sea of Qi (Lower Sea of Qi)

Ren 7 — Yin Crossing (Cinnabar Field, Crossroads of the Yin Forces)

Ren 8 — Spirit Deficiency (Spirit Gate, Spirit Palace Gate)

Ren 9 — Water Division (Water Balancer, Water Separation)

Ren 10 — Lower Duct (Lower Portion of the Stomach)

Ren 11 — Inner Strengthening (Established Mile)

Ren 12 — Central Duct (Supreme Granary, Middle Portion of the Stomach)

Ren 13 — Upper Duct (Upper Regulator, Upper Portion of the Stomach)

Ren 14 — Great Deficiency (Greatest Palace Gate)

Ren 15 — Dove Tail (Spirit Storehouse)

Ren 15 — Master Point

Ren 16 — Middle Hall (Central Palace, Middle Courtyard)

Ren 17 — Within the Breast (Upper Sea of Qi, Centre of the Chest, Central Hall)

Ren 18 — Jade Hall (Jade Court)

Ren 19 — Purple Palace (Purple Temple)

Ren 20 — Flower Covering (Magnificent Canopy)

Ren 21 — Pearl Jade (Fine Jade, Jade Pivot)

Ren 22 — Heaven Rushing Out (Celestial Chimney, Heavenly Process)

Ren 23 — Angle Spring (Pure Spring)

Ren 24 — Receiving Fluid (Precious Fluid, Heavenly Pond)

Du Mai Governor Vessel

Du 1 — Long Strength (Long and Strong)

Du 2 — Loins Correspondence (Lumbar Door)

Du 3 — Loins Yang Passageway (Loins Yang Border, Yang Gate, Lumbar Yang Gate)

Du 4 — Gate of Life (Gate of Destiny, Palace of Jing/Essence)

Du 5 — Suspended Pivot

Du 6 — Middle of the Spine (Spiritual Ancestor)

Du 7 — Middle Pivot (Central Pivot)

Du 8 — Contracted Muscle (Sinew Binder)

Du 9 — Utmost Yang (Extremity of Yang)

Du 10 — Supernatural Tower (Spirit Tower, Temple of the Soul)

Du 11 — Spirit Path

Du 12 — Body Pillar (Divine Column, Body Support)

Du 13 — Kiln Path (Road to Happiness)

Du 14 — Great Hammer (Big Vertebrae)

Du 15 — Gate of Dumbness

Du 16 — Wind Palace (Wind Treasury)

Du 17 — Brain Door

Du 18 — Strength Divider (Strong Gate)

Du 19 — Posterior Summit

Du 20 — One Hundred Meetings (Assembly of the One Hundred, Hundred Convergence)

Du 21 — Anterior Summit (In Front of the Summit)

Du 22 — Skull Meeting